CRITICAL CARE MEDICINE

An Algorithmic Approach

CRITICAL CARE MEDICINE

An Algorithmic Approach

Alexander Goldfarb-Rumyantzev, MD, PhD, PhD
Lecturer
Medicine
Harvard Medical School, Beth Israel Deaconess Medical Center
Boston, Massachusetts

Contributing Author

Robert Stephen Brown, MD
Associate Chief for Academic Affairs, Nephrology Division Medicine
Beth Israel Deaconess Medical Center
Boston, Massachusetts
Associate Professor of Medicine
Harvard Medical School
Boston, Massachusetts

Associate Editor

Martin Shao Foong Chong, MBBS, MA (Oxon), MRCP, FRCA, FFICM, FHEA
Magill Department of Anaesthesia
Chelsea and Westminster Hospital
London, UK

ELSEVIER

Elsevier
1600 John F. Kennedy Blvd.
Ste 1800
Philadelphia, PA 19103-2899

CRITICAL CARE MEDICINE: AN ALGORITHMIC APPROACH, FIRST EDITION   ISBN: 978-0-323-696074

Notice

Content Strategist: Michael Houston
Content Development Specialist: Erika Ninsin
Publishing Services Manager: Deepthi Unni
Project Manager: Radjan Lourde Selvanadin
Design Direction: Margaret Reid

Printed in India

Last digit is the print number: 9   8   7   6   5   4   3   2   1

 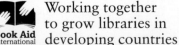

Dedication

*To my family, and specifically to my mom Tatiana, my late uncle Veniamin,
and my children Levi and Ben – my constant source of inspiration.*

Alexander Goldfarb-Rumyantzev

*To my wife Judy, son Bobby, and daughter Debbie
who have always supported my hours at work
and to the late Frank Epstein –
mentor, colleague, and friend for 40 years.*

Robert S. Brown

Dedicated in memory of Alexander Goldfarb-Rumyantzev, MD, PhD, PhD,
a colleague, co-author and friend,

This book is all Alex' doing – its conception, structure and writing. His unexpected
passing on January 18th, 2021 was a loss to us all – his innovative thinking,
logic, spirit, wit and humor will not be forgotten.

Robert S. Brown, MD

Contributing Author

Robert Stephen Brown, MD
Associate Chief for Academic Affairs, Nephrology Division Medicine
Beth Israel Deaconess Medical Center
Boston, Massachusetts
Associate Professor of Medicine
Harvard Medical School
Boston, Massachusetts

Associate Editor

Martin Shao Foong Chong, MBBS, MA (Oxon), MRCP, FRCA, FFICM, FHEA
Magill Department of Anaesthesia
Chelsea and Westminster Hospital
London, UK

Preface

Critical Care Medicine is a broad subject that covers many areas and almost all subspecialties of internal medicine. As one might remember from one's years in residency, the ICU rotation is exciting and the favorite of many. In this book we discuss practical issues of critical care medicine divided into chapters by subspecialty. Specifically, we separated the following aspects of critical care medicine: respiratory, cardiac and circulation, infectious disease, water and electrolytes and acid-base disorders, acute kidney injury and dialysis, gastroenterology, rheumatology, endocrinology, neurology, and COVID-19. Arguably, many aspects of critical care medicine are also relevant to general internal medicine. In effect, critical care is an internal medicine subspecialty focused on very sick people (plus invasive procedures). As such, the chapters in this book are applicable to the practice of general medicine as well. Therefore, the intended audience for this book includes critical care practitioners, as well as internal medicine physicians, and fellows and residents in critical care, internal medicine, and its subspecialties.

Let me point out what this book is NOT. First of all, it is important to note that the goal of this book is not to give comprehensive coverage of the topics, nor to provide a fundamental understanding of the physiology of the discussed conditions. Rather, we address the need for quick decision making in situations where timing is of essence. This book is intended to be a source of quick reference to provide help in approaching conditions frequently encountered in the intensive care unit, in formulating the plan of care, and in making a decision regarding the next step in management of a critical patient. In essence, this book allows the provider to alleviate the most urgent clinical matter and buy some time to regroup, think, call consults, and obtain more detailed and comprehensive information. By no means does it eliminates the need for a physician to read further and have a deeper understanding of the subject—of special importance is the understanding of the physiology of critical illnesses. Medicine is practiced in a rapidly changing environment and new information is coming daily. This book does not substitute the need to be on the top of contemporary literature. Understanding of the underlying disease process is very important, so, once the initial strategy is established and next steps are clear in general terms, the provider should probably step back and get additional information from more detailed sources. Along the same lines, this book cannot cover all topics, and the authors had to be selective. Because the purpose of the book is to be a source of quick reference, we selected topics representing common issues in critical care medicine, those that practitioners are dealing with on almost a daily basis, and those that require decisive steps.

The format of this book is different from most textbooks in that it is based mostly on graphical representation of information: diagrams, tables, algorithms. We believe that this format will be helpful to practitioners looking for concise data and references in an environment where decisions need to be made quickly.

Most of the references used for this book are open access sources. We specifically made an effort to select appropriate sources that would be easily available to readers, unless these sources were insufficient.

Four chapters in this book (Water and electrolyte disorders, Acid-base disorders, Acute kidney injury and dialysis, and COVID-19) were co-authored by Dr. Robert S. Brown.

We feel sure that you will find this book helpful in your daily practice and we are very much open to suggestions how to make the next edition better.

Alexander S. Goldfarb-Rumyantzev, MD, PhD, PhD

Contents

CHAPTER 1

Respiratory Failure

Alexander Goldfarb-Rumyantzev

Pulmonary

The chapter addresses two large areas of critical care medicine, specifically, acute respiratory failure and means of artificial gas exchange, such as mechanical ventilation and extracorporeal membrane gas exchange.

Diagnostic Tests

Chest X-Ray Assessment Algorithm

- Technical issues:
  - view (anterior-posterior/lateral), position/rotation
  - quality and penetration
  - inspiratory effort (number of ribs)
- Evaluate soft tissue
- Evaluate bones: ribs, vertebrae
- Heart, mediastinum, trachea
- Lungs contour: costo-diaphragmal angles, diaphragm, presence of pleural effusion/pneumothorax
- Lungs parenchyma:
  - dilated hila (dilated veins in congestive heart failure [CHF], dilated arteries in congenital defects, lymph nodes, tumor masses)
  - changes in lung parenchyma (e.g., infiltrate, pulmonary edema)

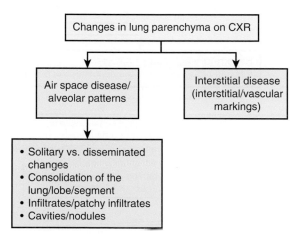

Pulmonary Function Test Interpretation

The pulmonary function test is used to diagnose and stage restrictive (caused by extrathoracic or intrathoracic problem) or obstructive lung disease. Restrictive lung diseases cause problems that impair lung expansion, which lead to decreased lung volume (e.g., obesity, interstitial lung disease). On the other hand, in obstructive lung disease, lung volume is usually preserved, but there is an impairment to air flow, potentially caused by bronchospasm or other airway obstruction.

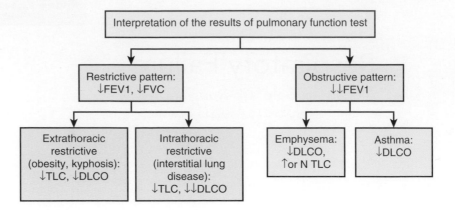

Arterial Blood Gas Analysis
Acid-base disorder diagnostic algorithm
The following diagram provides the algorithm of interpretation of arterial blood gases (ABGs) used in conjunction with plasma chemistry. To use this algorithm, first examine the pH and identify acidemia or alkalemia, then using the bicarbonate concentration from the serum electrolytes and pCO_2, identify whether the primary cause of the disorder is metabolic or respiratory. Finally, perform a calculation to examine if secondary metabolic compensation for a primary respiratory disorder or respiratory compensation for a primary metabolic disorder is appropriate. If not, there is a second primary disorder, considered to be a "complex" (meaning more than one) acid-base disorder, rather than a "simple" (meaning single) acid-base disorder underlying the observed changes.

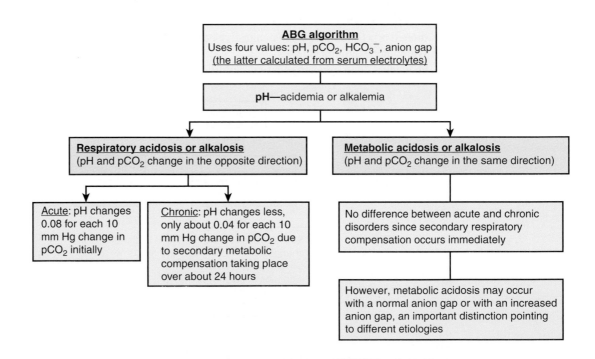

Pleural effusion

The normal amount of pleural fluid is about 10 mL. Pleural effusion might be formed due to several potential causes: increased fluid formation (increased amount of interstitial fluid in the lungs, increased intravascular pressure in the pleura, decreased pleural pressure, increased permeability of the pleura, increased pleural protein level, increased amount of peritoneal fluid disruption of blood vessels or lymphatics in the thorax) or decreased fluid absorption (obstruction of the lymphatics draining pleural fluid, disruption of the aquaporin system in the pleura, elevated systemic vascular pressure). The first diagnostic question of pleural fluid analysis is if it represents a transudate or an exudate.[2]

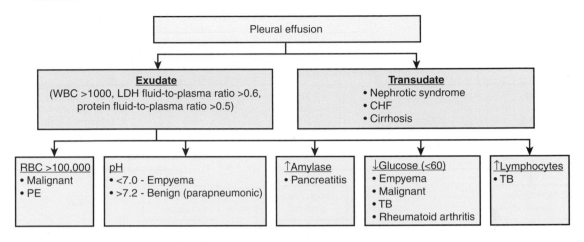

Acute Respiratory Failure

Acute respiratory failure is one of the most common conditions that requires patient to be treated in Intensive Care Unit (ICU). Unlike many other life-threatening conditions requiring ICU admission, respiratory failure presents immediate risk and needs to be addressed promptly. In a simplified format, respiration entails gas exchange with O_2 being absorbed and CO_2 excreted by the lungs. As a result, respiratory failure could be viewed either as a deficiency in oxygenation or as a failure to excrete CO_2. Some look at respiratory failure in sepsis as a separate entity, whereas others classify it within either hypoxemic or ventilatory failure. The next chart is a general algorithm describing types of respiratory failure and their mechanisms.[3] We provide more details about specific conditions below.

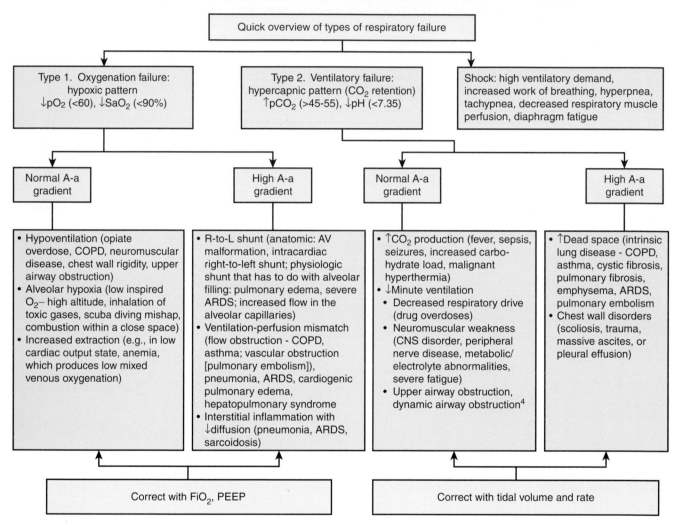

Quick overview of types of respiratory failure

Type 1. Oxygenation failure: hypoxic pattern ↓pO_2 (<60), ↓SaO_2 (<90%)

Type 2. Ventilatory failure: hypercapnic pattern (CO_2 retention) ↑pCO_2 (>45-55), ↓pH (<7.35)

Shock: high ventilatory demand, increased work of breathing, hyperpnea, tachypnea, decreased respiratory muscle perfusion, diaphragm fatigue

Normal A-a gradient

High A-a gradient

Normal A-a gradient

High A-a gradient

- Hypoventilation (opiate overdose, COPD, neuromuscular disease, chest wall rigidity, upper airway obstruction)
- Alveolar hypoxia (low inspired O_2– high altitude, inhalation of toxic gases, scuba diving mishap, combustion within a close space)
- Increased extraction (e.g., in low cardiac output state, anemia, which produces low mixed venous oxygenation)

- R-to-L shunt (anatomic: AV malformation, intracardiac right-to-left shunt; physiologic shunt that has to do with alveolar filling: pulmonary edema, severe ARDS; increased flow in the alveolar capillaries)
- Ventilation-perfusion mismatch (flow obstruction - COPD, asthma; vascular obstruction [pulmonary embolism]), pneumonia, ARDS, cardiogenic pulmonary edema, hepatopulmonary syndrome
- Interstitial inflammation with ↓diffusion (pneumonia, ARDS, sarcoidosis)

- ↑CO_2 production (fever, sepsis, seizures, increased carbo-hydrate load, malignant hyperthermia)
- ↓Minute ventilation
  - Decreased respiratory drive (drug overdoses)
  - Neuromuscular weakness (CNS disorder, peripheral nerve disease, metabolic/electrolyte abnormalities, severe fatigue)
  - Upper airway obstruction, dynamic airway obstruction[4]

- ↑Dead space (intrinsic lung disease - COPD, asthma, cystic fibrosis, pulmonary fibrosis, emphysema, ARDS, pulmonary embolism)
- Chest wall disorders (scoliosis, trauma, massive ascites, or pleural effusion)

Correct with FiO_2, PEEP

Correct with tidal volume and rate

Ventilatory Failure

Asthma and Chronic Obstructive Pulmonary Disease

Although pathophysiologies of asthma and chronic obstructive pulmonary disease (COPD) are different, the end result leading to ventilator failure is similar and is based on hypoventilation. Therefore whereas approaches to treatment of noncritical stable asthma and COPD might be different, once it reaches the stage of respiratory failure, the focus in both conditions is to relieve bronchospasm and provide adequate ventilation. However, one has to be cautious about gas trapping which can precipitate hemodynamic instability and barotrauma.[5,6]

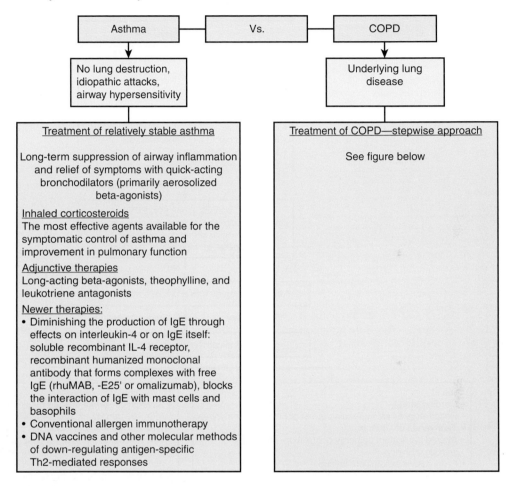

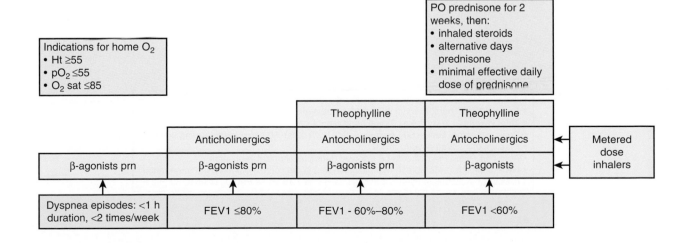

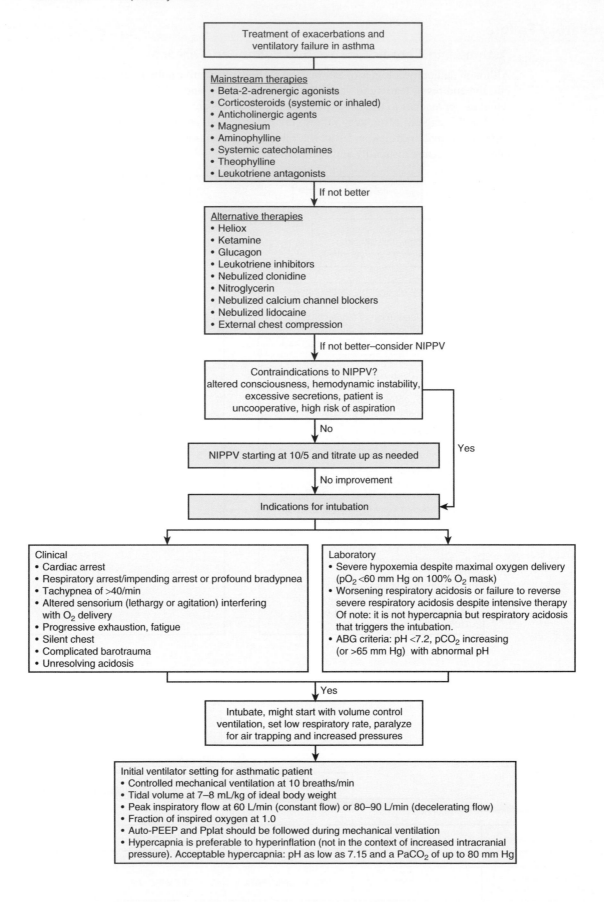

Treatment of exacerbations and
ventilatory failure in asthma

Mainstream therapies
• Beta-2-adrenergic agonists
• Corticosteroids (systemic or inhaled)
• Anticholinergic agents
• Magnesium
• Aminophylline
• Systemic catecholamines
• Theophylline
• Leukotriene antagonists

If not better

Alternative therapies
• Heliox
• Ketamine
• Glucagon
• Leukotriene inhibitors
• Nebulized clonidine
• Nitroglycerin
• Nebulized calcium channel blockers
• Nebulized lidocaine
• External chest compression

If not better–consider NIPPV

Contraindications to NIPPV?
altered consciousness, hemodynamic instability,
excessive secretions, patient is
uncooperative, high risk of aspiration

No

NIPPV starting at 10/5 and titrate up as needed

Yes

No improvement

Indications for intubation

Clinical
• Cardiac arrest
• Respiratory arrest/impending arrest or profound bradypnea
• Tachypnea of >40/min
• Altered sensorium (lethargy or agitation) interfering
  with O$_2$ delivery
• Progressive exhaustion, fatigue
• Silent chest
• Complicated barotrauma
• Unresolving acidosis

Laboratory
• Severe hypoxemia despite maximal oxygen delivery
  (pO$_2$ <60 mm Hg on 100% O$_2$ mask)
• Worsening respiratory acidosis or failure to reverse
  severe respiratory acidosis despite intensive therapy
  Of note: it is not hypercapnia but respiratory acidosis
  that triggers the intubation.
• ABG criteria: pH <7.2, pCO$_2$ increasing
  (or >65 mm Hg) with abnormal pH

Yes

Intubate, might start with volume control
ventilation, set low respiratory rate, paralyze
for air trapping and increased pressures

Initial ventilator setting for asthmatic patient
• Controlled mechanical ventilation at 10 breaths/min
• Tidal volume at 7–8 mL/kg of ideal body weight
• Peak inspiratory flow at 60 L/min (constant flow) or 80–90 L/min (decelerating flow)
• Fraction of inspired oxygen at 1.0
• Auto-PEEP and Pplat should be followed during mechanical ventilation
• Hypercapnia is preferable to hyperinflation (not in the context of increased intracranial
  pressure). Acceptable hypercapnia: pH as low as 7.15 and a PaCO$_2$ of up to 80 mm Hg

Issues with managing intubated patient with asthma

Assessing pulmonary hyperinflation

- Volume of gas exhaled during prolonged apnea (lung volume at inspiration V_{EI}). V_{EI} is affected by severity of airflow obstruction and ventilator settings. V_{EI} is the most reliable predictor of ventilator-related complications.
- Plateau airway pressure (Pplat; in acute severe asthma average 24–26 cm H_2O, acceptable up to 30)
- Auto-PEEP (10–15 cm H_2O in severe asthma) during volume-cycled ventilation.
- Peak airway pressure (Ppk), target <50 cm H_2O. Ppk depends on inspiratory flow-resistive properties in addition to hyperinflation. Ppk >50 cm H_2O does not predict increased risk of barotrauma.

Adjust ventilator settings based on severity of hyperinflation

- Minute ventilation. Increased minute ventilation increases the risk of hypotension and barotrauma (when increased from 10 to 16 to 26 L/min).
- Minimal PEEP ≤5 cm H_2) is recommended

Management of hypercapnia

- Consequence of dead space ventilation (caused by alveolar overdistension)
- Serious consequences of hypercapnia are uncommon
- Neuro: increased cerebral blood flow, intracranial pressure → cerebral edema and subarachnoid hemorrhage.
- Cardiac: decreased intracellular pH → reduced contractility
- Consider alkalinizing agent when pH is persistently below 7.15–7.2 (Na bicarbonate or tromethamine).

Medical management of asthma in the intubated patient
- Systemic corticosteroids: anti-inflammatory effect (2.5 mg/kg/day of methylprednisolone)
- Inhaled beta-agonists (MDI or nebulizer): albuterol 2.5 mg Q4 or Q6, ipratropium
- Other bronchodilators (IV theophylline)
- Deep sedation: combination of propofol (or benzodiazepine) and fentanyl
- Neuromuscular blocking agent is sometimes necessary (intermittent boluses rather than continuous infusion)

Additional measures (not supported by strong evidence):
- Heliox (a mixture of helium and oxygen)
- Inhalational anesthetics (isoflurane)–should the effect right away, and if not then discontinue
- Ketamine IV
- Bronchoscopic removal of impacted mucus
- Extracorporeal life support (membrane oxygenation and CO_2 removal)

See mechanical ventilation section for details on managing intubated and ventilated patient

---

Medical Management of Asthma in the Intubated Patient

- Systemic corticosteroids: antiinflammatory effect (2.5 mg/kg per day of methylprednisolone)
- Inhaled beta-agonists (MDI or nebulizer): albuterol 2.5 mg Q4 or Q6, ipratropium
- Other bronchodilators (IV theophylline)
- Deep sedation: combination of propofol (or benzodiazepine) and fentanyl
- Neuromuscular blocking agent is sometimes necessary (intermittent boluses rather than continuous infusion)

Additional Measures (not Supported by Strong Evidence)

- Heliox (a mixture of helium and oxygen)
- Inhalational anesthetics (isoflurane)—the effect should be right away; if not, then discontinue
- Ketamine IV
- Bronchoscopic removal of impacted mucus
- Extracorporeal life support (membrane oxygenation and CO_2 removal)

MDI, Metered dose inhaler.

See Mechanical Ventilation section for details on managing intubated and ventilated patient

Hypoxemic Respiratory Failure

A number of mechanisms can lead to hypoxemic respiratory failure, resulting either from oxygen delivery problems (acute respiratory distress syndrome [ARDS], pneumonia, pulmonary edema, high altitude) or lung perfusion problems (pulmonary embolism, shunting).

Below is the general approach to treatment of hypoxemic respiratory failure; we also discuss special cases (ARDS, pulmonary embolism) in more detail.

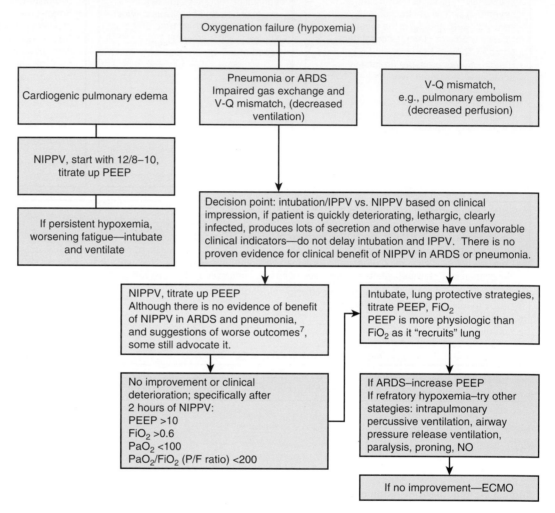

Other than ventilator failure and hypoxemic respiratory failure, some separate respiratory failure in sepsis into a separate entity, whereas in fact it is for the most part a multifactorial combination. Intubation and invasive positive pressure ventilation (IPPV) is the treatment of choice for the respiratory failure in sepsis.

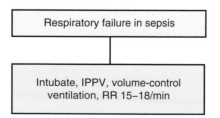

ARDS

ARDS is characterized by increased permeability of the alveolar capillary membrane, diffuse alveolar damage, and accumulation of proteinaceous alveolar edema. Mortality remains very high (>40%) and does not seem to decrease between 1994 and 2006.[8] That, in addition to high incidence and relatively limited therapeutic options, makes ARDS a serious and mostly unresolved issue in critical care.[1,3,9–12]

Establish the diagnosis: ARDS definition
1. Acute onset, presence of inciting event
2. $PaO_2/FiO_2 \leq 200$ (regardless of PEEP level)
3. Bilateral infiltrates seen on frontal chest radiograph
4. PCWP ≤ 18 mm Hg or no clinical evidence of left atrial hypertension

Classification by PaO_2/FiO_2 ratio
- Acute lung injury (ALI) or mild ARDS: <300
- Moderate >100–200
- Severe ≤ 100

Differential diagnosis and diagnostic steps
- Rule out other similar presentations: interstitial lung disease, malignancy presenting similar to ARDS, acute eosinophilic pneumonia, diffuse alveolar hemorrhage, hypersensitivity pneumonitis, and pulmonary alveolar proteinosis
- Consider BAL: identify infectious causes (e.g., bacterial or viral)
- Consider lung biopsy if
  o high clinical suspicion for a "contributive result" (results leading to additional therapy)[13]
  o the risk of empirical therapy is too high
  o when empirical therapy has been unsuccessful[14]
  o note that lung biopsy presents substantial risk in ventilated patient on high PEEP and benefits must clearly outweigh risks

---

Therapies

Effective therapies:
- Lung protective ventilation (lower tidal volume and airway pressures) (see mechanical ventilation box below)
- Neuromuscular blockade[15,16]
  cisatracurium should be considered for short-term use (<48 h) in patients with severe ARDS (defined as PaO_2/FiO_2 <120 mm Hg) until further studies are available[17]
- Esophageal pressure to adjust PEEP (improves oxygenation)
- Fluid conservative vs fluid-liberal therapy (see fluid management box below)
- Extracorporeal membrane oxygenaton (see ECMO section for details)

No proven benefit:
- High PEEP
- High frequency ventilation
- Early prone positioning
- Continuous administration of surfactant has no effect on 30-day survival, duration of mechanical ventilation, or physiologic function
- Activated protein C (APC)
- GM-CSF
- Pulmonary artery catheter
- Methylprednisolone/steroids (questionable benefit). Some recommend 7–14-day trial of 2–4 mg/kg prednisone in patients with severe ARDS who show no clinical signs of improvement. Rule out or treat systemic infections.
- Omega-3 fatty acid (may be harmful)
- Beta-2 agonists
- Antioxidants
- Vasodilator therapy (liposomal prostoglandin E1, nitric oxide). Liposomal PGE^1 blocks platelet aggregation, downregulates neutrophil-mediated inflammation, produce vasodilatation.
- Ketoconazole inhibits tromboxane synthesis and biosynthesis of leukotriens
- N-acetylcysteine

Details of some specific therapeutic approaches

Details of fluid management

- Excessive fluid administration may lead to an increased amount of pulmonary edema and a worsening of oxygenation. On the other hand, inadequate intravascular volume may create decreased cardiac output and inadequate perfusion of the organs. Monitor biochemical markers of organ dysfunction and lactate.
- If the patient is anemic (Hct <21), transfusion of packed RBC can be used as a volume expander.
- Otherwise crystalloids or colloids should be utilized.
- Volume depletion may be accomplished with diuretics.

Details of mechanical ventilation

- Optimize sedation and analgesia.
- Lower initial tidal volume (6–8 mL/kg), do not produce a transpulmonary pressure that exceeds 30–35 cm H_2O.
- Titrate PEEP to maintain an arterial oxygen saturation of >90% at an FiO_2 <60% (usually PEEP 5–12 cm H_2O).
- Low volume-low pressure ventilation (plateau pressure <30 cm H_2O) to reduce mechanical stretch improves outcome in ARDS, but might lead to hypoxemia, poor lung compliance, severe respiratory acidosis.[11]
- Avoid oxygen toxicity if possible (FiO_2 <0.6).
- Inverse ratio ventilation (strategy, when the amount of time the lungs are in inhalation is greater than the amount of time they are in exhalation) may enhance recruitment at the expense of ventilation. The resultant effect on $PaCO_2$ is "permissive hypercapnia" (keep static peak airway pressure <40 cm H_2O, maintain O_2 saturation >90%, while tolerating pH as low as 7.15 before initiating IV buffering agents bicarbonate or THAM. Higher doses of propofol are required to sedate patients managed with permissive hypercapnia).
- Consider mechanical ventilation in the prone position.[1]
- Inhaled nitric oxide at 10 parts per million to improve VQ matching and oxygenation but has not been shown to alter outcome
- High-frequency oscillatory ventilation (see[10] for specific severity criteria)
- Airway pressure (release) ventilation (alternative approach to open lung)
- ECMO

Outcome: resolution might be slow and mortality remains very high

Resolution mechanism

- reabsorbtion of alveolar edema
- repair of epithelial and endothelial barriers
- removal of inflammatory cells and exudate from distal airspaces

Causes of death[15]

- underlying illness or injury
- sepsis
- irreversible respiratory failure
- associated multi system organ failure due to unremitting hypoxia

Interstitial Lung Disease and Pulmonary Fibrosis

Underlying interstitial lung disease (ILD) might be a cause of hypoxemic respiratory failure. ILD refers to lung diseases affecting the interstitium of the lungs (alveolar epithelium, pulmonary capillary endothelium, basement membrane, and perivascular and perilymphatic tissues).[19] Detailed discussion of ILD management is outside the scope of this chapter; however, we briefly discuss the causes and diagnostic approach to ILD below.

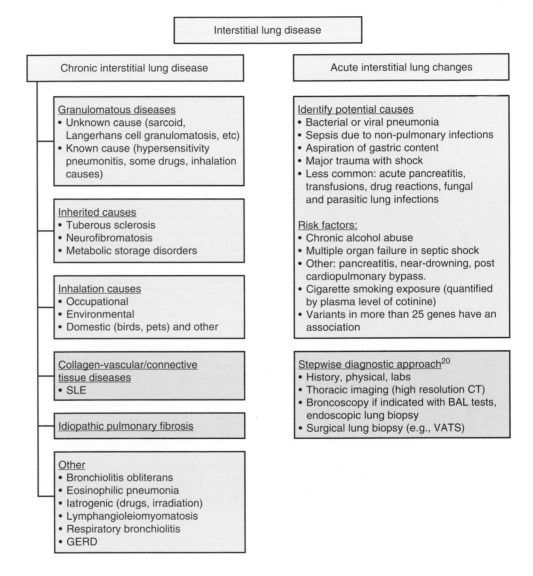

Interstitial lung disease

Chronic interstitial lung disease

Granulomatous diseases
- Unknown cause (sarcoid, Langerhans cell granulomatosis, etc)
- Known cause (hypersensitivity pneumonitis, some drugs, inhalation causes)

Inherited causes
- Tuberous sclerosis
- Neurofibromatosis
- Metabolic storage disorders

Inhalation causes
- Occupational
- Environmental
- Domestic (birds, pets) and other

Collagen-vascular/connective tissue diseases
- SLE

Idiopathic pulmonary fibrosis

Other
- Bronchiolitis obliterans
- Eosinophilic pneumonia
- Iatrogenic (drugs, irradiation)
- Lymphangioleiomyomatosis
- Respiratory bronchiolitis
- GERD

Acute interstitial lung changes

Identify potential causes
- Bacterial or viral pneumonia
- Sepsis due to non-pulmonary infections
- Aspiration of gastric content
- Major trauma with shock
- Less common: acute pancreatitis, transfusions, drug reactions, fungal and parasitic lung infections

Risk factors:
- Chronic alcohol abuse
- Multiple organ failure in septic shock
- Other: pancreatitis, near-drowning, post cardiopulmonary bypass.
- Cigarette smoking exposure (quantified by plasma level of cotinine)
- Variants in more than 25 genes have an association

Stepwise diagnostic approach[20]
- History, physical, labs
- Thoracic imaging (high resolution CT)
- Broncoscopy if indicated with BAL tests, endoscopic lung biopsy
- Surgical lung biopsy (e.g., VATS)

Treatment for specific forms of ILD[20]

Idiopathic pulmonary fibrosis:
Supportive care, anti-reflux measures,
N-acetylcysteine, lung transplantation

Sarcoidosis:
Corticosteroids, methotrexate, influximab,
lung transplantation

Nonspecific interstitial pneumonia:
Corticosteroids, mycophenolate, other immunosuppression,
lung transplantation

Cryptogenic organizing pneumonia:
Corticosteroids, other immunosuppression, macrolides

Hypersensitivity pneumonitis:
Corticosteroids, other immunosuppression,
lung transplantation

Eosinophilic pneumonia:
Corticosteroids, other immunosuppression

Connective tissue disease associated ILD:
Corticosteroids, mycophenolate, other
DMARD agents, anti-reflux therapy, treatment
of pulmonary hypertension, lung transplantation

Acute interstitial pneumonia/ Diffuse alveolar damage:
Corticosteroids, cytotoxic drugs

Pulmonary Embolism

After establishing the diagnosis of pulmonary embolism, therapeutic options are (1) anticoagulation, (2) thrombolysis/thrombectomy, or (3) if anticoagulation is contraindicated—placement of intravenous filter. Treatment of pulmonary embolism is discussed in the diagram below.[21]

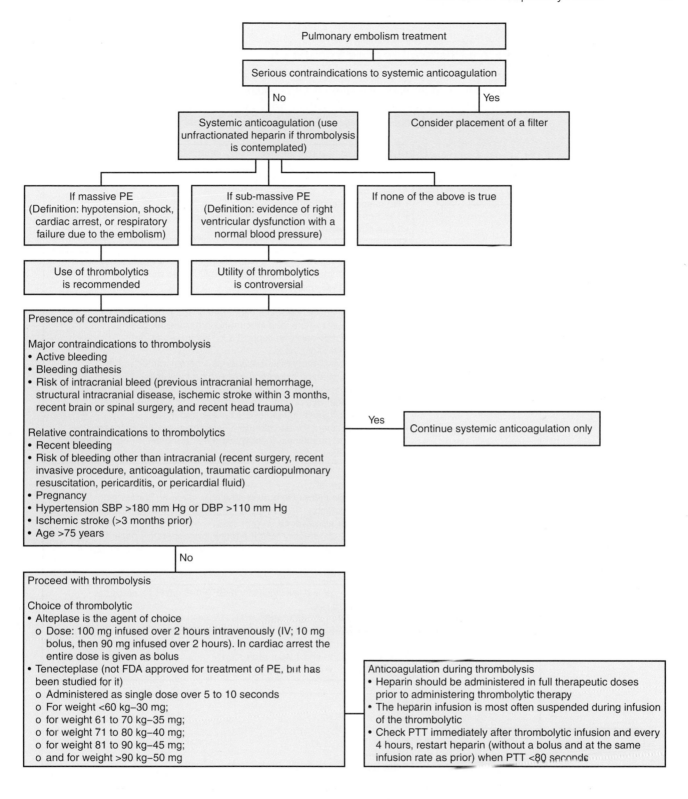

Mechanical Ventilation

Noninvasive Positive Pressure Ventilation

Noninvasive positive pressure ventilation (NIPPV) is an alternative to intubation and invasive ventilation that can be used for both ventilatory (COPD, asthma) and hypoxemic (cardiogenic pulmonary edema) failure.[22] It is a cost-effective and less invasive modality, but current evidence only supports its use in obstructive pulmonary disease and in cardiogenic pulmonary edema.

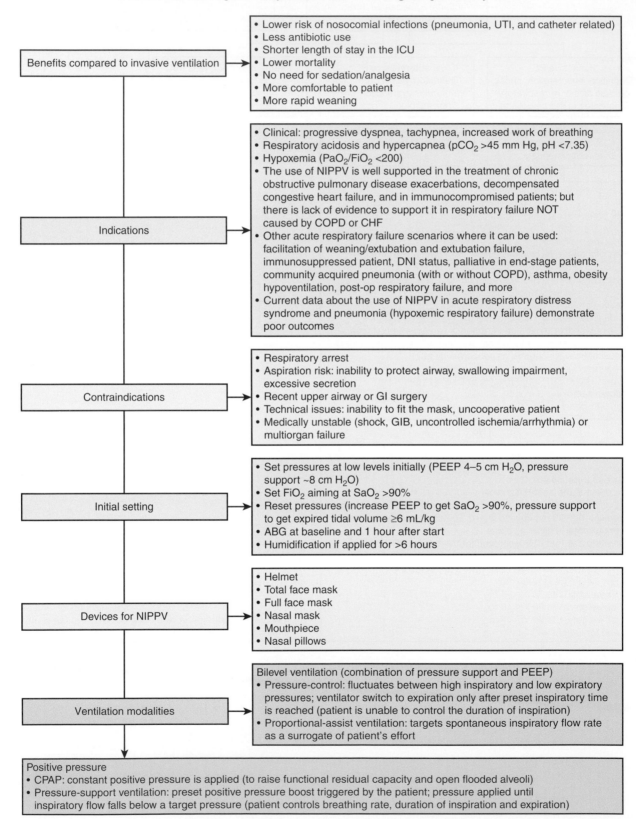

Benefits compared to invasive ventilation
- Lower risk of nosocomial infections (pneumonia, UTI, and catheter related)
- Less antibiotic use
- Shorter length of stay in the ICU
- Lower mortality
- No need for sedation/analgesia
- More comfortable to patient
- More rapid weaning

Indications
- Clinical: progressive dyspnea, tachypnea, increased work of breathing
- Respiratory acidosis and hypercapnea (pCO_2 >45 mm Hg, pH <7.35)
- Hypoxemia (PaO_2/FiO_2 <200)
- The use of NIPPV is well supported in the treatment of chronic obstructive pulmonary disease exacerbations, decompensated congestive heart failure, and in immunocompromised patients; but there is lack of evidence to support it in respiratory failure NOT caused by COPD or CHF
- Other acute respiratory failure scenarios where it can be used: facilitation of weaning/extubation and extubation failure, immunosuppressed patient, DNI status, palliative in end-stage patients, community acquired pneumonia (with or without COPD), asthma, obesity hypoventilation, post-op respiratory failure, and more
- Current data about the use of NIPPV in acute respiratory distress syndrome and pneumonia (hypoxemic respiratory failure) demonstrate poor outcomes

Contraindications
- Respiratory arrest
- Aspiration risk: inability to protect airway, swallowing impairment, excessive secretion
- Recent upper airway or GI surgery
- Technical issues: inability to fit the mask, uncooperative patient
- Medically unstable (shock, GIB, uncontrolled ischemia/arrhythmia) or multiorgan failure

Initial setting
- Set pressures at low levels initially (PEEP 4–5 cm H_2O, pressure support ~8 cm H_2O)
- Set FiO_2 aiming at SaO_2 >90%
- Reset pressures (increase PEEP to get SaO_2 >90%, pressure support to get expired tidal volume ≥6 mL/kg
- ABG at baseline and 1 hour after start
- Humidification if applied for >6 hours

Devices for NIPPV
- Helmet
- Total face mask
- Full face mask
- Nasal mask
- Mouthpiece
- Nasal pillows

Ventilation modalities
Bilevel ventilation (combination of pressure support and PEEP)
- Pressure-control: fluctuates between high inspiratory and low expiratory pressures; ventilator switch to expiration only after preset inspiratory time is reached (patient is unable to control the duration of inspiration)
- Proportional-assist ventilation: targets spontaneous inspiratory flow rate as a surrogate of patient's effort

Positive pressure
- CPAP: constant positive pressure is applied (to raise functional residual capacity and open flooded alveoli)
- Pressure-support ventilation: preset positive pressure boost triggered by the patient; pressure applied until inspiratory flow falls below a target pressure (patient controls breathing rate, duration of inspiration and expiration)

Endotracheal Intubation

Intubation is one of the most frequent procedures in critically ill patients. Whereas some indications are very clear, certain situations represent a gray area, where the decision might not be straightforward, mostly based on uncertainty whether the patient is going to deteriorate. As any invasive procedure, it carries a burden of complications and entails a commitment to mechanical ventilation, sedation, and sometimes paralysis, which should also be considered in the risk-benefit analysis.[5]

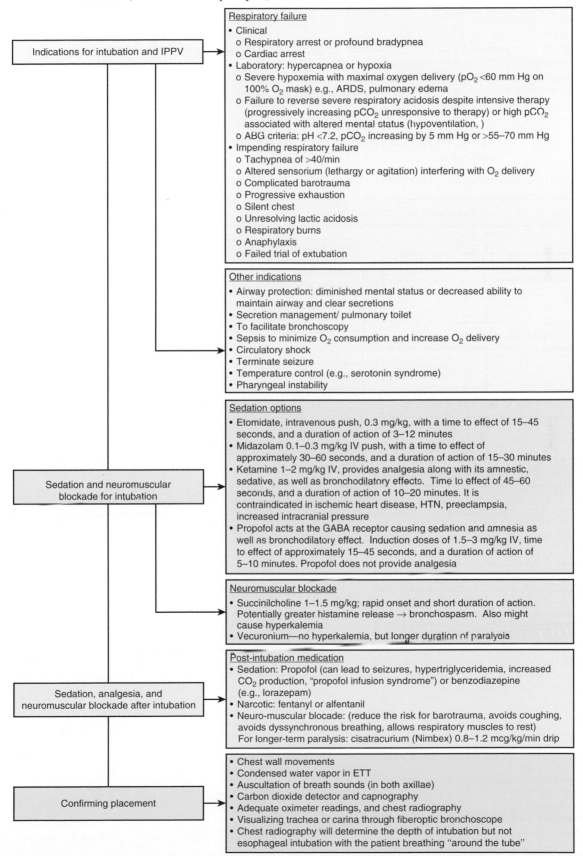

Indications for intubation and IPPV

Respiratory failure
- Clinical
  o Respiratory arrest or profound bradypnea
  o Cardiac arrest
- Laboratory: hypercapnea or hypoxia
  o Severe hypoxemia with maximal oxygen delivery (pO_2 <60 mm Hg on 100% O_2 mask) e.g., ARDS, pulmonary edema
  o Failure to reverse severe respiratory acidosis despite intensive therapy (progressively increasing pCO_2 unresponsive to therapy) or high pCO_2 associated with altered mental status (hypoventilation,)
  o ABG criteria: pH <7.2, pCO_2 increasing by 5 mm Hg or >55–70 mm Hg
- Impending respiratory failure
  o Tachypnea of >40/min
  o Altered sensorium (lethargy or agitation) interfering with O_2 delivery
  o Complicated barotrauma
  o Progressive exhaustion
  o Silent chest
  o Unresolving lactic acidosis
  o Respiratory burns
  o Anaphylaxis
  o Failed trial of extubation

Other indications
- Airway protection: diminished mental status or decreased ability to maintain airway and clear secretions
- Secretion management/ pulmonary toilet
- To facilitate bronchoscopy
- Sepsis to minimize O_2 consumption and increase O_2 delivery
- Circulatory shock
- Terminate seizure
- Temperature control (e.g., serotonin syndrome)
- Pharyngeal instability

Sedation and neuromuscular blockade for intubation

Sedation options
- Etomidate, intravenous push, 0.3 mg/kg, with a time to effect of 15–45 seconds, and a duration of action of 3–12 minutes
- Midazolam 0.1–0.3 mg/kg IV push, with a time to effect of approximately 30–60 seconds, and a duration of action of 15–30 minutes
- Ketamine 1–2 mg/kg IV, provides analgesia along with its amnestic, sedative, as well as bronchodilatory effects. Time to effect of 45–60 seconds, and a duration of action of 10–20 minutes. It is contraindicated in ischemic heart disease, HTN, preeclampsia, increased intracranial pressure
- Propofol acts at the GABA receptor causing sedation and amnesia as well as bronchodilatory effect. Induction doses of 1.5–3 mg/kg IV, time to effect of approximately 15–45 seconds, and a duration of action of 5–10 minutes. Propofol does not provide analgesia

Neuromuscular blockade
- Succinilcholine 1–1.5 mg/kg; rapid onset and short duration of action. Potentially greater histamine release → bronchospasm. Also might cause hyperkalemia
- Vecuronium—no hyperkalemia, but longer duration of paralysis

Sedation, analgesia, and neuromuscular blockade after intubation

Post-intubation medication
- Sedation: Propofol (can lead to seizures, hypertriglyceridemia, increased CO_2 production, "propofol infusion syndrome") or benzodiazepine (e.g., lorazepam)
- Narcotic: fentanyl or alfentanil
- Neuro-muscular blocade: (reduce the risk for barotrauma, avoids coughing, avoids dyssynchronous breathing, allows respiratory muscles to rest) For longer-term paralysis: cisatracurium (Nimbex) 0.8–1.2 mcg/kg/min drip

Confirming placement

- Chest wall movements
- Condensed water vapor in ETT
- Auscultation of breath sounds (in both axillae)
- Carbon dioxide detector and capnography
- Adequate oximeter readings, and chest radiography
- Visualizing trachea or carina through fiberoptic bronchoscope
- Chest radiography will determine the depth of intubation but not esophageal intubation with the patient breathing "around the tube"

Complications of Intubation and Mechanical Ventilation

Complications of IPPV

- Ventilator-associated pneumonia
- Sepsis
- Venous thromboembolism
- Barotrauma
- Hypotension (by decreasing venous return, increase in right ventricular afterload risk related to degree of hyperinflation): 30–60-second apnea trial is recommended, rapid infusion of fluid, then if not better consider pneumothorax or myocardial depression

- Central Nervous System (CNS) injury (cerebral anoxia due to cardiorespiratory arrest prior to intubation)
- Muscle weakness due to acute myopathy (possibly effect of glucocorticoids and neuromuscular paralysis or due to prolonged near-total muscle inactivity)
- Pneumothorax (chest tubes should be placed by blunt dissection to avoid piercing hyperinflated lung)

Some of the specific complications of intubation and mechanical ventilation are discussed in more detail below.

(With permission from Henderson JJ, Popat MT, Latto IP, Pearce AC, Difficult Airway Society 2004.)

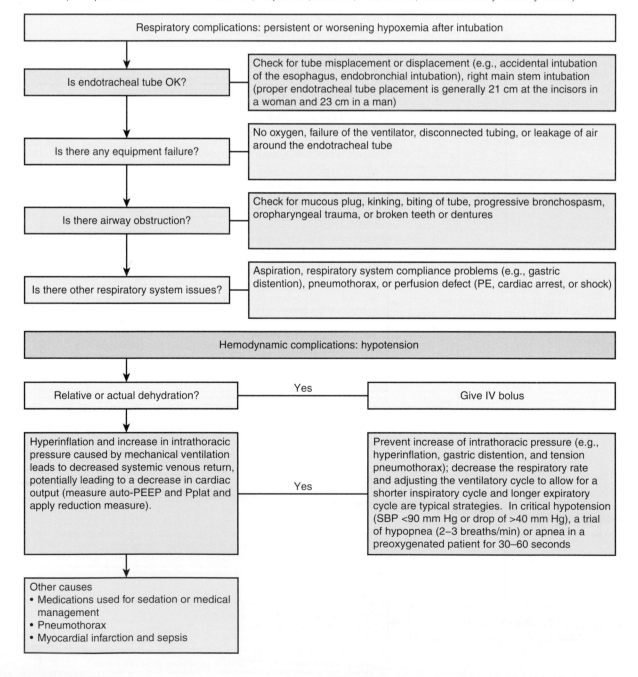

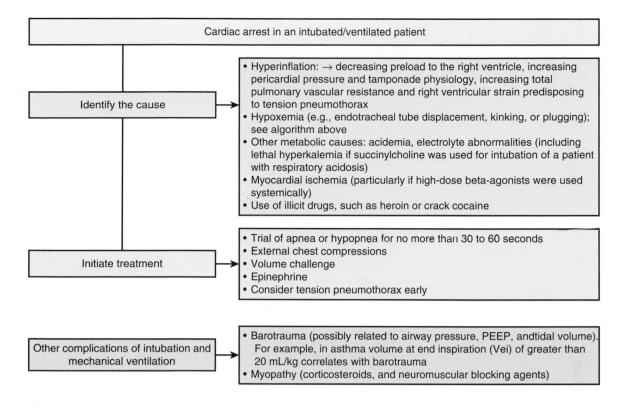

Cardiac arrest in an intubated/ventilated patient

Identify the cause
- Hyperinflation: → decreasing preload to the right ventricle, increasing pericardial pressure and tamponade physiology, increasing total pulmonary vascular resistance and right ventricular strain predisposing to tension pneumothorax
- Hypoxemia (e.g., endotracheal tube displacement, kinking, or plugging); see algorithm above
- Other metabolic causes: acidemia, electrolyte abnormalities (including lethal hyperkalemia if succinylcholine was used for intubation of a patient with respiratory acidosis)
- Myocardial ischemia (particularly if high-dose beta-agonists were used systemically)
- Use of illicit drugs, such as heroin or crack cocaine

Initiate treatment
- Trial of apnea or hypopnea for no more than 30 to 60 seconds
- External chest compressions
- Volume challenge
- Epinephrine
- Consider tension pneumothorax early

Other complications of intubation and mechanical ventilation
- Barotrauma (possibly related to airway pressure, PEEP, andtidal volume). For example, in asthma volume at end inspiration (Vei) of greater than 20 mL/kg correlates with barotrauma
- Myopathy (corticosteroids, and neuromuscular blocking agents)

Difficult Airway

Difficult airway refers to two different clinical scenarios: difficult mask ventilation and difficult endotracheal intubation.[7,23,24]

Difficult Tracheal Intubation

- Difficulty in visualization of the larynx (difficult direct laryngoscopy)

- Anatomic abnormalities (distortion or narrowing of larynx or trachea)

Prediction: Conditions Associated With Difficult Airway

- Abnormal facial anatomy/development
  o Small mouth, large tongue, dental abnormality
  o Obesity, advanced pregnancy, acromegaly
- Inability to open mouth
- Cervical immobility/abnormality
  o Short neck/obesity
  o Poor cervical mobility
- Pharyngeal and laryngeal abnormality
  o High or anterior larynx
  o Deep vallecula

  o Tumor
  o Subglottic stenosis
  o Anatomical abnormality of epiglottis

Other predictors
- Past airway difficulty
- Age >55 years
- Body mass index >26 kg/m^2
- Presence of beard
- Lack of teeth
- History of snoring

```
┌─────────────────────────────────────────────────────────────────────────────┐
│ Does patient have predictors of difficult intubation and airway is anticipated to be difficult │
└─────────────────────────────────────────────────────────────────────────────┘
                    │ Yes
                    ▼
┌─────────────────────────────────────────────────────────────────────┐
│ Options for anticipated difficult airway                              │
│ • Awake intubation                                                    │
│   o Fiberoptic (technique of choice)                                  │
│   o Retrograde intubation: introducing cannula and wire with ETT tube │
│     placed over the wire                                              │
│ • Under anesthesia without neuromuscular blockade                     │
└─────────────────────────────────────────────────────────────────────┘

        No, but found difficult airway in the process of intubation
                                                        │
                                                        ▼
┌─────────────────────────────────────────────────────────────────────┐
│ Strategy for unanticipated difficult airway—difficulty during intubation │
│ • Maintain oxygenation and avoid hypercapnia                          │
│ • Let patient recover consciousness                                   │
│ • Cricoid cartilage pressure or bimanual laryngoscopy                 │
│ • Using stylet (to shape the tube) or gum elastic bougie (place bougie │
│   first and introduce the ET tube over bougie)                        │
│ • Chose different laryngoscope blade                                  │
│ • Lighted stylet (blind tracheal intubation, light is visible through │
│   anterior soft tissues, ET tube introduced over stylet)             │
│ • Fiberoptic intubation                                               │
│ • Supraglottic airway devices (e.g., laryngeal mask airway)          │
│ • Cricothyrotomy (needle, wire-guided percutaneous, surgical)         │
└─────────────────────────────────────────────────────────────────────┘
```

Extubation

Early weaning seems to be beneficial. There is higher mortality, increased rate of pneumonia, and longer hospital stay observed in the group with delayed discontinuation of mechanical ventilation. Although there is still a possibility of selection bias, if the patient seems to be ready to be extubated and meets the criteria, the extubation and discontinuation of mechanical ventilation should not be delayed. While that is true, approximately 15% of all patients who have been extubated and in whom mechanical ventilation has been discontinued require reintubation within 48 hours. Below are the approaches to weaning and extubation.[25]

Strategies to Reduce the Duration of Mechanical Ventilation

• Low TV (6 mL/kg of ideal body weight) in patients with ARDS
• Sedation
  o Wake up (interrupt sedation) patient daily and prior to spontaneous breathing trial
  o No use of sedatives
• Early physical therapy
• Conservative fluid management
• Strategies to reduce ventilator-associated pneumonia

Typical Readiness Criteria

• Hemodynamic stability
• Ratio of PaO_2 (mm Hg) to FiO_2 >200 with PEEP of 5 or less
• Improvement in underlying condition causing respiratory failure

Other criteria

• Improved clinical status
• Adequate oxygenation
• pH 7.33–7.48 with acceptable $PaCO_2$
• Respiratory rate (RR) of 25 or less
• Vital capacity of 10 mL/kg or more
• Maxim inspiratory pressure force <−25 cm H_2O
• TV >5 mL/kg
  Ratio of RR (breaths/min) to TV (liters) 105 or less during 1-minute trial with T-piece (also called rapid shallow breathing index or RSBI)

PEEP, Positive end-expiratory pressure.

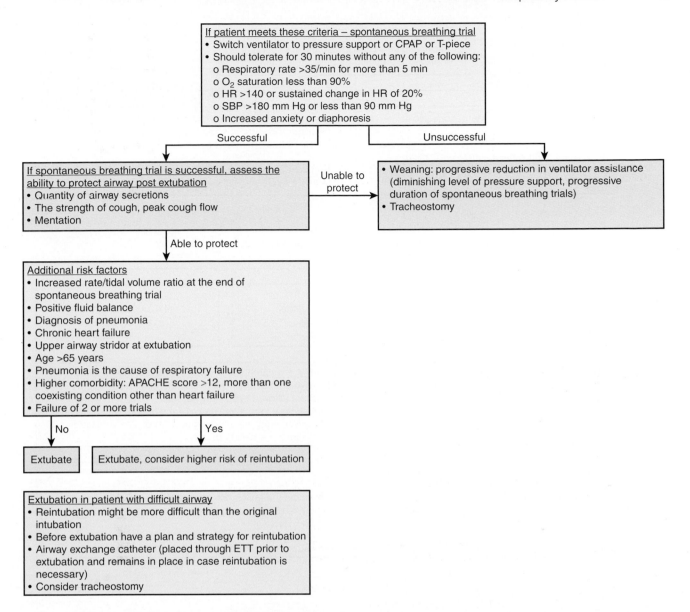

If patient meets these criteria – spontaneous breathing trial
- Switch ventilator to pressure support or CPAP or T-piece
- Should tolerate for 30 minutes without any of the following:
  o Respiratory rate >35/min for more than 5 min
  o O_2 saturation less than 90%
  o HR >140 or sustained change in HR of 20%
  o SBP >180 mm Hg or less than 90 mm Hg
  o Increased anxiety or diaphoresis

Successful

Unsuccessful

If spontaneous breathing trial is successful, assess the ability to protect airway post extubation
- Quantity of airway secretions
- The strength of cough, peak cough flow
- Mentation

Unable to protect

- Weaning: progressive reduction in ventilator assistance (diminishing level of pressure support, progressive duration of spontaneous breathing trials)
- Tracheostomy

Able to protect

Additional risk factors
- Increased rate/tidal volume ratio at the end of spontaneous breathing trial
- Positive fluid balance
- Diagnosis of pneumonia
- Chronic heart failure
- Upper airway stridor at extubation
- Age >65 years
- Pneumonia is the cause of respiratory failure
- Higher comorbidity: APACHE score >12, more than one coexisting condition other than heart failure
- Failure of 2 or more trials

No

Yes

Extubate

Extubate, consider higher risk of reintubation

Extubation in patient with difficult airway
- Reintubation might be more difficult than the original intubation
- Before extubation have a plan and strategy for reintubation
- Airway exchange catheter (placed through ETT prior to extubation and remains in place in case reintubation is necessary)
- Consider tracheostomy

Details of Mechanical Ventilation

Ventilation Modalities

The ventilation modality is determined by three factors[26]:
- Trigger: spontaneous (describes the patient effort) or machine (machine or patient initiates the breath): assist control (AC) or intermittent mandatory ventilation (IMV). Variable flow shapes indicate IMV.
- Target: pressure control (PC) (pressure is the target) or volume control (VC). If various pressures are in different breaths, then it is volume controlled; if volume is different in different breaths, it is pressure controlled (pressure should be stable in each breath).
- Cycle: what turns the breath off: time, volume, or flow criteria/pressure.

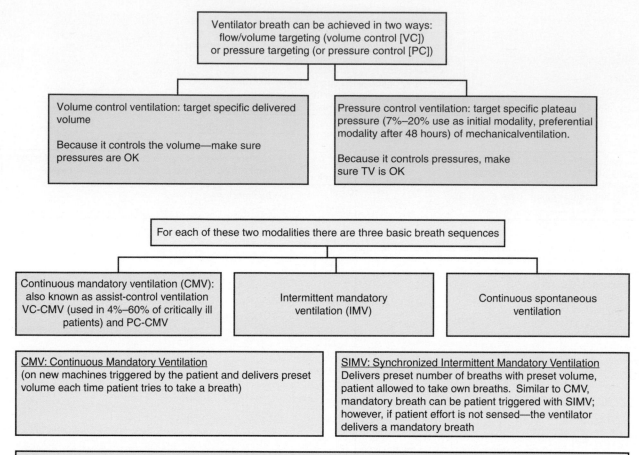

Other PC Modalities in Addition to PC-CMV and PC-IMV
- Pressure support ventilation: patient determines inflation volume and respiratory frequency (but not pressure, as this is pressure controlled), used to augment spontaneous breathing to overcome the resistance of ventilator, especially during weaning, or to augment spontaneous breathing. It is different from PCV in that in PCV breaths are initiated by the machine.
- Airway pressure release ventilation (APRV)
- Biphasic positive airway pressure
- Pressure-regulated VC ventilation (PRVC) is combination of two: PC and VC

PC-CMV, Pressure control–continuous mandatory ventilation.

PC vs. VC

	Pressure Control	Volume Control
Trigger	Patient triggered or time triggered	Patient triggered or time triggered
Set ventilatory variables	Inspiratory pressure Pressure rise time RR Inspiratory time (Ti) or fraction (I:E ratio) Set variables that affect oxygenation: PEEP and FiO_2	TV Vt, ventilator uses the same flow-time waveform in every breath RR Ti or fraction (I:E ratio) Set variables that affect oxygenation: PEEP and FiO_2
Dependent variables	Volume and flow; vary with both respiratory mechanics and patient effort	Airway pressure
Pressure and flow waveforms	The pressure waveform during inspiration is virtually constant (square) and the flow waveform is one of decelerating flow	Inspiratory flow pattern in VC-CMV is most frequently a square flow; other flow patterns can be used (e.g., ramp [accelerating or decelerating] or sinusoidal)
Cycling	Determined by time or flow	Time or volume
Ppk	With PC-CMV, the Ppk is guaranteed by the ventilator and will not exceed the preset pressure limit	Ppk in VC-CMV is the sum of the elastic and resistive pressures plus the initial pressure in the system during flow delivery
TV	Depends on driving pressure, resistance/compliance of respiratory system, and Ti	Preset

Ppk, Peak airway pressure; *VC-CMV*, volume control–continuous mandatory ventilation.

PC Ventilation
- Limits the maximum airway pressure delivered to the lung
- May result in variable tidal and minute volume
- Clinician titrates the inspiratory pressure to the measured tidal volume (TV)
- Inspiratory flow and flow waveform are determined by the ventilator (as it attempts to maintain a square inspiratory pressure profile)

VC Ventilation
- Safety of a preset TV and minute ventilation
- Clinician needs to appropriately set the inspiratory flow, flow waveform, and inspiratory time
- Airway pressure increases in response to reduced compliance, increased resistance, or active exhalation and may increase the risk of ventilator-induced lung injury

The beneficial characteristics of both volume-controlled ventilation (VCV) and pressure-controlled ventilation (PCV) may be combined in dual-control modes, which are volume targeted, pressure limited, and time cycled.[27]

	Pressure Control	Volume Control
Mechanism	Set inspiratory pressure level, PEEP, I:E ratio, RR, and FiO_2 The TV can be variable depending on patient characteristics (compliance, airway/tubing resistance) and driving pressures (difference between the plateau pressure of the airways at end-inspiration and PEEP; also be expressed as the ratio of TV to respiratory system compliance. Evidence suggests we should keep driving pressure below 14 cm H_2O)	Set TV, PEEP, RR, FiO_2 inspiratory pressure level, PEEP, I:E ratio, RR, and FiO_2
Advantages	PC favors the control of oxygenation[28] • Increased mean airway pressure, which improves oxygenation • Increased duration of alveolar recruitment (alveoli are opened earlier and remain open for longer) • Protective against barotrauma (prevents exposure to extremely high pressures) • Work of breathing and patient comfort may be improved (initial high flow rate prevents the "flow starvation") • Limits the maximum airway pressure delivered to the lung • PCV may offer lower work of breathing and improved comfort for patients with increased and variable respiratory demand[27]	VC favors the control of ventilation[28] • Guaranteed TVs produce a more stable minute volume • The minute volume remains stable over a range of changing pulmonary characteristics • The initial flow rate is lower than in pressure-controlled modes, i.e., it avoids a high resistance-related early pressure peak[28]
Disadvantages	• TV and minute volume are variable and dependent on respiratory compliance • Uncontrolled volume may result in "volutrauma" (overdistension) • A high early inspiratory flow may breach the pressure limit if airway resistance is high[28] • PCV offers no advantage over VCV in patients who are not breathing spontaneously[27]	• The mean airway pressure is lower • Recruitment may be poorer in lung units with poor compliance • In the presence of a leak, the mean airway pressure may be unstable • Insufficient flow may give rise to patient-ventilator dyssynchrony[28]
Specific cases when to use		

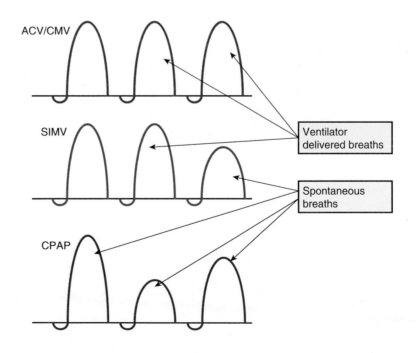

Clinical Objectives of Mechanical Ventilation

- To reverse hypoxemia
- To reverse acute respiratory acidosis
- To relieve respiratory distress
- To prevent or reverse atelectasis
- To reverse respiratory muscle fatigue

- To permit sedation and/or neuromuscular blockage
- To decrease systemic or myocardial oxygen consumption
- To reduce intracranial pressure
- To stabilize the chest wall

Initial Ventilator Setting for Ventilatory Failure Patient

- Controlled mechanical ventilation, e.g., assist controlled, occasionally other modes (e.g., PRVC, CMV)
- Rate: 10 breaths/min (8–16 is acceptable rate initially), depending on desired $PaCO_2$ ($PaCO_2$ target/$PaCO_2$real = Rate_target/Rate_real)
- TV = 6–8 mL/kg of ideal body weight, calculate ideal body weight first: males: 50 + 2.3* (height in inches: 60); females: 45.5 + 2.3* (height in inches: 60)
- High peak inspiratory flow such as 80–90 L/min to minimize inspiratory time and enhance expiratory time

- Fraction of inspired oxygen at 1.0 initially, and then adjust to provide adequate oxygenation
- PEEP—supports expiratory pressure to prevent closure of edematous small airways, indicated when oxygenation is inadequate (start at 5, increase by 2–5 to maintain oxygenation PaO_2[3] 60 mm Hg, PEEP >12 sometimes requires an S-G catheter)
- Pressure support = supports inspiratory pressure (=peak airway pressure/3)

S-G, Swan-Ganz.

Troubleshooting of Common Ventilator Issues

Desaturation	D—displacement of the tube, air leak/broken cuff (difference in TV in and out) O—obstruction (tube or filter): elevated peak pressure P—pneumothorax (feel pressure while bagging, elevated peak, and plateau pressure), PE, parenchymal disease (worsening of CXR), intrapulmonary shunt E—equipment failure (rare) R—rigidity of chest wall (increased pressures) Action: examine the tube, pressure cuff, check ventilator parameters (peak and plateau pressures, TV in and TV out), disconnect ventilator and bag, see if there is resistance (tube obstruction, pneumothorax, rigidity), and if O_2 saturation improves with bagging (suggests machine setting issues). If ARDS is the cause—prone and paralyze

Elevated peak pressure[29,30]	• If patient is hypotensive—think elevated intrathoracic pressure: critical auto-PEEP or tension pneumothorax. Remove ventilator and bag (if auto-PEEP) hypotension improves. If patient does not improve –think tube obstruction or pneumothorax: consider needle decompression and then chest tube
	• If hemodynamically stable
	  o If high difference between peak and plateau (>5 cm H_2O)—increase resistance of airways (e.g., bronchospasm, ET tube obstruction, ventilator circuit obstruction, anaphylaxis, or inappropriately high inspiratory flow >60 L/min): inline suctioning, bronchodilators
	  o If low difference—acute decrease in lung compliance (e.g., pneumothorax, ARDS, evolving pneumonia, pulmonary edema, auto-PEEP caused by "breath staking," chest wall rigidity, abdominal distention, right main stem intubation)

Hypotension in ventilated patient[31]	• Relative hypovolemia (reduction in venous return exacerbated by positive intrathoracic pressure) • Drug-induced vasodilation and myocardial depression (all anesthetic induction agents have some short-lived vasodilatory/myocardial depressant effects) • Gas trapping (dynamic hyperinflation) • Tension pneumothorax
Patient-ventilator dyssynchrony	See below

ET, Endotracheal tube.

Troubleshooting for Ventilator Issues

- Air leak: discrepancy between set TV and delivered TV: check tubing for leak
- Disconnected airway: check for continuity of tubing
- TV issues in PC mode (TV drops): check for decreased compliance or increased resistance
- Increased pressures in VC mode:

  o If both peak and plateau pressure increased—decreased compliance (e.g., pneumothorax, tube migrated to right bronchus, pulmonary edema)
  o If only peak pressure elevated—increased resistance (e.g., mucous plug)

Quick Algorithm and Checklist of Ventilator Setting Assessment/Adjustment

- If settings are adequate: look at ABG: PaO_2 goal 55–80 mm Hg or SpO_2 88%–95%, pH goal 7.3–7.45. FiO_2 and PEEP affect pO_2, while TV and rate affect pCO_2.
  o If pH 7.15–7.3 (respiratory acidosis): increase RR until pH >7.3 or $PaCO_2$ <25 (max RR 35)
  o If pH <7.15 (respiratory acidosis): increase RR to 35; if pH remains <7.15: increase TV in 1-mL/kg steps until pH >7.15 (maintain Pplat not higher than 30)
  o If ↓ pCO_2—hyperventilation—decrease rate or TV
  o If ↑ pCO_2—CO_2 retention—increase rate or TV
  o If hypoxemic—increase FiO_2 or PEEP
  o I:E ratio: duration of inspiration ≤ expiration
- If settings are safe: look at the
  - TV (not more than 6 mL/kg), calculate ideal body weight first: males: 50 + 2.3* (height in inches: 60); females: 45.5 + 2.3* (height in inches: 60). If you are concerned about TV, then control the flow/volume.

- Pressures:
  - Peak pressure reflect resistance in the entire circuit from ventilator to alveolus
  - Pplat (goal <30 cm H_2O) reflects on resistance to lung inflation (e.g., restrictive lung disease, too high TV)
  - Transpulmonary pressure (Pplat minus Pesoph) of 25–30 cm H_2O
  - Driving pressure (Pplat minus PEEP), should be 15–18, if higher—reduce TV[32]
  - O_2 and PEEP: pO_2 goal 55–80 mm Hg or SpO_2 88%–95%, use a minimal PEEP of 5 cm H_2O
  - Is there potentially intrinsic PEEP (auto-PEEP)
- If patient is comfortable (look for tachypnea, asynchrony): one way to improve comfort and synchrony—control pressure. More on asynchrony—see below
- If possible, extubate

I:E ratio, Inspiratory-to-expiratory ratio; *Pesoph,* esophageal pressure; *Pplat,* plateau pressure.

Ventilator Asynchrony Management

Disrupted or poor interaction between the patient and ventilator leads to asynchrony between ventilator-delivered breaths and patient's breathing. This eventually results in patient discomfort and fatigue.[33] Asynchronous ventilator pattern should be avoided.

```
┌─────────────────────────────┐
│   Asynchrony management      │
└─────────────────────────────┘
```

Abnormal triggering the ventilator
- Missed triggers or delayed trigger: patient effort not recognized by the ventilator secondary to intrinsic PEEP, weak effort, or inappropriate sensitivity setting (if the patient is having difficulty triggering the ventilator despite a sensitive setting—consider that auto-PEEP causing dynamic hyperinflation is the problem)
- Auto-triggering: breaths delivered in the absence of patient effort secondary to leaks or inappropriate sensitivity setting
- Double triggering: continued patient effort following breath delivery, resulting in a second triggered breath: volume control continuous mandatory ventilation and neurally adjusted ventilatory assist (NAVA)
- Reverse triggering: activation of respiratory muscles by mandatory, time triggered breaths

→

Solutions for trigger asynchrony
In volume assist-control (VAC):
- In the older generation ventilators flow trigger would, at times, reduce trigger asynchrony.
- Increase sensitivity
- Reduce auto PEEP
- Apply extrinsic PEEP

Flow delivery problems
- Flow mismatch or flow asynchrony (patient demand does not match ventilator output): volume control
- Insufficient pressurization rate (rise time too slow): pressure support
- Mode asynchrony: active effort during adaptive pressure ventilation, resulting in insufficient support: use of intermittent mandatory ventilation with interspersed volume and pressure breaths, precluding sufficient respiratory muscle unloading

→

Solutions for flow asynchrony
- VAC
  o Increase set flow (decrease Ti)
  o Switch to a pressure target mode
  o Square wave of flow (decrease Ti)
- Pressure assist-control (PAC)/PSV
  o Adjust the rise time
  o Increase the inspiratory pressure (watch for increase in Vt)

Timing/cycle asynchrony
- Premature cycling: neuromechanical asynchrony: mechanical inspiratory time shorter than neural inspiratory time
- Late cycling: neuromechanical asynchrony: mechanical inspiratory time longer than neural inspiratory time
- I:E ratio: 1:2 ratio is close to a normal breathing pattern and is more comfortable

→

Solutions for Cycle Asynchrony
Premature cycling in VAC
- Decrease flow/Vt in VAC
Premature cycling in PAC
- Increase Ti
- Switch to PSV
Premature cycling in PSV
- Adjust flow termination %
- Mode of ventilation
  o Spontaneous modes are more comfortable than control modes
  o BIPAP might be more comfortable and improves synchrony

Adjustment of Ventilator Parameters Based on Compliance and Resistance

Decreased compliance and increased resistance might give additional insight and dictate further adjustment of ventilator parameters.[5,6]

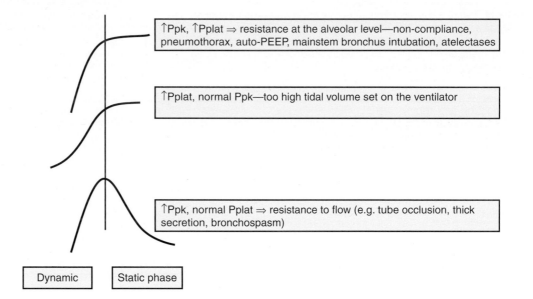

Diagnostic value of compliance and resistance[34]

Compliance
- Definition
  - Static compliance = TV/(Pplat – PEEP) normally 60 and below cm H_2O
  - Dynamic compliance = TV/(Ppeak – PEEP) normally 100 and below cm H_2O
- Diagnostic value: decreased compliance presents as increased both peak pressure and plateau pressure: ≥30 mL/cm H_2O
- Stiffer lungs will show shallow volume curve
- Decreased compliance is observed in:
  - Pulmonary edema
  - Fibrosis
  - ARDS
  - Pneumothorax

Resistance
- Definition: Resistance = (Paw – Pplat)/Peak inspiratory flow rate
- Diagnostic value: increased resistance presents as increased peak pressure and increased difference between peak and plateau): ≥6 cm H_2O
- Increased resistance will "lose" tidal volume; check TV in pressure control ventilation
- Increased resistance:
  - Bronchospasm
  - Mucous plugging

Ppk—peak inspiratory pressure (<25–35 cm H_2O)
Pplat—plateau pressure (<30 cm H_2O)

↑Ppk, ↑Pplat ⇒ resistance at the alveolar level—non-compliance, pneumothorax, auto-PEEP, mainstem bronchus intubation, atelectases

↑Pplat, normal Ppk—too high tidal volume set on the ventilator

↑Ppk, normal Pplat ⇒ resistance to flow (e.g. tube occlusion, thick secretion, bronchospasm)

Dynamic   Static phase

More Details on Managing Intubated/Ventilated Patient in Specific Conditions

Mechanical Ventilation in Obstructive Lung Disease (COPD, Asthma)[5,6]

Potential Issues With Ventilating Patient With Obstructive Disease	
Assess for pulmonary hyperinflation (see below)	Assess compliance and resistance and adjust ventilator parameters
Manage hypercapnia (see below)	
Address asynchrony	

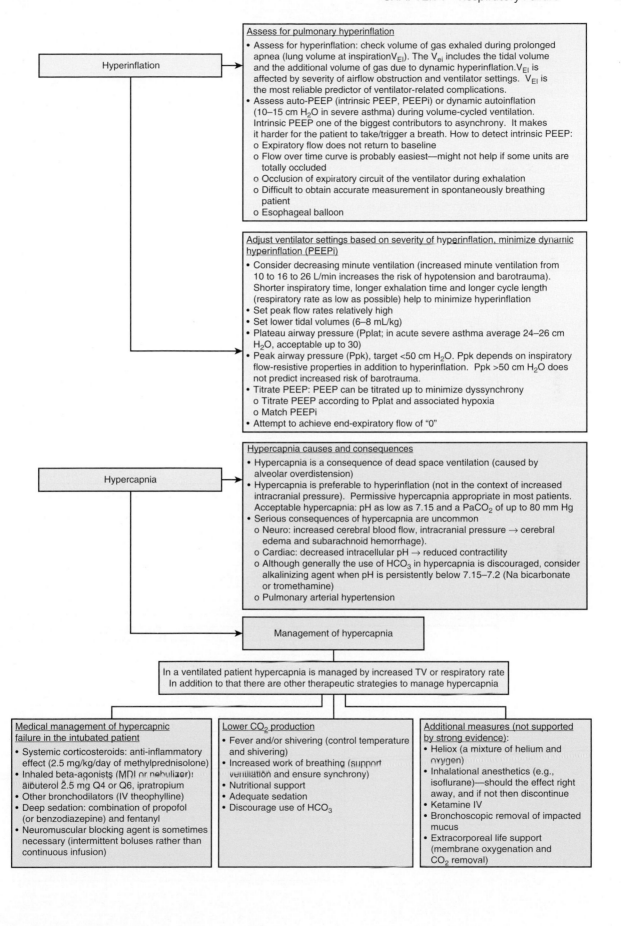

Hyperinflation

Assess for pulmonary hyperinflation

- Assess for hyperinflation: check volume of gas exhaled during prolonged apnea (lung volume at inspiration V_{EI}). The V_{ei} includes the tidal volume and the additional volume of gas due to dynamic hyperinflation. V_{EI} is affected by severity of airflow obstruction and ventilator settings. V_{EI} is the most reliable predictor of ventilator-related complications.
- Assess auto-PEEP (intrinsic PEEP, PEEPi) or dynamic autoinflation (10–15 cm H_2O in severe asthma) during volume-cycled ventilation. Intrinsic PEEP one of the biggest contributors to asynchrony. It makes it harder for the patient to take/trigger a breath. How to detect intrinsic PEEP:
  - o Expiratory flow does not return to baseline
  - o Flow over time curve is probably easiest—might not help if some units are totally occluded
  - o Occlusion of expiratory circuit of the ventilator during exhalation
  - o Difficult to obtain accurate measurement in spontaneously breathing patient
  - o Esophageal balloon

Adjust ventilator settings based on severity of hyperinflation, minimize dynamic hyperinflation (PEEPi)

- Consider decreasing minute ventilation (increased minute ventilation from 10 to 16 to 26 L/min increases the risk of hypotension and barotrauma). Shorter inspiratory time, longer exhalation time and longer cycle length (respiratory rate as low as possible) help to minimize hyperinflation
- Set peak flow rates relatively high
- Set lower tidal volumes (6–8 mL/kg)
- Plateau airway pressure (Pplat; in acute severe asthma average 24–26 cm H_2O, acceptable up to 30)
- Peak airway pressure (Ppk), target <50 cm H_2O. Ppk depends on inspiratory flow-resistive properties in addition to hyperinflation. Ppk >50 cm H_2O does not predict increased risk of barotrauma.
- Titrate PEEP: PEEP can be titrated up to minimize dyssynchrony
  - o Titrate PEEP according to Pplat and associated hypoxia
  - o Match PEEPi
- Attempt to achieve end-expiratory flow of "0"

Hypercapnia

Hypercapnia causes and consequences

- Hypercapnia is a consequence of dead space ventilation (caused by alveolar overdistension)
- Hypercapnia is preferable to hyperinflation (not in the context of increased intracranial pressure). Permissive hypercapnia appropriate in most patients. Acceptable hypercapnia: pH as low as 7.15 and a $PaCO_2$ of up to 80 mm Hg
- Serious consequences of hypercapnia are uncommon
  - o Neuro: increased cerebral blood flow, intracranial pressure → cerebral edema and subarachnoid hemorrhage).
  - o Cardiac: decreased intracellular pH → reduced contractility
  - o Although generally the use of HCO_3 in hypercapnia is discouraged, consider alkalinizing agent when pH is persistently below 7.15–7.2 (Na bicarbonate or tromethamine)
  - o Pulmonary arterial hypertension

Management of hypercapnia

In a ventilated patient hypercapnia is managed by increased TV or respiratory rate
In addition to that there are other therapeutic strategies to manage hypercapnia

Medical management of hypercapnic failure in the intubated patient

- Systemic corticosteroids: anti-inflammatory effect (2.5 mg/kg/day of methylprednisolone)
- Inhaled beta-agonists (MDI or nebulizer): albuterol 2.5 mg Q4 or Q6, ipratropium
- Other bronchodilators (IV theophylline)
- Deep sedation: combination of propofol (or benzodiazepine) and fentanyl
- Neuromuscular blocking agent is sometimes necessary (intermittent boluses rather than continuous infusion)

Lower CO_2 production

- Fever and/or shivering (control temperature and shivering)
- Increased work of breathing (support ventilation and ensure synchrony)
- Nutritional support
- Adequate sedation
- Discourage use of HCO_3

Additional measures (not supported by strong evidence):

- Heliox (a mixture of helium and oxygen)
- Inhalational anesthetics (e.g., isoflurane)—should the effect right away, and if not then discontinue
- Ketamine IV
- Bronchoscopic removal of impacted mucus
- Extracorporeal life support (membrane oxygenation and CO_2 removal)

Mechanical Ventilation in Parenchymal Lung Disease (e.g., ARDS)

Strategies to adjust PEEP
- Optimal PEEP in patients with ARDS remains an area of active investigation
- The easiest approach to select PEEP might be according to the severity of the disease: 5–10 cm H_2O PEEP in mild ARDS, 10–15 cm H_2O PEEP in moderate ARDS, and 15–20 cm H_2O PEEP in severe ARDS[35]
- Several methods of selecting optimal PEEP are available: increasing or decreasing PEEP trial (see below), ARDSnet study tables (see below)[36]
- Consider recruitment maneuvers[37]
- Optimal PEEP may depend on the tidal volume (so if TV is changed optimal PEEP might need to be established again)[38]
- Increase PEEP and check plateau pressure, if increased by less than PEEP addition, then it means some lung volume has been recruited
- Be cognizant of RV function: PEEP affects RV function in acute respiratory failure patients[39]
- Use measurements to adjust PEEP:
  - Stress index (a parameter derived from the shape of the pressure-time curve, can identify injurious mechanical ventilation)
  - Esophageal pressure
  - Pressure volume curve

PEEP trial
- Establish level of PEEP at which oxygen delivery is optimal or that maximizes lung compliance
- If a pulmonary artery catheter is in place, oxygen delivery (DO_2) is calculated with each change in PEEP: $DO_2 = (Hb \times SaO_2 \times 1.34 + PaO_2 \times 0.003) \times CO$
  - Note: DO_2 declines if the drop in CO caused by PEEP outweighs the rise in arterial O_2 content. Therefore, the best PEEP may be less than the amount that achieves the highest SaO_2
- If a pulmonary artery catheter is not available, the best PEEP may be approximated by determining the level which results in the highest compliance for a given tidal volume, using the formula: compliance = TV / (Ppl - PEEP)
  - Note: cardiac output may fall independently of changes in thoracic compliance

ARDSnet study tables[40]
OXYGENATION GOAL: PaO_2 55–80 mm Hg or SpO_2 88%–95%
Use a minimum PEEP of 5 cm H_2O. Consider use of incremental FiO_2/PEEP combinations such as shown below (not required) to achieve goal

Lower PEEP/higher FiO_2

FiO_2	0.3	0.4	0.4	0.5	0.5	0.6	0.7	0.7
PEEP	5	5	8	8	10	10	10	12

FiO_2	0.7	0.8	0.9	0.9	0.9	1.0
PEEP	14	14	14	16	18	18.24

Higher PEEP/lower FiO_2

FiO_2	0.3	0.3	0.3	0.3	0.3	0.4	0.4	0.5
PEEP	5	8	10	12	14	14	16	16

FiO_2	0.5	0.5–0.8	0.8	0.9	1.0	1.0
PEEP	18	20	22	22	22	24

Lung recruitment maneuvers[35]
- Multiple methods have been described
- 40 cm H_2O for 40–60 seconds
- 3 consecutive sighs/min with a plateau pressure of 45 cm H_2O
- 2 minutes of peak pressure of 50 cm H_2O and PEEP above upper inflection point (obese/trauma patients may require >60–70 cm H_2O)
- Long slow increase in inspiratory pressure up to 40 cm H_2O (RAMP)
- Stepped increase in pressure (e.g., staircase recruitment maneuver)

General Principles

- Mode of mechanical ventilation is not important
- Provide adequate oxygenation (PO_2 55–80 mm Hg) with nontoxic FiO_2 levels (<0.5–0.7), and lung protective ventilation
- Low TV, low pressure: plateau <30 cm H_2O to avoid VALI
- Keep lung recruited (PEEP). Some suggest that PEEP does not cause barotrauma

- Decrease O_2 consumption (e.g., treat fever, tachycardia, and inflammation)
- Adequate hemodynamic support and hemoglobin

VALI, Ventilator-associated lung injury.

Mechanical Ventilation and Acute Renal Failure

Renal failure is not uncommon in ventilated patients. Aside from an underlying disease, mechanical ventilation can cause or worsen renal failure through several mechanisms either through ischemic or toxic effect on the kidneys. Specifically, permissive hypercapnia, hypoxemia, and diminished renal blood flow might precipitate tubular damage through ischemic effect. At the same time, mechanical ventilation might trigger or worsen inflammatory reaction with direct toxic effects on renal parenchyma.[41]

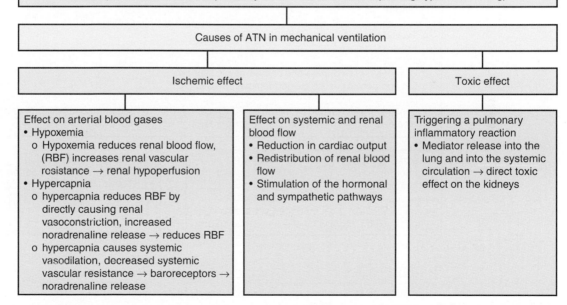

Complications of Mechanical Ventilation[5,6]

- Ventilator-associated pneumonia
- Sepsis
- Venous thromboembolism
- Barotrauma
- Hypotension (by decreasing venous return, increase in right ventricular afterload risk related to degree of hyperinflation): 30–60-second apnea trial is recommended, rapid infusion of fluid, then if not better consider pneumothorax or myocardial depression

- CNS injury (cerebral anoxia due to cardiorespiratory arrest prior to intubation)
- Muscle weakness due to acute myopathy (possibly effect of glucocorticoids and neuromuscular paralysis or due to prolonged near-total muscle inactivity)
- Pneumothorax (chest tubes should be placed by blunt dissection to avoid piercing hyperinflated lung)

Extracorporeal Membrane Oxygenation

Extracorporeal membrane oxygenation (ECMO) is based on a gas exchange through a semipermeable membrane. Venous blood comes to the oxygenator and oxygenated blood is returned into either the artery or the large vein.[11,42,43]

> The goal of ECMO is to support gas exchange and oxygen delivery to the tissues

Indications

Respiratory
- Respiratory failure hypoxic (e.g., ARDS) or hypercapnic
- Bridge to lung transplantation or during graft dysfunction
- Massive air leak syndromes (bronchopleural fistula)
- Status asthmaticus
- Diffuse alveolar hemorrhage
- Pulmonary embolism

Cardiac
- Cardiogenic shock ischemic (acute MI) or non-ischemic (e.g., fulminant myocarditis, post-cardiotomy)
- Sepsis-associated cardiomyopathy
- Pulmonary hypertensive crisis
- Extracorporeal cardio-pulmonary resuscitation
- Graft failure after heart transplantation
- Bridge to VAD or heart transplantation

Only ARDS is supported by some randomized controlled studies, for other indications evidence is from cohort studies

Contraindications

There are no absolute contraindications
Relative contraindications:
- Recent central nearvous system
- Hemorrhage and other contraindications to anticoagulation
- Advanced vascular disease

Technique
- Veno-venous (blood drained from central vein and returned to central vein)
  - Typical cannulas range from 23 to 29F
  - Provides gas exchange only
- Veno-arterial
  - Provides gas exchange and hemodynamic support
  - Extracorporeal carbon dioxide removal (ECCO2R)

Oxygenation is determined by: blood flow, FiO_2 delivered by oxygenator, contribution of native lungs
CO_2 removal is determined by: rate of gas flow through oxygenator, blood flow rate.

Potential complications
- Hemorrhage
- Thromboses
- Infection
- Limb ischemia and compartment syndrome
- Hemolysis, thrombocytopenia, DIC, air embolism

Predictors of poor outcome
- Renal failure predicts poor prognosis
- Longer duration of mechanical ventilation before ECMO (specifically >7 days)

REFERENCES

1. Sud S, Sud M, Friedrich JO, Adhikari NK. Effect of mechanical ventilation in the prone position on clinical outcomes in patients with acute hypoxemic respiratory failure: a systematic review and meta-analysis. *CMAJ (Can Med Assoc J)*. 2008;178(9):1153–1161.
2. Na MJ. Diagnostic tools of pleural effusion. *Tuberc Respir Dis*. 2014;76(5):199–210.
3. Mosier JM, Hypes C, Joshi R, Whitmore S, Parthasarathy S, Cairns CB. Ventilator strategies and rescue therapies for management of acute respiratory failure in the emergency department. *Ann Emerg Med*. 2015;66(5):529–541.
4. Pradhan D, Berger K. Images in clinical medicine. Dynamic extrathoracic airway obstruction. *N Engl J Med*. 2012;367(1):e2.
5. Brenner B, Corbridge T, Kazzi A. Intubation and mechanical ventilation of the asthmatic patient in respiratory failure. *J Emerg Med*. 2009;37(suppl 2):S23–S34.
6. Leatherman J. Mechanical ventilation for severe asthma. *Chest*. 2015;147(6):1671–1680.
7. Lavery GG, McCloskey BV. The difficult airway in adult critical care. *Crit Care Med*. 2008;36(7):2163–2173.
8. Phua J, Badia JR, Adhikari NK, et al. Has mortality from acute respiratory distress syndrome decreased over time?: a systematic review. *Am J Respir Crit Care Med*. 2009;179(3):220–227.

9. Liu LL, Aldrich JM, Shimabukuro DW, et al. Special article: rescue therapies for acute hypoxemic respiratory failure. *Anesth Analg*. 2010;111(3):693–702.
10. Hemmila MR, Napolitano LM. Severe respiratory failure: advanced treatment options. *Crit Care Med*. 2006;34(suppl 9):S278–S290.
11. Ventetuolo CE, Muratore CS. Extracorporeal life support in critically ill adults. *Am J Respir Crit Care Med*. 2014;190(5):497–508.
12. Matthay MA, Ware LB, Zimmerman GA. The acute respiratory distress syndrome. *J Clin Invest*. 2012;122(8):2731–2740.
13. Papazian L, Doddoli C, Chetaille B, et al. A contributive result of open-lung biopsy improves survival in acute respiratory distress syndrome patients. *Crit Care Med*. 2007;35(3):755–762.
14. Palakshappa JA, Meyer NJ. Which patients with ARDS benefit from lung biopsy? *Chest*. 2015;148(4):1073–1082.
15. Papazian L, Forel JM, Gacouin A, et al. Neuromuscular blockers in early acute respiratory distress syndrome. *N Engl J Med*. 2010;363(12):1107–1116.
16. Hall JB. Point: should paralytic agents be routinely used in severe ARDS? Yes. *Chest*. 2013;144(5):1440–1442.
17. Hall JB, Sessler CN, Hall JB, Sessler CN. Counterpoint: should paralytic agents be routinely used in severe ARDS? No. *Chest*. 2013;144(5):1442–1445.
18. Montgomery AB, Stager MA, Carrico CJ, Hudson LD. Causes of mortality in patients with the adult respiratory distress syndrome. *Am Rev Respir Dis*. 1985;132(3):485–489.
19. Antoniou KM, Margaritopoulos GA, Tomassetti S, Bonella F, Costabel U, Poletti V. Interstitial lung disease. *Eur Respir Rev*. 2014;23(131):40–54.
20. Meyer KC. Diagnosis and management of interstitial lung disease. *Transl Respir Med*. 2014;2(1):4.
21. Bartel B. Systemic thrombolysis for acute pulmonary embolism. *Hosp Pract*. 2015;43(1):22–27.
22. Nava S, Hill N. Non-invasive ventilation in acute respiratory failure. *Lancet*. 2009;374(9685):250–259.
23. Apfelbaum JL, Hagberg CA, Caplan RA, et al. Practice guidelines for management of the difficult airway: an updated report by the American Society of Anesthesiologists Task force on management of the difficult airway. *Anesthesiology*. 2013;118(2):251–270.
24. Henderson JJ, Popat MT, Latto IP, Pearce AC. Difficult Airway Society. Difficult Airway Society guidelines for management of the unanticipated difficult intubation. *Anaesthesia*. 2004;59(7):675–694.
25. McConville JF, Kress JP. Weaning patients from the ventilator. *N Engl J Med*. 2012;367(23):2233–2239.
26. Rittayamai N, Katsios CM, Beloncle F, Friedrich JO, Mancebo J, Brochard L. Pressure-controlled vs volume-controlled ventilation in acute respiratory failure: a physiology-based narrative and systematic review. *Chest*. 2015;148(2):340–355.
27. Campbell R, Davis B. Pressure-controlled versus volume-controlled ventilation: does it matter? *Respir Care*. 2002;47(4):416–424; discussion 424-426.
28. Practical differences between pressure and volume controlled ventilation. In: Deranged Physiology. https://derangedphysiology.com/main/cicm-primary-exam/required-reading/respiratory-system/Chapter 542/practical-differences-between. Accessed June 26, 2020.
29. Jain M, Sznajder JI. Bench-to-bedside review: distal airways in acute respiratory distress syndrome. *Crit Care*. 2007;11(1):206.
30. Covert T, Niu NT. Differential diagnosis of high peak airway pressures. *Dimens Crit Care Nurs*. 2015;34(1):19–23.
31. Troubleshooting mechanical ventilation. www.aic.cuhk.edu.hk/web8/Mech vent troubleshooting.htm. Accessed April 8, 2020.
32. Bugedo G, Retamal J, Bruhn A. Driving pressure: a marker of severity, a safety limit, or a goal for mechanical ventilation? *Crit Care*. 2017;21(1):199.
33. Branson RD, Blakeman TC, Robinson BR. Asynchrony and dyspnea. *Respir Care*. 2013;58(6):973–989.
34. Grinnan DC, Truwit JD. Clinical review: respiratory mechanics in spontaneous and assisted ventilation. *Crit Care*. 2005;9(5):472–484.
35. Hess DR. Recruitment maneuvers and PEEP titration. *Respir Care*. 2015;60(11):1688–1704.
36. Al Masry A, Boules ML, Boules NS, Ebied RS. Optimal method for selecting PEEP level in ALI/ARDS patients under mechanical ventilation. *J Egypt Soc Parasitol*. 2012;42(2):359–372.
37. Hodgson C, Goligher EC, Young ME, et al. Recruitment manoeuvres for adults with acute respiratory distress syndrome receiving mechanical ventilation. *Cochrane Database Syst Rev*. 2016;11:CD006667.
38. McKown AC, Semler MW, Rice TW. Best PEEP trials are dependent on tidal volume. *Crit Care*. 2018;22(1):115.
39. Dambrosio M, Fiore G, Brienza N, et al. Right ventricular myocardial function in ARF patients. PEEP as a challenge for the right heart. *Intensive Care Med*. 1996;22(8):772–780.
40. ARDSnet: NIH NHLBI ARDS Clinical Network Mechanical Ventilation Protocol Summary. http://www.ardsnet.org/files/ventilator_protocol_2008-07.pdf. Accessed July 23, 2019.
41. Kuiper JW, Groeneveld AB, Slutsky AS, Plotz FB. Mechanical ventilation and acute renal failure. *Crit Care Med*. 2005;33(6):1408–1415.
42. Abrams D, Combes A, Brodie D. Extracorporeal membrane oxygenation in cardiopulmonary disease in adults. *J Am Coll Cardiol*. 2014;63(25 Pt A):2769–2778.
43. Combes A, Brodie D, Bartlett R, et al. Position paper for the organization of extracorporeal membrane oxygenation programs for acute respiratory failure in adult patients. *Am J Respir Crit Care Med*. 2014;190(5):488–496.

CHAPTER 2

Critical Care Cardiology and Hypertension

Alexander Goldfarb-Rumyantzev

Chest Pain

Chest pain is an important symptom of cardiac ischemia; however, in most of the patients presenting with chest pain, it has a noncardiac origin. The diagram below describes different etiologies of chest pain. The distinction between cardiac and noncardiac chest pain is not always obvious, but clinically important. Several indicators and prediction scores of chest pain related to acute coronary syndrome (ACS) are described below.[1]

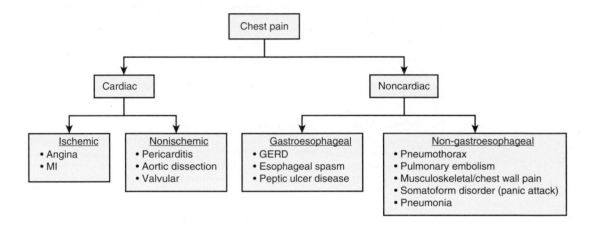

Does Patient Have ACS[2,3]

The clinical factors most suggestive of ACS: prior abnormal stress test, peripheral arterial disease, and pain radiation to both arms

The most useful electrocardiogram (ECG) findings: ST-segment depression or any evidence of ischemia

TIMI Risk Score (Predicting ACS in Patients With Undifferentiated Chest Pain)[4]

Thrombolysis in Myocardial Infarction (TIMI) risk score
- Age ≥65 years
- ≥3 coronary artery disease (CAD) risk factors
- Known CAD (stenosis ≥50%)
- Aspirin (ASA) use in the past 7 days
- Severe angina (≥2 episodes in 24 hours)
- ECG ST changes ≥0.5 mm
- Positive cardiac marker
- Each "yes" answer adds one point to the score

HEART Risk Score (Predicts 6-Month Risk of Major Cardiac Events)[5]

History (highly suspicious +2, moderately suspicious +1, slightly suspicious 0)
ECG (significant ST depression +2, nonspecific repolarization disturbance +1, normal 0)
Age (≥65 + 2, 45–65 + 1, <45 years)
Risk factors:
- hypercholesterolemia
- hypertension
- diabetes mellitus
- cigarette smoking
- family history
- obesity (≥3 risk factors or history of atherosclerotic disease +2, 1–2 risk factors +1)

Troponin (>3x normal limit +2, 1-3x normal limit +1, < upper limit of normal limit 0)
HEART scores 0 to 3: major adverse cardiac events (MACE) occurred in 1.7%
HEART scores 4 to 6: MACE was diagnosed in 16.6%
HEART scores 7 to 10: MACE occurred in 50.1%

GRACE Risk Score (Mortality Prediction)[6]

Global Registry of Acute Coronary Events (GRACE) risk score
- Age
- Increased heart rate (HR)
- Lower systolic blood pressure (SBP)
- Creatinine
- Cardiac arrest at admission
- ST-segment deviation on ECG
- Elevated/abnormal cardiac enzymes
- Killip class (signs/symptoms): signs of congestive heart failure (CHF) (class 1), rales and/or jugular vein distention (JVD) (class 2), pulmonary edema (class 3), cardiogenic shock (class 4)
- The c-statistic of the HEART score is 0.83, of TIMI is 0.75, and of GRACE is 0.70.[5]

Pathogenesis of ACS

Several etiologies and mechanisms of ACS are indicated in the diagram below. ACS is caused by insufficient amount of blood flow in relation to the demand of the myocardium. It can be caused by mechanical obstruction (e.g., ruptured plaque), coronary vasoconstriction, or increased demand (e.g., tachycardia) while supply cannot be upregulated.

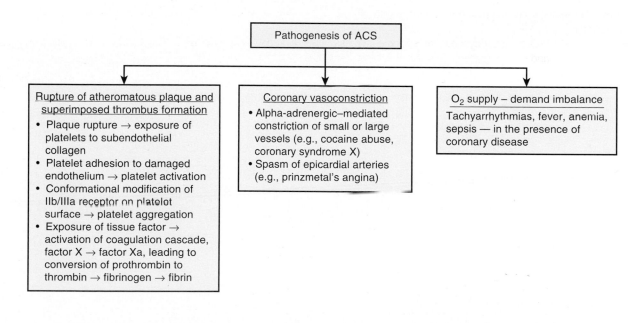

Acute Coronary Syndrome

ACS is further classified based on ECG findings, specifically, presence of ST-segment elevation and presence of cardiac enzymes: ST-elevation myocardial infarction (MI), non–ST-elevation MI (NSTEMI), unstable angina.

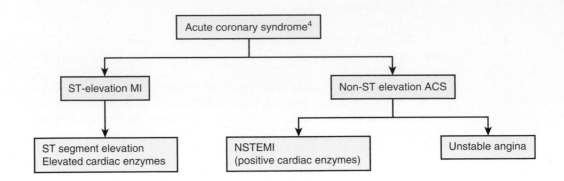

Additional Diagnostic Tests in ACS

As it was indicated earlier, ACS is classified based on ECG features and presence of abnormal cardiac enzymes. The next tier of tests includes echocardiogram and other imaging modalities, additional biochemical markers, and ECG signs.

ECG

- ST-segment depression (persistent or transient)
- Deep, symmetrical T-wave inversions are compatible with ACS but not diagnostic

Biomarkers

- Cardiac troponins (I or T) reflect myonecrosis, elevated in NSTEMI; two negative results 6–9 hours apart usually rule out NSTEMI
- Elevated CRP (inflammation marker) associated with increased long-term risk
- BNP or proBNP reflects hemodynamic stress, increased risk
- Elevated HbA$_{1c}$ and Cr—increased risk of event and adverse outcome

Imaging

- Echo: assess ventricular function, regional wall motion abnormalities (cannot distinguish old vs. recent)
- 99m-Tc-sestamibi myocardial perfusion: areas of hypoperfusion (cannot distinguish old vs. recent)
- Contrast CT can identify vulnerable plaques, coronary stenosis
- Cardiac MRI: global and reginal left ventricular function, perfusion, viability
- Coronary angiography

BNP, B-type natriuretic peptide; *CRP*, C-reactive protein; *CT*, computed tomography; *MRI*, magnetic resonance imaging.

Q-Wave Myocardial Infarction ECG Presentation.		
	Coronary Artery	ECG
Anterior	Left main or anterior descending	Q waves in V_2–V_4
Inferior	Right main or posterior descending	Q waves in II, III, AVF
Posterior	Circumflex	Broad R waves in V_1 and V_2

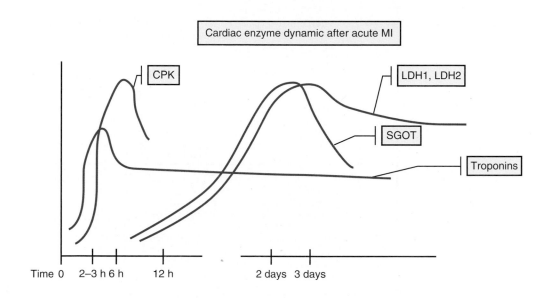

Cardiac enzyme dynamic after acute MI

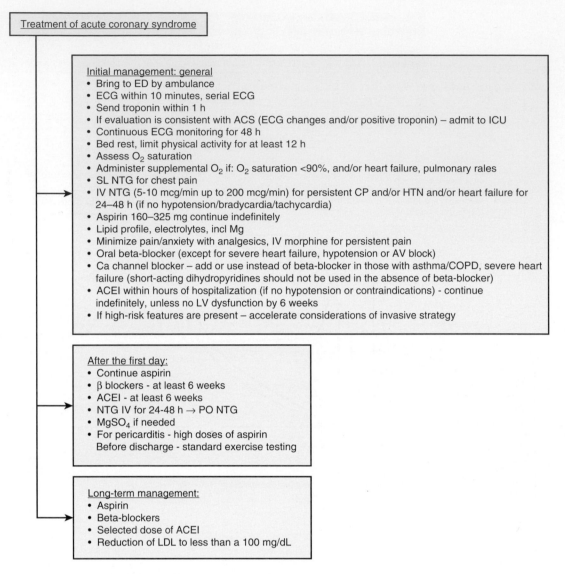

Management of ACS and aggressiveness with revascularization strategy depends on the negative outcome risk. Risk is stratified based on the factors listed below.

High-Risk Features (Identifies Those Benefiting From Early Invasive Strategy)	
Recurrent angina or ischemia	Hemodynamic instability
Elevated cardiac enzymes	Sustained ventricular tachycardia
New ST depression	PCI within 6 months of event or prior CABG
Signs of heart failure, reduced LV function (EF < 40%) or mitral regurgitation (new or worsening)	High-risk score (TIMI or GRACE)

CABG, Coronary artery bypass grafting; *EF,* ejection fraction; *LV,* left ventricular; *PCI,* percutaneous coronary intervention.

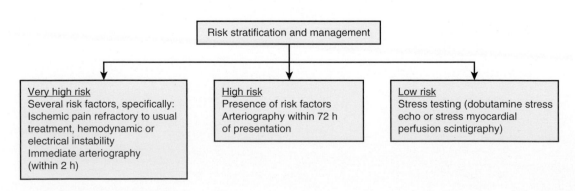

The choice of revascularization strategy (coronary artery bypass grafting [CABG] vs. percutaneous coronary intervention [PCI]) is based upon the anatomy of coronary disease and left ventricular (LV) function.

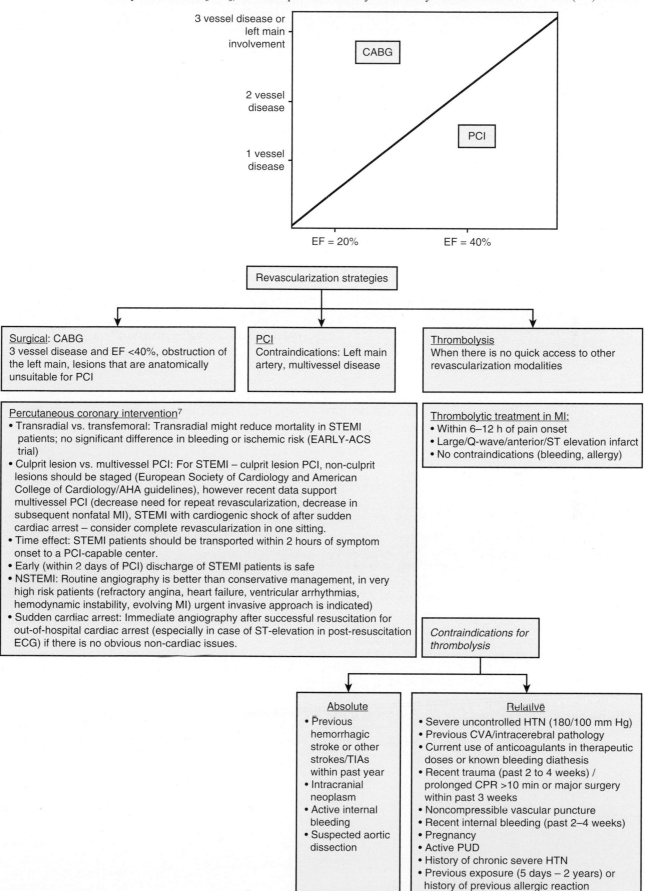

Revascularization strategies

Surgical: CABG
3 vessel disease and EF <40%, obstruction of the left main, lesions that are anatomically unsuitable for PCI

PCI
Contraindications: Left main artery, multivessel disease

Thrombolysis
When there is no quick access to other revascularization modalities

Percutaneous coronary intervention[7]
- Transradial vs. transfemoral: Transradial might reduce mortality in STEMI patients; no significant difference in bleeding or ischemic risk (EARLY-ACS trial)
- Culprit lesion vs. multivessel PCI: For STEMI – culprit lesion PCI, non-culprit lesions should be staged (European Society of Cardiology and American College of Cardiology/AHA guidelines), however recent data support multivessel PCI (decrease need for repeat revascularization, decrease in subsequent nonfatal MI), STEMI with cardiogenic shock of after sudden cardiac arrest – consider complete revascularization in one sitting.
- Time effect: STEMI patients should be transported within 2 hours of symptom onset to a PCI-capable center.
- Early (within 2 days of PCI) discharge of STEMI patients is safe
- NSTEMI: Routine angiography is better than conservative management, in very high risk patients (refractory angina, heart failure, ventricular arrhythmias, hemodynamic instability, evolving MI) urgent invasive approach is indicated)
- Sudden cardiac arrest: Immediate angiography after successful resuscitation for out-of-hospital cardiac arrest (especially in case of ST-elevation in post-resuscitation ECG) if there is no obvious non-cardiac issues.

Thrombolytic treatment in MI:
- Within 6–12 h of pain onset
- Large/Q-wave/anterior/ST elevation infarct
- No contraindications (bleeding, allergy)

Contraindications for thrombolysis

Absolute
- Previous hemorrhagic stroke or other strokes/TIAs within past year
- Intracranial neoplasm
- Active internal bleeding
- Suspected aortic dissection

Relative
- Severe uncontrolled HTN (180/100 mm Hg)
- Previous CVA/intracerebral pathology
- Current use of anticoagulants in therapeutic doses or known bleeding diathesis
- Recent trauma (past 2 to 4 weeks) / prolonged CPR >10 min or major surgery within past 3 weeks
- Noncompressible vascular puncture
- Recent internal bleeding (past 2–4 weeks)
- Pregnancy
- Active PUD
- History of chronic severe HTN
- Previous exposure (5 days – 2 years) or history of previous allergic reaction

Antiplatelet and Anticoagulation Therapy[8,9]

Antiplatelet and anticoagulation therapy are critical components of ACS management.

Antiplatelet Therapy

ASA: irreversibly blocks COX-1 and prevents platelet activation and synthesis of thromboxane A2. Loading dose of 162–325 mg followed by 75–100 mg/day. Higher dose is not necessary (OASIS-7 trial). Contraindicated in allergy/intolerance, active bleeding, active peptic ulcer, another source of GI bleeding

$P2Y_{12}$ blockers: thienopyridines (clopidogrel, prasugrel) irreversible blockers of $P2Y_{12}$ receptor, triazolopyrimidine (ticagrelor) reversible blocker. Cangrelor administered IV.

- Clopidogrel. Addition of clopidogrel to ASA improves outcome (CURE trial). Loading dose 300 (acts in 4–6 hours) or 600 mg (acts in 2–3 hours) followed by 150 mg/day for 7 days, followed by 75 mg/day
- Prasugrel—Acts in 30 minutes. More powerful inhibitor than clopidogrel. In patients receiving PCI improved outcome compared to clopidogrel (TRITON-TIMI 38 trial). Contraindicated in those with stroke/TIA, age >75 years, body weight <60 kg, with risk of bleeding

- Ticagrelor. Rapid onset of action. 180 mg loading dose followed by 90 mg BID. Improved outcome compared to clopidogrel (PLATO trial)

Dual antiplatelet therapy (ASA + $P2Y_{12}$ blocker) for 1 year after ACS episode and after drug-eluting stent, and then only ASA for indefinite period. Add PPI (other than omeprazole) in those with risk of GI bleeding.

GP IIb/IIIa Blockers

Block fibrinogen-mediated cross-linkage of platelets through the GP IIb/IIIa receptor

Tirofiban, eptifibatide, abciximab

Routine early use in addition to ASA and clopidogrel—not recommended

May add to ASA and clopidogrel at the time of PCI in high-risk patients

PAR (protease activated receptor) Antagonists

Atopaxar
Vorapaxar

COX-1, Cyclooxygenase-1; *GI*, gastrointestinal; *GP*, glycoprotein; *PPI*, proton pump inhibitor; *TIA*, transient ischemic attack; *TRITON-TIMI*, Trial to Assess Improvement in Therapeutic Outcomes by Optimizing Platelet Inhibition with Prasugrel–Thrombolysis in Myocardial Infarction.

Anticoagulation Therapy

- Unfractionated heparin (activates antithrombin, blocks circulating factors IIa and Xa) IV infusion 60–70 U/kg bolus followed by 12–15 U/kg/hour titrated to Partial thromboplastin time (PTT) 1.5–2 times normal for 2–5 days
- Low-molecular-weight heparins (enoxaparin subcutaneous 1 mg/kg BID)
- Bivalirudin (direct inhibitor of thrombin) 0.75 mg/kg bolus followed by 1.75 mg/kg/hr infusion during PCI: outcome

similar to use of heparin, but less bleeding. Not cleared by the kidneys
- Fondaparinux (inactivates of factor Xa) subcutaneous 2.5 mg/day, cleared by the kidneys, outcome similar to enoxaparin, less bleeding, but more catheter-related thrombosis (to avoid can be used with a small amount of heparin)
- Rivaroxaban (inhibits action of factor Xa) oral 2.5 mg BID

Diagnostic Algorithm for Hypotension and/or Shock

Shock is usually defined as diminished blood supply to the organs; there are several mechanisms of shock. Here we will focus more on cardiogenic shock, while septic shock will be discussed in detail in Chapter 6.

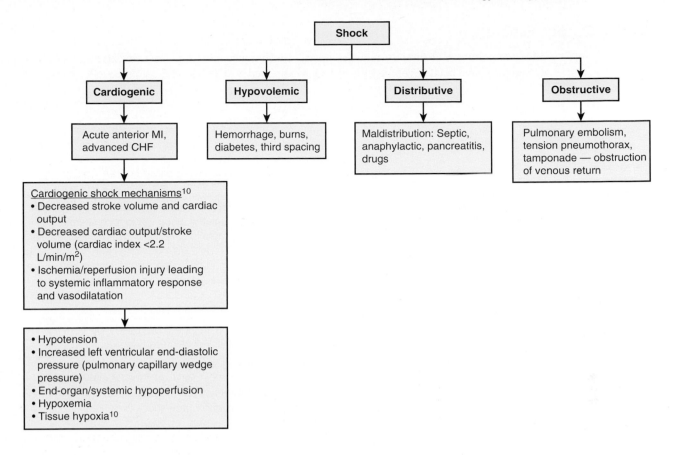

Cardiac Monitoring of Shock

Hemodynamic measurements (e.g., blood pressure [BP], cardiac output [CO]) are extremely helpful in determining the etiology of shock and in monitoring the effect of treatment.[11] These methods include the following techniques.

- BP monitoring (e.g., mean arterial pressure [MAP] <65 mm Hg considered pathological, associated with diminished perfusion and higher mortality)
- Pulmonary artery (PA) catheterization: provides an entire set of hemodynamic data (CO, central venous pressure [CVP], pulmonary artery wedge pressure [PAWP], right atrial and ventricular pressures, PA pressure). Use of PA catheter for hemodynamic monitoring is controversial but might be reasonable in selected patients
- Other CO monitoring methods including minimally or noninvasive CO monitoring devices (see table below)
- CVP measures (elevated in obstructive or cardiogenic shock, decreased in septic or hypovolemic shock). Positive end-expiratory pressure (PEEP) can falsely elevate CVP. Its value has been questioned, some suggest that it should not be used to guide management[12]
- Passive leg raising to estimate volume status and the effect of fluid bolus
- Echocardiography: provides information about diagnosis, changes in contractile function, volume status (inferior vena cava [IVC] diameter and collapsibility index)

Cardiac Output Estimation

Measurement of CO directly requires invasive technique; therefore least invasive or noninvasive techniques have been developed.[11,13,14] CO is expressed as: CO = systolic volume (SV) × HR

Method	Description
Fick formula	CO = $VO_2/(SaO_2 - SvO_2)$, where SaO_2 is arterial oxygen content as measured on ABG, SvO_2 is mixed venous blood oxygen content as measured on mixed venous gas from PA catheter; VO_2 is oxygen consumption calculated based on BSA, age, hemoglobin concentration
Dilution techniques (thermodilution or lithium dilution)[14]	• Transcardiac thermodilution: done by means of a PA catheter. The cold fluid mixes with the blood -> blood temperature change detected by thermistor at the distal tip of the catheter in the PA • Transpulmonary thermodilution: the central venous injection of cold saline → temperature changes, measured by the arterial thermistor • Lithium dilution/transpulmonary lithium dilution
Thoracic electrical bioimpedance-bioreactance	CO is calculated based on change in bioimpedance, from the global conduction velocity of electrical stimulus
Venous O_2 saturation[11]	• Mixed venous oxygen saturation (SvO_2: percentage saturation of hemoglobin in the PA = distal tip of the PA catheter) correlates with CO. The SvO_2 drops in cardiogenic shock (<70% in cardiogenic, >70% in distributive shock to failure of tissues to extract O_2). • Central venous oxygen saturation ($ScvO_2$) correlates with SvO_2 but not necessarily equivalent to SvO_2
Estimating CO by BP or pulse wave analysis	Different systems are available to transform BP wave into SV and CO
Estimating CO from BP and HR[13,15]	CO = (SV × HR), SV correlates with BP (PP, MAP, SBP, DBP). While this formulae might not be very precise to determine absolute value of CO, they are convenient and practical to estimate changes in the same patient. Below k is the linear coefficient, unique for each individual formula: • CO is directly proportional to PP: CO = k × (PP × HR) • CO = k × MAP × HR • Liljestrand and Zander formula: CO = (PP/[SBP + DBP]) × HR × k

Echocardiography and Doppler	• Volumetric method (echocardiography)
	• Doppler technology
	  ○ Transthoracic Doppler
	  ○ Transesophageal Doppler

ABG, Arterial blood gas; *BSA*, body surface area; *DBP*, diastolic blood pressure; *PP*, pulse pressure.

Use of Pulmonary Artery Catheterization

PA catheter allows to measure pressures in the right chambers of the heart and PA, while PAWP is interpreted as being almost equal to LV diastolic pressure. Using thermodilution PA catheter also allows to measure CO.

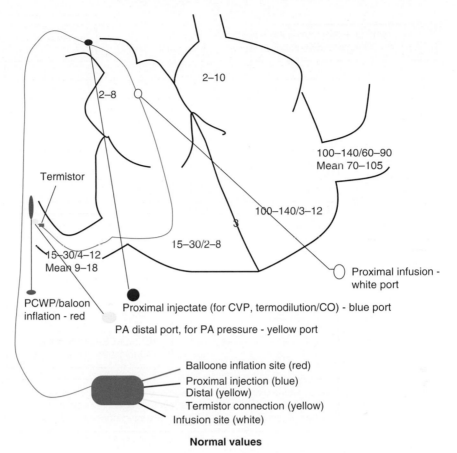

2–10

2–8

100–140/60–90
Mean 70–105

100–140/3–12

Termistor

15–30/2–8

15–30/4–12
Mean 9–18

Proximal infusion -
white port

PCWP/baloon
inflation - red

Proximal injectate (for CVP, termodilution/CO) - blue port

PA distal port, for PA pressure - yellow port

Balloone inflation site (red)
Proximal injection (blue)
Distal (yellow)
Termistor connection (yellow)
Infusion site (white)

Normal values

Cardiac index - 2.4 – 3.8 L/min/m^2 Systemic vascular resistance - 700–1600
Cardiac Output - 3.5 – 7 L/min   Total pulmonary resistance - 100–300
Stroke index - 30–65 mL/beat/m^2 Pulmonary vascular resistance - 30–130

Diagnostic Algorithm for the Mechanism of Hypotension and/or Shock

The most important initial clinical determinant of the cause of shock in a hypotensive patient is volume status (defined by the presence of JVD, CVP measurement, other elements of physical exam, IVC ultrasound, and B-type natriuretic peptide [BNP] level). Two other indicators are obtained from PA catheterization, which is not done routinely most of the time. Therefore it is not always easy to distinguish between distributive/septic shock and hypovolemia. While history and additional clinical data might be helpful, the initial therapeutic approach is frequently volume resuscitation in any case. The distinguishing feature of cardiogenic shock is hypervolemia, though the history and other clinical data should be very helpful to make this diagnosis.[11,16]

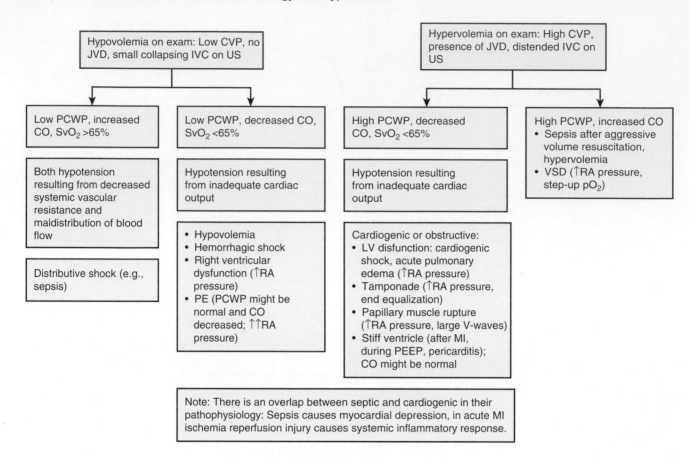

Therapeutic Algorithm for Hypotension and/or Shock

Treatment for every shock except for cardiogenic (clinically presented as hypervolemia) starts with IV fluids (IVFs). In other words, if the patient with shock does not demonstrate signs of hypervolemia, initial administration of IVFs on empiric basis is reasonable. The goal is euvolemia, which could be defined as a pulmonary capillary wedge pressure (PCWP) of 12 to 18 or CVP of 10 to 12. In case of cardiogenic shock, the use of inotropic drugs is indicated as the initial approach.

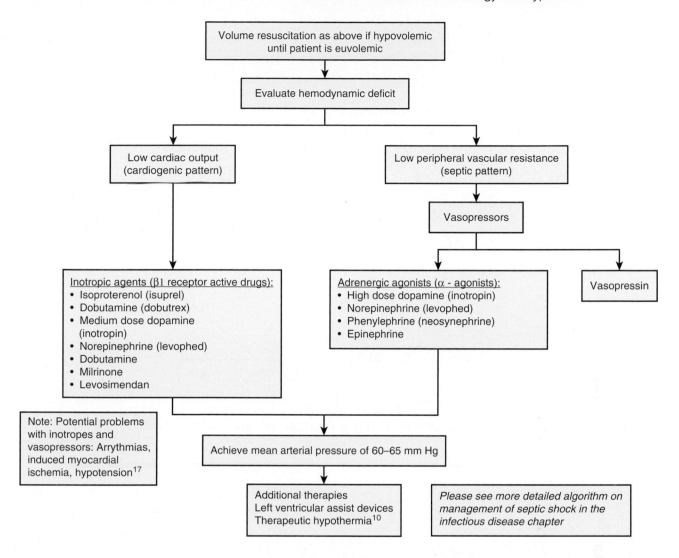

The mechanism of adrenergic medications (alpha- and beta-agonists) causes vasoconstriction (alpha) and increased CO (beta). Adrenergic medications exert different effects on alpha- and beta-receptors, causing inotropic and vasopressive effects to a different degree.[16] In the diagram below, adrenergic medications are listed in the order of decreasing alpha-adrenergic effect and increasing beta-adrenergic effect (e.g., phenylephrine is predominantly an alpha-agonist, while isoproterenol is predominantly a beta-agonist).

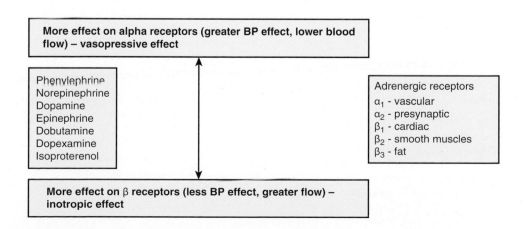

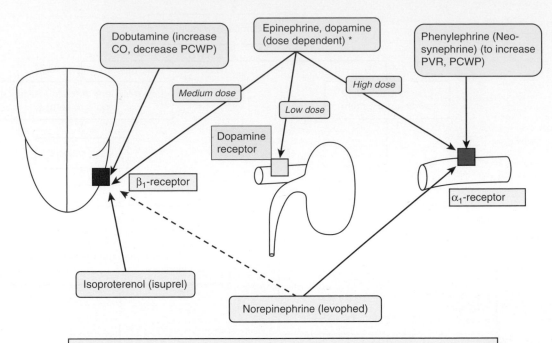

Illustration of mechanism of action of selected inotropes and vasopressors

Dobutamine (increase CO, decrease PCWP)

Epinephrine, dopamine (dose dependent) *

Phenylephrine (Neo-synephrine) (to increase PVR, PCWP)

Medium dose

High dose

Low dose

Dopamine receptor

β₁-receptor

α₁-receptor

Isoproterenol (isuprel)

Norepinephrine (levophed)

* Dopamine - dose dependent action:
1–3 µg/kg/min - selective renal and mesenteric vasodilation via dopaminergic receptors
2–5 µg/kg/min - positive inotropic effect via β1 receptors
5–10 µg/kg/min - α1 stimulation (prerenal vasoconstriction, ↑SVR)

More details on selected inotropes and vasopressors

Dobutamine

Direct agonist effect on beta-1- and beta-2-adrenergic receptors with no vasoconstrictor properties, less tachycardia

Raises BP solely by increasing CO
Infusions lasting longer than 72 hours were associated with pharmacodynamics tolerance[18]
Side effects: tachycardia, myocardial ischemia, and arrhythmia

Dopamine

The immediate precursor to norepinephrine in the catecholamine synthetic pathway
Low doses (<3 mg/kg/min): activates dopaminergic (D1) receptors → vasodilation in various vascular beds (e.g., coronary and renal arteries)
Intermediate doses (3–10 mg/kg/min): activate beta-adrenergic

receptors → increased inotropy and HR, promote release, and inhibit reuptake of norepinephrine in presynaptic sympathetic nerve terminals
Higher doses (10–20 mg/kg/min): alpha-adrenergic agonist → peripheral vasoconstriction
Increased incidence of arrhythmias compared with norepinephrine[19]

Milrinone

Non-catecholamine (phosphodiesterase [PDE] inhibitor)

It is both a positive inotropic agent and a peripheral vasodilator; also has lusitropic properties (improvement in diastolic function)

It raises HR, but not to the same extent as dobutamine

Mostly it is used in patients with advanced systolic heart failure to improve cardiac performance[20]; in some patients who have markedly elevated PA pressure; may be the preferred inotropic drug for patients receiving beta-adrenergic blocking drugs (it does not use the beta-adrenergic receptor)

It can lead to hypotension, especially in patients with low filling pressure. It should be avoided in patients with impaired renal function, as milrinone is renally cleared

Norepinephrine

Alpha- and beta-adrenergic receptor agonist properties including increased chronotropy, heightened inotropy, and increased peripheral vasoconstriction

Can be associated with tachycardia, myocardial ischemia, and arrhythmia

Norepinephrine increases BP as well as CO and renal, splanchnic, cerebral, and microvascular blood flow, while minimally increasing HR[21]

Norepinephrine causes alpha-1–adrenergic receptor–mediated venoconstriction; this increases the mean systemic pressure with a significant increase in venous return and cardiac preload

Typically, norepinephrine is infused at 0.05-1 mcg/kg/min

In situations in which norepinephrine is not available, epinephrine is a suitable alternative agent

Phenylephrine

Selective alpha-1–adrenergic agonist increases BP by vasoconstriction in vasodilatory shock

Effect of Selective Inotropes and Vasopressors on Hemodynamic Parameters.[16]

	Chronotropic effect	Inotropic effect	Vasoconstriction	Vasodilatation
Norepinephrine	1	2	4	0
Dopamine	1–2	1–3	0–3	0–1
Epinephrine	4	4	4	3
Phenylephrine	0	0	3	0
Vasopressin	0	0	4	0
Dobutamine	2	3–4	0	2
Milrinone	1	3	0	2
Levosimendan	1	3	0	2

Dose Ranges for Selected Inotropes and Vasopressors.[16]

Norepinephrine	0.05-1 mcg/kg/min
Dopamine	1–20 mcg/kg/min
Epinephrine	0.01-1 mcg/kg/min
Phenylephrine	20–200 mcg/min
Vasopressin	0.01-0.04 units/min
Dobutamine	2-20 mcg/kg/min
Milrinone	0.375–0.75 mcg/kg/min
Levosimendan	0.05–0.2 mcg/kg/min

Intra-Aortic Balloon Pump

Intra-aortic balloon pump (IABP) counterpulsation increases myocardial oxygen perfusion while at the same time increasing CO.

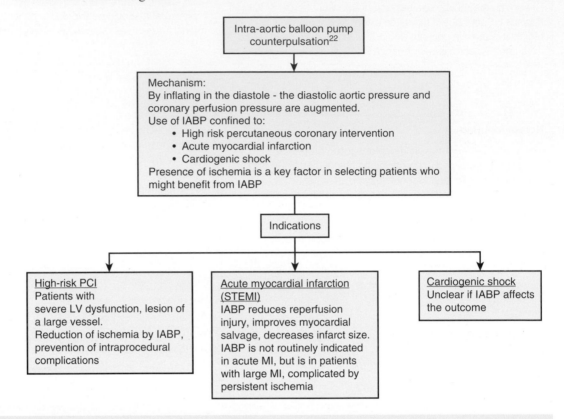

Cardiac Arrest

Therapeutic Hypothermia

Cooling is initiated as soon as possible after return of spontaneous circulation is associated with improved outcome.[23]

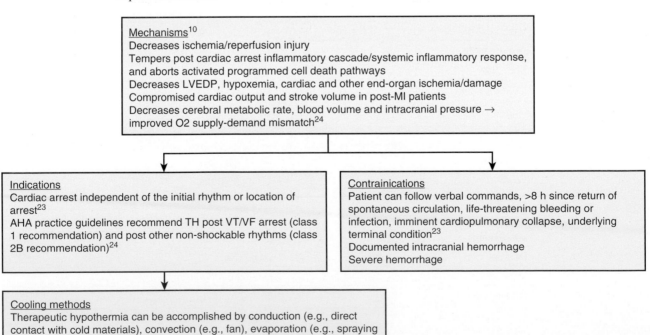

Phases of Therapeutic Hypothermia[25]				
	TH Phase: Induction	TH Phase: Maintenance	TH Phase: De-cooling	TH Phase: Normothermia
General goals	Prevent shivering and sedate Potassium repletion Cooling: surface cooling or intravascular cooling (infusion of 4°C fluids)	Maintain core temperature of 33°C for 18–24 hours Maintain normal electrolytes, glucose, and pH (by adequate ventilation), MAP (see below), consider antibiotics	Rewarm at 0.25–0.33°C per hour Maintain T <37.5°C until 72 hours after event Volume repletion Potassium Maintain MAP Extubate	Reevaluate for brain death 72 hours after event
Prevent shivering and sedate	Low-dose continuous infusion of short-acting sedatives (propofol, midazolam) and analgesics (fentanyl or hydromorphone) Magnesium sulfate to raise shivering threshold Neuromuscular blocking agents (cisatracurium 0.15 mg/kg ×3 every 10 minutes)		Stop paralytic Wean sedation after T >36°C	
Hemodynamics	Tachycardia and hypertension (result of shivering) When patient begins to cool: bradycardia, PR prolongation, junctional or ventricular rhythm. Bradycardia should be only treated if associated with hypotension	Hypotension (during cooling or rewarming) should be aggressively reversed (to avoid cerebral hypoperfusion). Goal MAP >65 (ideally 80–100) Goal CVP 10–12 mm Hg		
Ventilation	O_2 saturation goal 94%–96%. Avoid prolonged O_2 saturation of 100%. Maintain normocarbia			
Glucose control	Hyperglycemia is common during cooling (do not treat unless over 200 mg/mL); maintain 100–150 mg/dL		Hypoglycemia may occur during rewarming	
Potassium level	Hypokalemia during cooling: supplement levels to maintain above 3.5–3.8 mEq/L and reassess every 3–4 hours. Do not supplement 4 hours prior to start of rewarming		Hyperkalemia during rewarming	
Infection	Infections are common—so need surveillance cultures, consider empiric antibiotics			

Arrhythmias

Pathophysiology

There are two potential scenarios of arrhythmia development.[26]

1. A result of congenital combination of anatomical and electrophysiological changes. The range is from no structural cardiac abnormality (e.g., long QT syndrome), a minimal structural abnormality (e.g., an accessory pathway leading to Wolff-Parkinson-White syndrome [WPW]), or a severe structural abnormality (e.g., endocardial cushion defect with heart block).
2. A result of acquired disease (e.g., ventricular tachycardia [VT] after myocardial infarction) or aging (atrial fibrillation [AF]). Genetic susceptibility might play a role as well.

The underlying mechanism of arrhythmias is the impairment of automaticity, conductivity, and excitability.

1. Disorder of automaticity (impulse formation) may cause sinus tachycardia and some ectopic tachycardias. It is also involved in the development of junctional arrhythmias (idioventricular rhythm) and triggered activity.
2. Problems with conductivity lead to blocks (unidirectional block, bidirectional block), functional and anatomical reentry, reflection, and concealed conduction, which may be an underlying problem in arrhythmias.

3. Excitability might depend on ion imbalance. Ion gradient across myocyte membrane (sodium, potassium, calcium, and magnesium, which is necessary for sodium pump function) is very important for myocardial cell function. Higher gradient (low extracellular potassium, high extracellular sodium and calcium, high activity of membrane ATPases) leads to increased polarization potential and to increased excitability (e.g., tachycardia, fast conduction). On the other hand, lower gradient (high extracellular potassium, low intracellular potassium, low extracellular sodium and calcium, overdose of digitalis and glycosides, overdoses of some of antiarrhythmics) leads to decreased polarization potential and subsequently to junctional arrhythmias and blocks.

4. Other factors may play a role in the development of arrhythmias: ischemia, autonomic nervous system impairment, vagotonia, anatomical abnormalities (accessory pathways), and overdoses of antiarrhythmic drugs. Any kind of structural cardiac diseases may cause arrhythmia.

A brief summary of the mechanism of arrhythmias is represented in the diagram below.

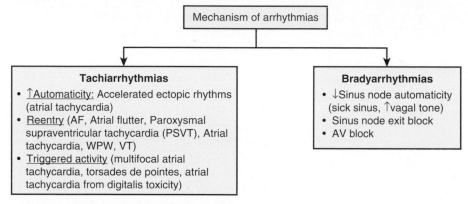

Electrolyte changes predisposing to arrhythmias

	Tachi-arrhythmias, fast conduction	Blocks, escapes
Extracellular electrolytes	$\downarrow K^+ (\uparrow \Delta K^+)$ $\uparrow Na^+ (\uparrow \Delta Na^+)$ $\uparrow Ca^{++} (\uparrow \Delta Ca^{++})$	$\uparrow K^+ (\downarrow \Delta K^+)$ $\downarrow Na^+$ $\downarrow Ca^{++}$

Δ - intracellular/extracellular difference

Illustration of Reentry Mechanism

Abnormal propagation of impulse or reentry is probably the most frequent cause of rhythm abnormality. Different types of reentry path and associated arrhythmia are represented in the diagram below.

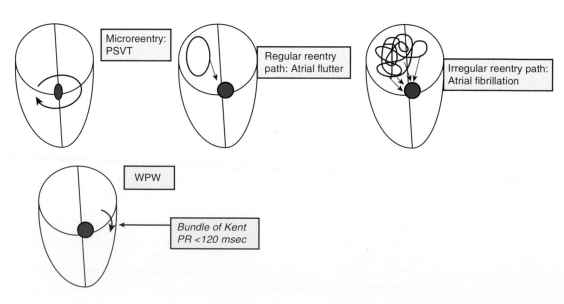

Evaluation of Arrhythmia

The initial step in evaluation is to see if the QRS complex is wide (e.g., VT, supraventricular tachycardia with aberrancy or preexcitation) or narrow (e.g., paroxysmal supraventricular tachycardia [PSVT], AF of flutter, atrial tachycardia).[27]

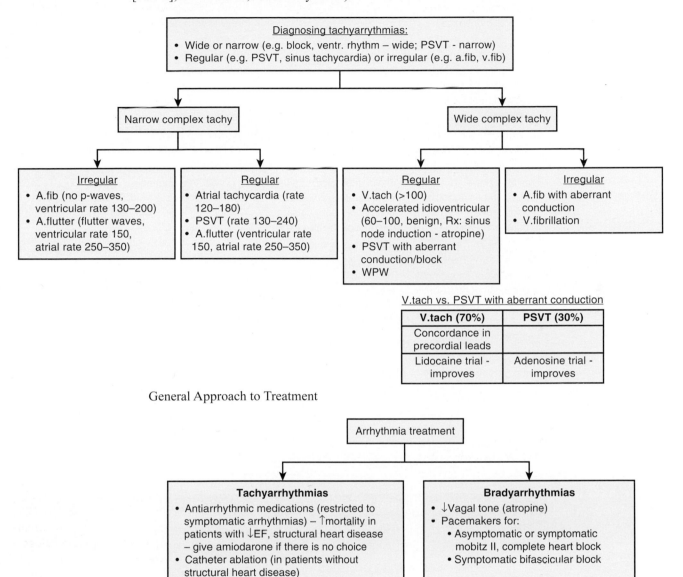

General Approach to Treatment

Antiarrhythmic Drugs

The classification of antiarrhythmic medications (Singh-Vaughan Williams classification) is presented in the table. There is an overlap in mechanism of action and also in the indications for use. One has to be aware of the proarrhythmic effect of most of the antiarrhythmic drugs.

Class	Examples	Indications	Potential Complications
Class 1—Membrane stabilizing agent (fast Na⁺ channel blockers, decrease upslope of action potential)			

Class	Examples	Indications	Potential Complications
Class 1a—Block sodium channels and delay repolarization, ↑ duration of action potential	Quinidine, disopyramide, procainamide	Ventricular arrhythmias, paroxysmal AF to maintain sinus rhythm, WPW syndrome (procainamide)	Prolong QT interval
Class 1b—Block sodium channel and accelerate repolarization, ↓ duration of action potential	Lidocaine, tocainide, phenytoin	Treatment of arrhythmias after acute MI	Increased risk of asystole, VT
Class 1c—Block sodium channel, with little effect on repolarization	Encainide, flecainide propafenone moricizine	AF or recurrent tachyarrhythmias to maintain sinus rhythm	Contraindicated after acute MI
Class 2—Anti-sympathetic agents (mostly beta-adrenoreceptor blockers)	Atenolol, metoprolol, carvedilol, esmolol, timolol, propranolol (also class 1 effect), sotalol (also class 3 effect)	Rate control in recurrent tachyarrhythmias	Hypotension
Class 3—Drugs increasing duration of action potential, potassium channel blockers	Amiodarone (also has class 1, 2, and 4 activity), bretylium, sotalol (also has class 2 activity), ibutilide	WPW syndrome, VT (amiodarone, sotalol), AF (amiodarone, sotalol, ibutilide), atrial flutter (ibutilide)	
Class 4—Calcium channel blockers	Verapamil, diltiazem	Rate control in AF, PSVTs	Hypotension
Class 5—Other	Adenosine, digoxin, magnesium sulfate	Supraventricular arrhythmias with CHF (digoxin), rate control, torsades de pointes (magnesium sulfate)	Contraindicated in ventricular arrhythmias

WPW, Wolff-Parkinson-White.

Classes of Calcium Channel Blockers.		
Class	Agents	
Diphenylalkylamines	Verapamil HCl	Negative chronotropes: affect sinoatrial and AV nodes—slow conduction, ↓ rate. Avoid in angina and impaired ventricular function
Benzothiazepines	Diltiazem HCl	Negative chronotropes: affect sinoatrial and AV nodes—slow conduction, ↓ rate. Avoid in angina and impaired ventricular function
Dihydropyridines	Nifedipine, nicardipine, isradipine, nimodipine, nisoldipine, felodipine, amlodipine	Negative inotropes, vasodilators. In systolic dysfunction—no nifedipine, but OK amlodipine, felodipine
Tetralols	Mibefradil	Affect sinoatrial and AV nodes, but not negatively inotropic
Other	Bepridil	Prolong the QT interval → proarrhythmic

AV, Atrioventricular.

Combinations of Calcium Channel Blockers With Beta-Blockers

"Good" combinations: dihydropyridine Ca blocker + beta-blocker (compensatory tachycardia of dihydropyridine is opposed by beta-blocker)

"Bad" combinations: verapamil + beta-blocker, diltiazem + beta-blocker, mibefradil + beta-blocker (common side effects, e.g., bradycardia)

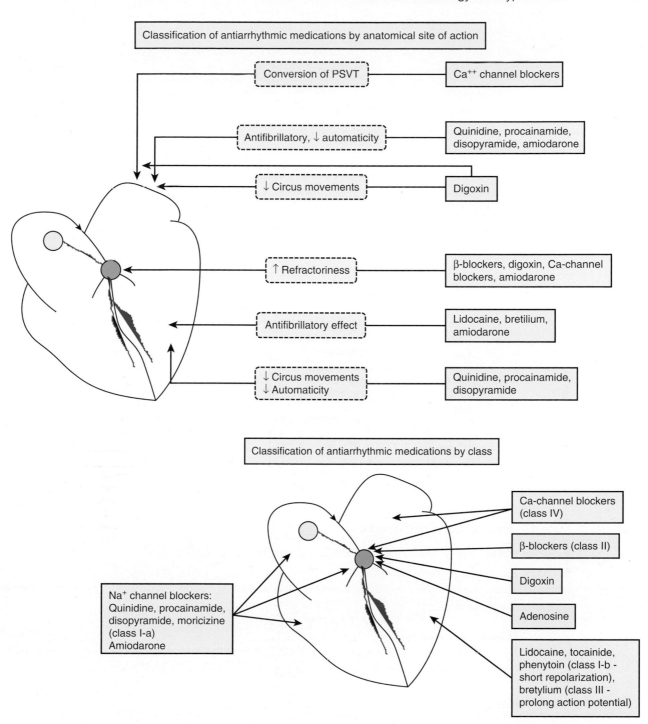

Classification of antiarrhythmic medications by anatomical site of action

Conversion of PSVT — Ca++ channel blockers

Antifibrillatory, ↓ automaticity — Quinidine, procainamide, disopyramide, amiodarone

↓ Circus movements — Digoxin

↑ Refractoriness — β-blockers, digoxin, Ca-channel blockers, amiodarone

Antifibrillatory effect — Lidocaine, bretilium, amiodarone

↓ Circus movements ↓ Automaticity — Quinidine, procainamide, disopyramide

Classification of antiarrhythmic medications by class

Ca-channel blockers (class IV)

β-blockers (class II)

Digoxin

Adenosine

Na+ channel blockers: Quinidine, procainamide, disopyramide, moricizine (class I-a) Amiodarone

Lidocaine, tocainide, phenytoin (class I-b - short repolarization), bretylium (class III - prolong action potential)

Suggested First Drug for Various Arrhythmias.	
Rapid AF	Beta-blocker, Ca blocker, amiodarone, but depends on the underlying problem
PSVT	Adenosine, verapamil, Ia antiarrhythmics
Rapid atrial flutter	Beta-blocker, digoxin, quinidine
PVC	No Rx if asymptomatic, if symptomatic—class 1 or 3; in post-MI/ischemic—amiodarone, beta-blockers
PAC	No Rx if asymptomatic, symptomatic—Ca blocker/beta-blocker
MAT	Ca blocker

WPW	Procainamide, amiodarone, shock
VT	Class 1 or 3, in post-MI/ischemic—amiodarone, beta-blockers
Ventricular fibrillation	Shock, ACLS protocol
Sudden cardiac death	Sotalol, amiodarone
Torsade de pointes	Mg++, isoproterenol, shock (last resort)

For digitalis-toxic arrhythmias, ventricular arrhythmias, torsades de pointes, premature contractions—intravenous Mg++.

Note: type 1 antiarrhythmics—increase mortality in CHF.

ACLS, Advanced cardiac life support; *MAT,* multifocal atrial tachycardia; *PAC,* premature atrial contractions; *PVC,* premature ventricular contraction.

Catheter Ablation

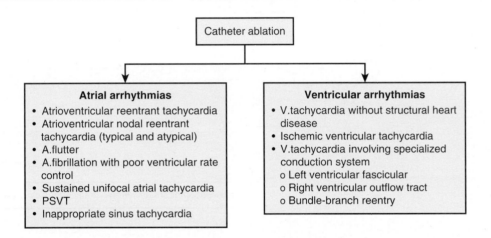

Implantable Cardioverter Defibrillator

Indications for Implantable Cardioverter Defibrillator[28]

Secondary Prevention
Ventricular arrhythmia causing hemodynamic instability + expected survival >1 year with good functional status.

Primary Prevention
Symptomatic heart failure (HF) and ejection fraction (EF) ≤35% despite >3 months of treatment with optimal pharmacological therapy, expected survival >1 year with good functional status.

Specific Arrhythmias

Ventricular Arrhythmias and Sudden Cardiac Death[29]

Initial Evaluation of Ventricular Arrhythmia

- ECG
- Echocardiogram
- Myocardial perfusion (if suspected that ischemia triggers ventricular arrhythmia)
- Coronary angiography (life-threatening ventricular arrhythmias or survivors of SCD)
- Electrophysiological testing (to document inducibility of VT, guide ablation, evaluate drug effects, assess the risks of recurrent VT or SCD, assess the indications for ICD)

ICD, Implantable cardioverter defibrillator; *SCD,* sudden cardiac death.

Classification

- Hemodynamically stable or unstable (e.g., syncope, SCD, sudden cardiac arrest)
- Symptomatic (e.g., palpitations, syncope) or asymptomatic

- Sustained or non-sustained
- Monomorphic or polymorphic
- ECG features (VT, ventricular fibrillation, torsades de pointes, bidirectional VT, bundle branch reentrant tachycardia)

General Principles of Acute Management

- Wide-QRS tachycardia should be presumed to be VT if the diagnosis is unclear
- Manage reversible factors (hypoxia, electrolytes, volume depletion, mechanical factors, stop offending drug)

- If VT or SCD associated with ischemia—aggressive attempts should be made to treat myocardial ischemia
- Non-pharmacological modalities: revascularization, ICD, catheter ablation, surgical resection
- Pharmacological therapy
- No role for class 1C drugs in those with Hx of MI

Management of specific scenarios

Cardiac arrest
Cardiopulmonary resuscitation, ACLS, shock, amiodarone is preferred antiarrhythmic drug to maintain rhythm after defibrillations
Precordial thump if witnessed cardiac arrest

Stable or unstable
Stable sustained VT – IV procainamide or lidocaine, no role for Ca-blockers especially in those with myocardial dysfunction
VT with hemodynamic compromise – cardioversion

Monomorphic or polymorphic
Repetitive monomorphic VT in the context of coronary disease - IV amiodarone, beta blockers, procainamide or sotalol
Recurrent polymorphic VT – IV beta-blockers, amiodarone, lidocaine

Intractable VT
Intravenous amiodarone or procainamide followed by VT ablation.
In those with myocardial ischemia - revascularization and beta blockade followed by intravenous antiarrythmic drugs (e.g., procainamide or amiodarone).
Intravenous amiodarone and intravenous beta blockers separately or together may be reasonable in patients with VT storm (three episodes of ventricular tachycardia in 24 h).

Torsades de Pointes
Withdrawal of any offending drugs, acute and long-term pacing (in those with block and symptomatic bradycardia)
Intravenous magnesium sulfate (not likely to be effective in patients with a normal QT interval)
Beta-blockers combined with pacing in those with sinus bradycardia
Isoproterenol (acute patients with recurrent pause dependent torsades de pointes who do not have congenital LQTS)
Potassium repletion, lidocaine in those with LQTS

Symptomatic VT with post-MI, LV dysfunction
Beta-blockers
Amlodarone
Sotalol
ICD, catheter ablation, surgical resection

Prolonged QT Interval

Prolongation of the QT interval is associated with the development of a torsades de pointes. It is not only prolongation, but also change in morphology of the QT interval that predicts the development of arrhythmia: deformity of the QT interval, manifested as prominent "U waves."[30]

Causes of Prolonged QT Interval

Metabolic factors
- Hypokalemia
- Hypomagnesemia
- Hypocalcemia

Drugs
- Antiarrhythmic agents (quinidine, procainamide, disopyramide, sotalol)
- Antibiotics (erythromycin, amantadine, chloroquine, pentamidine)
- Antihistamine (terfenadine [Seldane])
- Psychiatric agents (haloperidol, amitriptyline, doxepin)
- Other drugs (bepridil, cisapride)

Other
- Liquid protein diets

Treatment of Prolonged QT Interval
- Removal of offending agent
- Magnesium sulfate IV
- Potassium ion repletion
- Atrial or ventricular pacing
- Isoproterenol

Atrial Fibrillation

New-Onset AF[31,32]

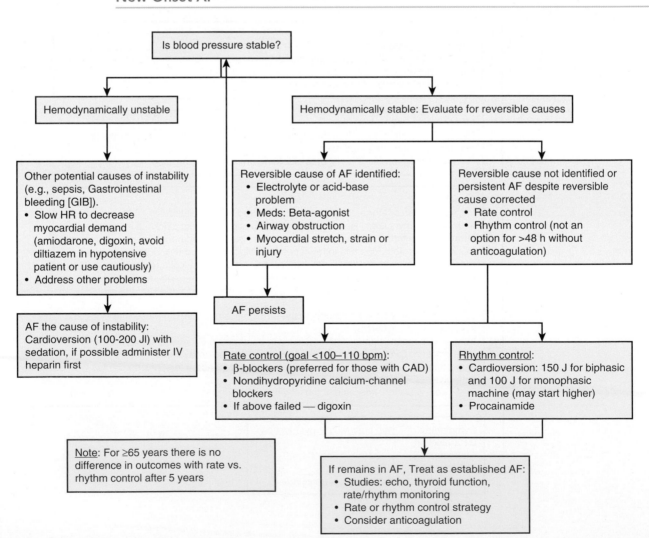

Established AF/Atrial Flutter

Pathophysiology

- Primary arrhythmia without identifiable heart disease
- Secondary arrhythmia without structural heart disease and with systemic abnormality (hyperthyroidism)
- Secondary arrhythmia with heart disease that affects the atria

Electrophysiology: multiple reentrant impulses of various sizes wandering through the atria, creating continuous electrical activity.

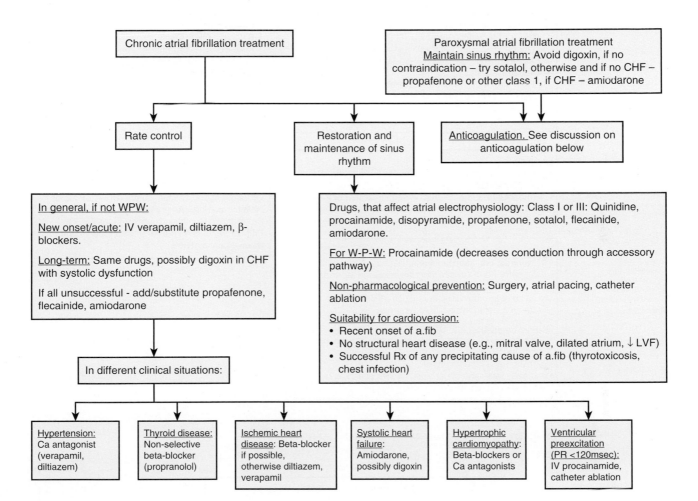

Anticoagulation Issues in AF[33]

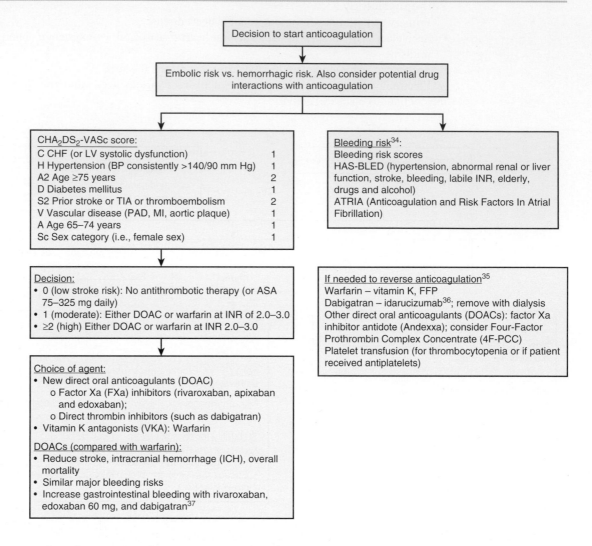

```
                        ┌─────────────────────────────────────┐
                        │  Decision to start anticoagulation   │
                        └─────────────────────────────────────┘
                                          │
                                          ▼
                ┌───────────────────────────────────────────────────┐
                │ Embolic risk vs. hemorrhagic risk. Also consider   │
                │ potential drug interactions with anticoagulation   │
                └───────────────────────────────────────────────────┘
```

CHA$_2$DS$_2$-VASc score:
C CHF (or LV systolic dysfunction)	1
H Hypertension (BP consistently >140/90 mm Hg)	1
A2 Age ≥75 years	2
D Diabetes mellitus	1
S2 Prior stroke or TIA or thromboembolism	2
V Vascular disease (PAD, MI, aortic plaque)	1
A Age 65–74 years	1
Sc Sex category (i.e., female sex)	1

Bleeding risk[34]:
Bleeding risk scores
HAS-BLED (hypertension, abnormal renal or liver function, stroke, bleeding, labile INR, elderly, drugs and alcohol)
ATRIA (Anticoagulation and Risk Factors In Atrial Fibrillation)

Decision:
- 0 (low stroke risk): No antithrombotic therapy (or ASA 75–325 mg daily)
- 1 (moderate): Either DOAC or warfarin at INR of 2.0–3.0
- ≥2 (high) Either DOAC or warfarin at INR 2.0–3.0

If needed to reverse anticoagulation[35]
Warfarin – vitamin K, FFP
Dabigatran – idarucizumab[36]; remove with dialysis
Other direct oral anticoagulants (DOACs): factor Xa inhibitor antidote (Andexxa); consider Four-Factor Prothrombin Complex Concentrate (4F-PCC)
Platelet transfusion (for thrombocytopenia or if patient received antiplatelets)

Choice of agent:
- New direct oral anticoagulants (DOAC)
    o Factor Xa (FXa) inhibitors (rivaroxaban, apixaban and edoxaban);
    o Direct thrombin inhibitors (such as dabigatran)
- Vitamin K antagonists (VKA): Warfarin

DOACs (compared with warfarin):
- Reduce stroke, intracranial hemorrhage (ICH), overall mortality
- Similar major bleeding risks
- Increase gastrointestinal bleeding with rivaroxaban, edoxaban 60 mg, and dabigatran[37]

Role of Anticoagulation Prior to Cardioversion in AF

If AF lasted >48 h prior to cardioversion – need to have INR 2–3

If on warfarin: Need to have INR 2–3 for 3–4 weeks prior to cardioversion

If on DOACs: Anticoagulation for ≥3 weeks prior and continued for ≥4 weeks post-cardioversion

Alternatively: Transesophageal echocardiography prior to cardioversion (though transesophageal echocardiography did not reduce the rate of thromboembolic events in clinical trial[38])

Heart Blocks

Presentation of the Bundle Branch Blocks and Hemiblocks on 12-Lead ECG.						
	I, AVL	II, III, AVF	V_1	V_6	Axis	QRS
Right bundle branch block (RBBB)	Wide S		Late prominent positive R wave, slurred QRS	Wide, deep S		Prolonged
Left bundle branch block (LBBB)	Monophasic R, no Q		QS or rS, deep S	No Q, monophasic R, slurred QRS		Prolonged
Left anterior superior fascicular block	Small Q, prominent R	Small R, prominent S			Left deviation (−60 degrees)	Slightly prolonged, increased voltage in limb leads
Left posterior inferior fascicular block	Small R, prominent S	Small Q, prominent R			Right deviation (+120 degrees)	Slightly prolonged, increased voltage in limb leads
Septal fascicular block			Q waves in V_1, V_2			Normal duration

How to Differentiate A-V Block From A-V Dissociation

- Number of Ps > number of QRS—block

- Number of QRSs > number of Ps (Ps marching into QRSs)—A-V dissociation without block (VPCs, sinus brady with junctional escape, etc.)

VPC, Ventricular premature complex.

Presentation of Premature Ventricular Complexes on 12-Lead ECG.			
	V_1	V_6	V_4
Right VPC (looks like LBBB)	VPC predominantly negative. Wide initial R	VPC has typical positive morphology	Deeper (rS or QS) complex in V_4 than in V_1
Left VPC (looks like RBBB)	VPC predominantly positive, monophasic R or diphasic qR. QRS often has two peaks	Diphasic (rS) or monophasic (QS) complex	

Classification of Atrioventricular Block (by Degree)

First degree: prolongation of PR interval (fixed PR interval of at least 0.2 seconds)

Type 1 second degree (Wenckebach): gradual prolongation of PR before dropped QRS

Type 2 second degree: constant PR interval and occasional missing QRS
Third degree: complete dissociation between P wave and QRS complex

Pacemakers[39]

Indications for permanence pacemakers

Sinus node dysfunctions with symptomatic bradyarrhythmias

- Persistent sinus bradycardia (<40 bpm), persistent sinus arrest with escape rhythm and symptoms:
  - intermittent symptoms consistent with bradycardia
  - syncope of unexplained origin with sinus node abnormalities diagnosed
- Chronotropic incompetence (inability to increase the rate to increased demand)

AV Block

- Third-degree AV block
- Type 2 second-degree AV block
- Controversial in type 1 second-degree AV block (Wenckebach)
- Rare indications in first-degree AV block

Other Indications

- Hypersensitive carotid sinus syndrome — evidence is lacking, but older patients with syncope might benefit
- CHF NYHA class 2–4 with QRS >150 ms (cardiac resynchronization therapy) might combine with ICD

AV, Atrioventricular. *NYHA*, New York Heart Association.

Permanent Pacemakers Coding			
Chamber(s) Paced	Chamber(s) Sensed	Mode(s) of Response	Programmable Capabilities
V—Ventricle	V—Ventricle	T—Triggered	R—Rate modulated
A—Atrium	A—Atrium	I—Inhibited	P—Programmable
D—Dual	D—Dual	D—Dual	
	O—None	O—None	

Congestive Heart Failure[40]

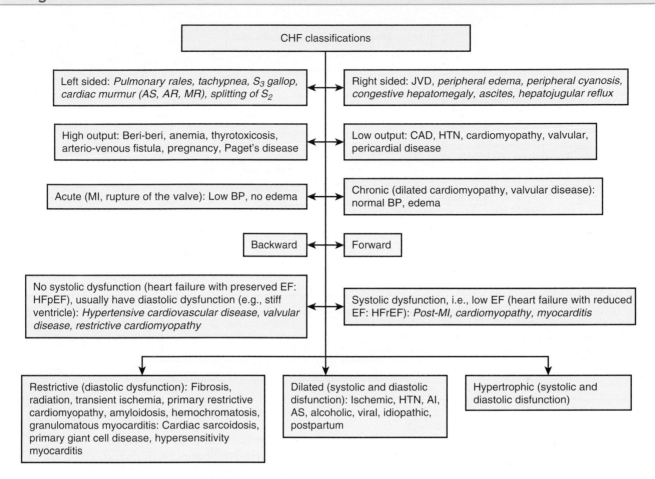

Causes of Cor Pulmonale

1. Pulmonary vascular disease
   - repeated pulmonary emboli
   - pulmonary vasculitis
   - pulmonary vasoconstriction secondary to high altitude

- congenital heart disease with left-to-right shunting
- pulmonary veno-occlusive disease

2. Parenchymal disease
   - Cor pulmonale may be caused by both obstructive and restrictive lung diseases, more frequently the former

Treatment Approach to CHF Based on Comorbidities and Clinical Scenarios

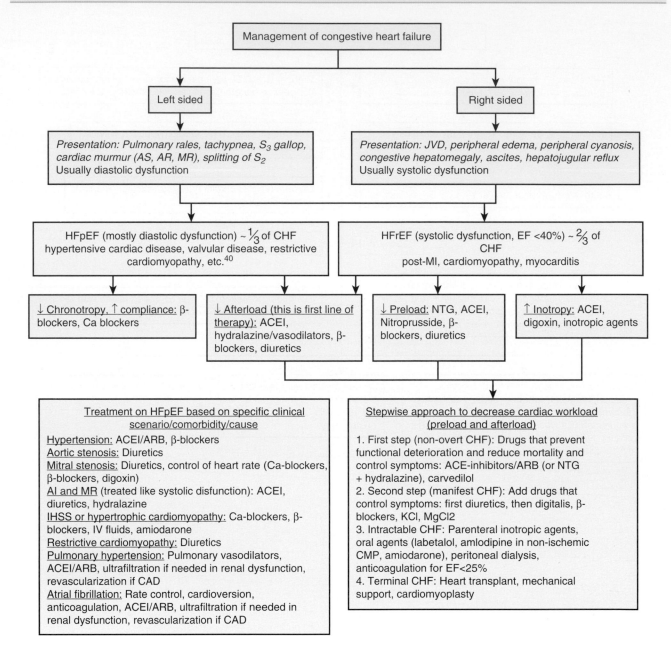

Pharmacologic Agents Used in the Treatment of CHF

	Morbidity	Mortality	Data Source
ACEI	↓	↓	V-HeFT I, II, SOLVD, SAVE, CONSENSUS, etc.
ARB	↓	↓	ELITE
Hydralazine + isosorbide dinitrate	↓	↓	SOLVD
Carvedilol	↓	↓	US Carvedilol Heart Failure Trials
Digoxin	↓	0	PROVED RADIANCE
Amlodipine	↓ in nonischemic CHF		PRAISE
Amiodarone	↓	↓	
Inotropes	↓	↑ (arrhythmogenic)	

- Rationale for beta-blockers in systolic dysfunction: reduce ischemia, negative chronotropic effect, increase coronary flow, carvedilol was shown to increase survival

- Ca blockers contraindicated in systolic dysfunction because of negative inotropic effect
- Digoxin

Acute Heart Failure Syndromes[41,42]

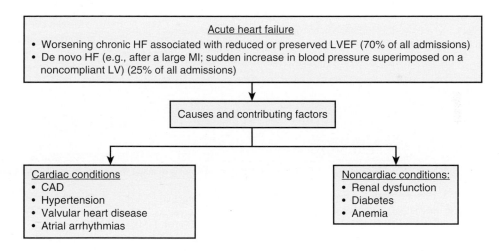

Clinical Presentations

- Elevated SBP
- Low SBP (low CO with signs of organ hypoperfusion)
- Cardiogenic shock (complicating acute MI, fulminant myocarditis)

- ACSs
- Pulmonary edema ("flash," rapid, or gradual onset)
- Isolated right HF (e.g., acute cor pulmonale, right ventricular infarct)
- Post–cardiac surgery HF (often related to worsening diastolic function and volume overload after surgery)

Targets for Therapy

- High LV filling pressure (excess salt intake, renal dysfunction, neurohormonal and cytokine activation, and medications may contribute to fluid retention)
- Decreased CO
- Elevated BP
- Myocardial damage/injury
- Renal dysfunction
- Adverse drug effects. Multiple medications can cause or exacerbate HF[43] (loop diuretics—renal function decline, inotropes—increased oxygen consumption, vasodilators—low BP—renal hypoperfusion, myocardial ischemia)

Treatment[41]

Prehospitalization (emergency) phase

- Loop diuretics
- Vasodilators (NTG)
- IV ACEI (controversial: IV enalapril may have deleterious effects in patients with acute MI)
- IV beta-blockers in those with HTN, rapid AF
- Other: morphine, O_2 supplement, noninvasive ventilation

In-hospital management (once patient is stabilized and dyspnea is improved)

- ACEIs, angiotensin receptor blockers, beta-blockers, or aldosterone antagonists
- Diuretics
- Inotropes (controversial, poorer outcome with dobutamine and milrinone)

ACEI, Angiotensin converting enzyme inhibitor; *HTN*, hypertension; *NTG*, nitroglycerin.

Prognostic Factors[41]

- SBP (high admission BP is associated with lower post-discharge mortality)
- CAD (a two-fold increase in post-discharge mortality compared with patients with primary cardiomyopathy)
- Troponin release (a two-fold increase in post-discharge mortality and a three-fold increase in rehospitalization)
- BUN and BUN/creatinine ratio (better predictor than creatinine)
- Hyponatremia (two- to three-fold increase in in-hospital and post-discharge mortality)
- Natriuretic peptides (higher post-discharge mortality and repeated hospitalizations)
- PCWP
- Functional capacity
- Other prognostic factors LVEF, anemia, diabetes mellitus, new sustained arrhythmias, and nonuse of neurohormonal antagonists

BUN, Blood urea nitrogen.

REFERENCES

1. McConaghy JR, Oza RS. Outpatient diagnosis of acute chest pain in adults. *Am Fam Physician*. 2013;87(3):177–182.
2. Fanaroff AC, Rymer JA, Goldstein SA, Simel DL, Newby LK. Does this patient with chest pain have acute coronary syndrome?: the rational clinical examination systematic review. *J Am Med Assoc*. 2015;314(18):1955–1965.
3. D'Ascenzo F, Biondi-Zoccai G, Moretti C, et al. TIMI, GRACE and alternative risk scores in acute coronary syndromes: a meta-analysis of 40 derivation studies on 216,552 patients and of 42 validation studies on 31,625 patients. *Contemp Clin Trials*. 2012;33(3):507–514.
4. Antman EM, Cohen M, Bernink PJ, et al. The TIMI risk score for unstable angina/non-ST elevation MI: a method for prognostication and therapeutic decision making. *J Am Med Assoc*. 2000;284(7):835–842.
5. Backus BE, Six AJ, Kelder JC, et al. A prospective validation of the HEART score for chest pain patients at the emergency department. *Int J Cardiol*. 2013;168(3):2153–2158.
6. Eagle KA, Lim MJ, Dabbous OH, et al. A validated prediction model for all forms of acute coronary syndrome: estimating the risk of 6-month postdischarge death in an international registry. *J Am Med Assoc*. 2004;291(22):2727–2733.
7. Meier P, Lansky AJ, Baumbach A. Almanac 2013: acute coronary syndromes. *Acta Cardiol*. 2014;69(1):100–108.
8. Bhatt DL, Hulot JS, Moliterno DJ, Harrington RA. Antiplatelet and anticoagulation therapy for acute coronary syndromes. *Circ Res*. 2014;114(12):1929–1943.
9. Clark MG, Beavers C, Osborne J. Managing the acute coronary syndrome patient: evidence based recommendations for anti-platelet therapy. *Heart Lung*. 2015;44(2):141–149.
10. Stegman BM, Newby LK, Hochman JS, Ohman EM. Post-myocardial infarction cardiogenic shock is a systemic illness in need of systemic treatment: is therapeutic hypothermia one possibility? *J Am Coll Cardiol*. 2012;59(7):644–647.

11. Simmons J, Ventetuolo CE. Cardiopulmonary monitoring of shock. *Curr Opin Crit Care*. 2017;23(3):223–231.
12. Marik PE, Baram M, Vahid B. Does central venous pressure predict fluid responsiveness? A systematic review of the literature and the tale of seven mares. *Chest*. 2008;134(1):172–178.
13. Koenig J, Hill LK, Williams DP, Thayer JF. Estimating cardiac output from blood pressure and heart rate: the liljestrand & zander formula. *Biomed Sci Instrum*. 2015;51:85–90.
14. García X, Mateu L, Maynar J, Mercadal J, Ochagavía A, Ferrandiz A. Estimating cardiac output. Utility in the clinical practice. Available invasive and non-invasive monitoring. *Med Intensiva (English Ed.)*. 2011;35(9):552–561.
15. Zhang J, Critchley LAH, Huang L. Five algorithms that calculate cardiac output from the arterial waveform: a comparison with Doppler ultrasound. *Br J Anaesth*. 2015;115(3):392–402.
16. Hollenberg SM. Vasoactive drugs in circulatory shock. *Am J Respir Crit Care Med*. 2011;183(7):847–855.
17. Francis GS, Bartos JA, Adatya S. Inotropes. *J Am Coll Cardiol*. 2014;63(20):2069–2078.
18. Unverferth DA, Blanford M, Kates RE, Leier CV. Tolerance to dobutamine after a 72 hour continuous infusion. *Am J Med*. 1980;69(2):262–266.
19. Lampard JG, Lang E. Vasopressors for hypotensive shock. *Ann Emerg Med*. 2013;61(3):351–352.
20. Overgaard CB, Dzavik V. Inotropes and vasopressors: review of physiology and clinical use in cardiovascular disease. *Circulation*. 2008;118(10):1047–1056.
21. Marik PE. Early management of severe sepsis: concepts and controversies. *Chest*. 2014;145(6):1407–1418.
22. van Nunen LX, Noc M, Kapur NK, Patel MR, Perera D, Pijls NH. Usefulness of intra-aortic balloon pump counterpulsation. *Am J Cardiol*. 2016;117(3):469–476.
23. Nolan JP, Morley PT, Hoek TL, Hickey RW. Advancement life support task force of the international liaison committee on resuscitation. Therapeutic hypothermia after cardiac arrest. An advisory statement by the advancement life support task force of the international liaison committee on resuscitation. *Resuscitation*. 2003;57(3):231–235.
24. Scirica BM. Therapeutic hypothermia after cardiac arrest. *Circulation*. 2013;127(2):244–250.
25. Seder DB, Van der Kloot TE. Methods of cooling: practical aspects of therapeutic temperature management. *Crit Care Med*. 2009;37(suppl 7):S211–S222.
26. Albert CM, Stevenson WG. The future of arrhythmias and electrophysiology. *Circulation*. 2016;133(25):2687–2696.
27. Goldberger ZD, Rho RW, Page RL. Approach to the diagnosis and initial management of the stable adult patient with a wide complex tachycardia. *Am J Cardiol*. 2008;101(10):1456–1466.
28. Szwejkowski BR, Wright GA, Connelly DT, Gardner RS. When to consider an implantable cardioverter defibrillator following myocardial infarction? *Heart*. 2015;101(24):1996–2000.
29. Zipes DP, Camm AJ, Borggrefe M, et al. ACC/AHA/ESC 2006 guidelines for management of patients with ventricular arrhythmias and the prevention of sudden cardiac death—executive summary: a report of the American College of Cardiology/American Heart Association Task Force and the European Society of Cardiology Committee for Practice Guidelines (writing committee to develop guidelines for management of patients with ventricular arrhythmias and the prevention of sudden cardiac death) developed in collaboration with the European Heart Rhythm Association and the heart rhythm society. *Eur Hear J*. 2006;27(17):2099–2140.
30. Kannankeril P, Roden DM, Darbar D. Drug-induced long QT syndrome. *Pharmacol Rev*. 2010;62(4):760–781.
31. Walkey AJ, Hogarth DK, Lip GY. Optimizing atrial fibrillation management: from ICU and beyond. *Chest*. 2015;148(4):859–864.
32. Atzema CL, Barrett TW. Managing atrial fibrillation. *Ann Emerg Med*. 2015;65(5):532–539.
33. Kovacs RJ, Flaker GC, Saxonhouse SJ, et al. Practical management of anticoagulation in patients with atrial fibrillation. *J Am Coll Cardiol*. 2015;65(13):1340–1360.
34. Roldan V, Marín F, Fernández H, et al. Predictive value of the HAS-BLED and ATRIA bleeding scores for the risk of serious bleeding in a 'real-world' population with atrial fibrillation receiving anticoagulant therapy. *Chest*. 2013;143(1):179–184.
35. Treml B, Oswald E, Schenk B. Reversing anticoagulation in the hemorrhaging patient. *Curr Opin Anaesthesiol*. 2019;32(2):206–212.
36. Pollack Jr CV, Reilly PA, van Ryn J, et al. Idarucizumab for dabigatran reversal—full cohort analysis. *N Engl J Med*. 2017;377(5):431–441.
37. Ruff CT, Giugliano RP, Braunwald E, et al. Comparison of the efficacy and safety of new oral anticoagulants with warfarin in patients with atrial fibrillation: a meta-analysis of randomised trials. *Lancet*. 2014;383(9921):955–962.
38. Nagarakanti R, Ezekowitz MD, Oldgren J, et al. Dabigatran versus warfarin in patients with atrial fibrillation: an analysis of patients undergoing cardioversion. *Circulation*. 2011;123(2):131–136.
39. Donay KL, Johansen M. Common questions about pacemakers. *Am Fam Physician*. 2014;89(4):279–282.
40. Shah SJ, Kitzman DW, Borlaug BA, et al. Phenotype-specific treatment of heart failure with preserved ejection fraction: a multiorgan roadmap. *Circulation*. 2016;134(1):73–90.
41. Gheorghiade M, Zannad F, Sopko G, et al. Acute heart failure syndromes: current state and framework for future research. *Circulation*. 2005;112(25):3958–3968.
42. Weintraub NL, Collins SP, Pang PS, et al. Acute heart failure syndromes: emergency department presentation, treatment, and disposition: current approaches and future aims: a scientific statement from the American Heart Association. *Circulation*. 2010;122(19):1975–1996.
43. Page 2nd RL, O'Bryant CL, Cheng D, et al. Drugs that may cause or exacerbate heart failure: a scientific statement from the American Heart Association. *Circulation*. 2016;134(6):e32–e69.

CHAPTER 3

Renal Failure and Renal Replacement Therapy

Robert Stephen Brown and Alexander Goldfarb-Rumyantzev

Definition of Acute Kidney Injury[1]

- Increase in serum creatinine (S_{Cr}) by ≥0.3 mg/dL within 48 hours
- Increase in S_{Cr} to ≥1.5 times baseline, which is known or presumed to have occurred within the prior 7 days
- Urine volume <0.5 mL/kg/h for 6 hours after any indicated volume replacement

Staging of Acute Kidney Injury[1]

The following definition of stages of acute kidney injury (AKI) was proposed by the Kidney Disease: Improving Global Outcomes (KDIGO) group as a single definition to replace similar staging systems by Risk, Injury, Failure, Loss of kidney function, and End-stage kidney disease (RIFLE)[2] and Acute Kidney Injury Network (AKIN).[3] Remember that formulae designed for calculating estimated glomerular filtration rate (eGFR) or creatinine clearance from S_{Cr} levels must not be used in patients with AKI or any case in which the serum level is unstable.

Stage	Serum Creatinine	Urine Output
1	1.5–1.9 times baseline OR ≥0.3 mg/dL (≥26.5 mmol/L) increase	<0.5 mL/kg/h for 6–12 hours
2	2.0–2.9 times baseline	<0.5 mL/kg/h for ≥12 hours
3	3.0 times baseline OR Increase in S_{Cr} to ≥4.0 mg/dL OR Initiation of renal replacement therapy OR In patients <18 years, decrease in eGFR to <35 mL/min/1.73 m^2	<0.3 mL/kg/h for ≥24 hours OR Anuria for ≥12 hours

Incidence and Mortality Rate of AKI

It appears that the incidence of AKI in hospitalized patients has been rising over the past two decades. In one study of a representative nationwide sample of over 5 million inpatients discharged with acute renal failure (ARF) or ARF that required dialysis (ARF-D) between 1988 and 2002, the incidence of ARF increased from 61 to 288 per 100,000 population, and ARF-D increased from 4 to 27 per 100,000 population. However, over the same 15 years, the mortality rate of ARF declined from 40.4% to 20.3% and that of ARF-D declined from 41.3% to 28.1%, as shown in the graphs below.

Furthermore, there is a substantial increase in the rate of hospitalizations for AKI in men and women in the United States from 2000 to 2014.[4]

The significant increase in inpatients requiring dialysis suggests that the increased incidence of ARF is not explained by a change of diagnostic criteria over time, but a real rise of kidney injuries, likely caused by multiple factors described in this chapter in the setting of better resuscitative medical management and increased use of nephrotoxic agents. Moreover, it has been recognized that even small increments in the S_{Cr}, as little as a ≥0.3 to 0.5-mg/dL rise, in general hospital patients or after cardiac surgery are associated with several-fold increases in the mortality rate, and this increase may persist for up to 10 years following acute myocardial infarction.

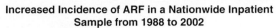

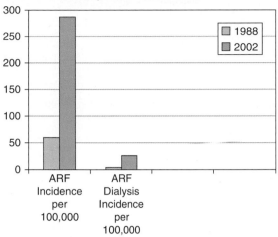

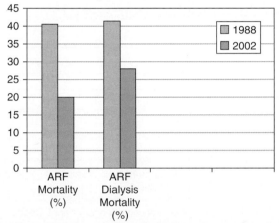

Modified from Lameire N, Van Biesen W, Vanholder R. The rise of prevalence and the fall of mortality of patients with acute renal failure: what the analysis of two databases does and does not tell us. J Am Soc Nephrol. 2006 Apr;17(4):923-5. doi: 10.1681/ASN.2006020152. Epub 2006 Mar 15. PMID: 16540555.

Factors Predicting AKI in ICU Patients[5,6]

Risk Factor	Odds Ratio (95% CI)
Disease severity	9.08 (4.57–13.60)
Age	4.95 (3.79–6.12)
Use of vasopressors	4.52 (2.03–10.05)
Sepsis/systemic immune response syndrome (SIRS)	4.15 (2.36–7.32)
Hypotension/shock	3.33 (1.70–6.52)
High risk/urgent surgery	2.34 (1.23–4.49)
Heart failure	2.05 (1.77–2.38)
Diabetes	1.58 (1.36–1.84)
Use of nephrotoxic medication	1.53 (1.09–2.14)
Hypertension	1.43 (1.08–1.89)
Baseline creatinine	0.14 (0.01–0.27)

Initial Diagnostic Approach to AKI

Initial step in diagnostic approach to patient with kidney insufficiency is to determine if the injury is acute or chronic.

Source of Information	Acute	Chronic
Medical history (prior records)	Abrupt ↑ in S_{Cr} over days	Slow increase in S_{Cr} over weeks to months
Symptoms	Recent onset of symptoms, e.g., fever, flank pain, decreased and/or discolored urine	No symptoms or slow onset of fatigue, anorexia, weakness, nausea, and/or pruritus
Labs	Further ↑ in S_{Cr} after initial evaluation	Relatively stable S_{Cr}
Anemia	Less typical or secondary to other than renal causes	More typical although not very specific
Ultrasound	Normal or enlarged kidney size	Small kidneys with increased echogenicity commonly, although may be of normal or even increased size, particularly with diabetes, amyloidosis, or polycystic kidney disease

Diagnostic Steps to Establish the Cause of AKI

Diagnostic steps

- History, prior medical records, physical exam
- Urine output measurement: Oliguria, defined as <400 mL/24h, or anuria, defined as <100 mL/24h (no urine or absolute anuria is diagnostically significant and usually caused by hypotensive shock, complete urinary tract obstruction, bilateral renovascular occlusion, or HUS/TTP with renal cortical necrosis)
- Foley catheter to measure urine output if oligo/anuric
- Urinalysis
- Urinary indices (see below)
- Ultrasound of urinary tract ± Doppler
- Rate of rise in S_{Cr} over time (i.e., 0.4–2.0 mg/dL per day rise in acute tubular necrosis (ATN); less and often variable in prerenal azotemia)

- Evaluation of intravascular volume and cardiac output
- Additional blood tests (complement levels, hepatitis B and C viral tests, lupus serology, serum and urine protein electrophoresis for myeloma)
- Renal vascular studies (radioisotope scan, MR angiography, radiocontrast angiography if vascular occlusion suspected)
- Gallium scan—positive with strong uptake in acute interstitial nephritis (AIN), negative in ATN
- Therapeutic trials as indicated: volume expansion, inotropic agents, relief of ureteral obstruction (i.e., S_{Cr} improves within 24–72 h with improved renal perfusion in prerenal azotemia, but does not in ATN), note that diuretics may increase urine output but do not increase GFR

- Kidney biopsy
- Empiric therapy for suspected disease, e.g., corticosteroids for AIN

Diagnostic Algorithm for AKI

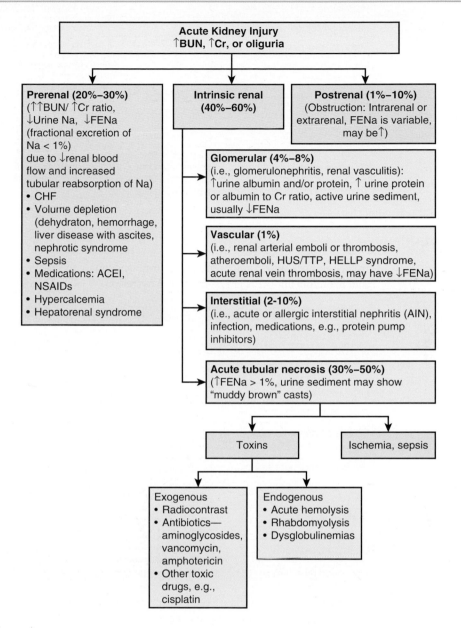

Red Flags

Whereas most of the cases of AKI are due to either prerenal conditions or acute tubular necrosis (ATN), one should be able to identify "red flags" for other potential etiologies of AKI. In addition, do not miss urinary obstruction, kidney ultrasound should be done in a majority of AKI cases.

Signs and Symptoms	Potential Etiology
Proteinuria and hematuria	Glomerulonephritis, acute interstitial nephritis (AIN)
Heavy proteinuria (>3 g/day)	Glomerulonephritis, renal vein thrombosis
Thrombocytopenia	HUS/TTP, HELLP, DIC
Lung infiltrates/nodules, hemoptysis, ARF	Pulmonary-renal syndromes—see below
Purpura (palpable purpura)	HSP, other forms of vasculitis, cryoglobulinemia
Skin rash	AIN, SLE
Very high blood pressure	Scleroderma crisis, malignant hypertension
Joint pain	SLE, rheumatoid arthritis, HSP

AIN, Acute interstitial nephritis; *DIC*, disseminated intravascular coagulation; *HELLP*, hemolysis, elevated liver enzyme levels, low platelet count; *HSP*, Henoch-Schönlein purpura; *HUS/TTP*, hemolytic uremic syndrome/thrombotic thrombocytopenic purpura; *SLE*, systemic lupus erythematosus.

Urinary Indices in Acute Renal Failure

Urinary indices on a random or "spot" urine specimen and other signs to differentiate between prerenal azotemia and ATN (FE = fractional excretion).

Lab Test	Prerenal Azotemia	ATN
Urine-to-plasma Cr ratio	>40	<20
BUN/Cr ratio	>20	<10–15
$U_{Urea\ nitrogen}$/BUN	>8	<3
UNa (mEq/L)	<20 (usually <10)	>40
FENa (%)	<1	>2
FE uric acid (%)—useful when on loop diuretics	<7	>15
Urinalysis sediment exam	Hyaline casts or negative sediment	Abnormal: muddy brown granular and epithelial cell casts, free epithelial cells
Specific gravity	>1.020	1.006–1.012 if no radiocontrast nor glucose
Uosm (mOsm/kg)	>500	<350–450

BUN, Blood urea nitrogen; *FENa*, fractional excretion of sodium; *UNa*, urinary sodium; *Uosm*, urine osmolality.

None of the above criteria of prerenal disease may be present in patients with underlying chronic renal disease since their ability to concentrate the urine might be impaired by chronic kidney disease (CKD).

Fractional Excretion of Sodium

FENa, which is the fractional excretion of sodium (expressed as a percentage), is probably the urinary index most commonly used in the work-up of AKI:

$$FE_{Na} = \frac{\text{Clearance of Na}}{\text{Clearance of Cr}} = \frac{\text{Na excreted}}{\text{Na filtered}}$$

$$FE_{Na} = \frac{U_{Na}/P_{Na}}{U_{Cr}/P_{Cr}} = \frac{(U_{Na} \times P_{Cr} \times 100\%)}{(P_{Na+} \times U_{Cr})}$$

where P is plasma or serum and U is urine.

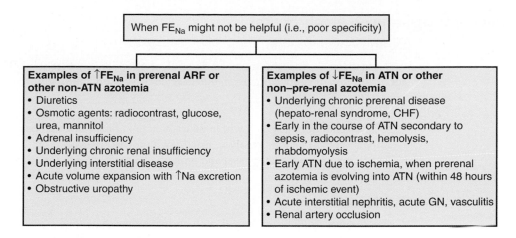

Blood Urea Nitrogen/Creatinine Ratio

Another index that is easily calculated is the blood urea nitrogen/creatinine (BUN/Cr) ratio. Normally it ranges from about 10 to 20. However, in certain conditions, BUN and Cr levels might change disproportionately.

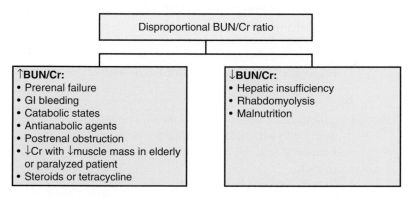

Acute Tubular Necrosis

CAUSES OF ATN	
Ischemia	**Toxicity**
- Sepsis - Hypovolemia (GI, renal or skin losses, bleeding), hypotension - Decreased renal plasma flow in edematous states (CHF, cirrhosis, hepatorenal syndrome, nephrotic syndrome) - Medications (ACEI, ARB, calcineurin inhibitors, NSAIDs, amphotericin, radiocontrast) - Renal vascular disease (renal artery thrombosis, stenosis, or embolization; atheroemboli; HUS/TTP, other forms of vasculitis; or small vessel injury including transplant rejection, sickle cell anemia, preeclampsia, malignant HTN)	- Aminoglycosides (e.g., gentamicin), vancomycin,[8] amphotericin, other drugs (see below) - Radiocontrast - Hemoglobin (intravascular hemolysis) - Myoglobin (rhabdomyolysis) - Other toxins (e.g., heavy metals, ethylene glycol) - Chemotherapy agents (see below)

ACEI, Angiotensin converting enzyme inhibitors; *ARB*, arterial blood gas; *CHF*, congestive heart failure; *GI*, gastrointestinal; *HTN*, hypertension; *NSAIDs*, nonsteroidal antiinflammatory drugs.

Radiocontrast-Induced Nephropathy[9]

Definition

Increase in the S_{Cr} concentration of 0.5 mg/dL or a 25% increase from baseline within 3 days after the administration of contrast media in the absence of an alternative cause.

Natural History

- S_{Cr} concentration increases within 24 to 48 hours of exposure and peaks at 3 to 5 days
- Impaired renal function resolves, usually within 7 to 10 days
- Renal impairment of later onset and prolonged duration: Look for other causes (e.g., atheroemboli after arteriography)

Incidence

- Approximately 0.5% of patients with normal kidney function
- 10% to 40% of patients with preexisting renal insufficiency with arteriography[10,11]

Pathophysiology

- Compromised renal blood flow which results in medullary ischemia
- Alterations in the metabolism of nitric oxide (NO), adenosine, angiotensin II, and prostaglandins
- Contrast induces osmotic diuresis, and active transport increases renal metabolic activity and oxygen consumption
- Contrast media stimulate a rapid influx of extracellular calcium leading to prolonged constriction of renal vasculature
- Contrast generates reactive oxygen species, which may also reduce the regional blood flow
- Contrast can also have direct toxic renal tubular effects
- High osmolarity results in reduction of renal blood flow

Risk Factors[12]

- Diminished baseline renal function (exponential increase in risk of radiocontrast-induced nephropathy [CIN] with rising creatinine)
- Peripheral vascular disease
- Diabetes
- Congestive heart failure (CHF)
- Cardiogenic shock
- Volume depletion
- Chronic liver disease
- Volume of contrast agent
- Potentially nephrotoxic drugs (e.g., nonsteroidal antiinflammatory drugs [NSAIDs])
- Proteinuria, especially myeloma proteins
- Hypertension

Prevention or Risk Reduction[13]

- Limit the dose of contrast
- Use alternative imaging techniques whenever possible
- Volume expansion with either isotonic sodium chloride or sodium bicarbonate solutions
- Pretreatment with n-acetylcysteine (NAC)—conflicting data
- Use of iso-osmolar contrast

Biomarkers

Numerous biomarkers potentially useful in the diagnosis of ATN have been proposed. Clinical use of these biomarkers to this day is limited to research as the clinical implementation of these diagnostics remains controversial. The most promising biomarkers are summarized in the following table. Most are normally expressed in the proximal tubule, some also by the distal tubule (except for cystatin C—expressed by all nucleated cells), and are measured by enzyme-linked immunosorbent assay (ELISA) (except for N-acetyl-beta-glucosaminidase [NAG]).

Biomarker	Function
Urine/serum neutrophil gelatinase–associated lipocalin (NGAL)	Growth differentiation factor, also participates in iron trafficking, upregulated in ischemic injury and released into urine
Urine kidney injury molecule-1 (KIM-1)	Membrane glycoprotein, shed into urine during acute injury, production increased in response to injury
Urine/serum IL-18	Immunomodulation, inflammation, upregulated in ischemic injury and released into urine
Urine/serum cystatin C	Protein produced by nucleated cells, cysteine protease inhibitor, during injury filtration decreased and proximal tubule metabolism decreases with increased serum levels
Urine liver fatty acid–binding protein (L-FABP)	Fatty acid trafficking protein, which translocates from cytosol to tubular lumen during ischemic injury increased in urine
Plasma IL-6	Immunomodulation, inflammation, the production increased and clearance decreased in association with AKI with increased plasma levels
Urine alpha-glutathione S-transferase (alpha-GST)	Cytosolic enzymes released into urine during injury
Urine NAG	Lysosomal enzyme (glucosidase) expressed in proximal tubules increased in urine with injury

IL-18, Interleukin-18.

Acute Kidney Injury Due to Glomerular Disease

ACUTE GLOMERULONEPHRITIS CAUSING AKI	
Primary GN	**Secondary Glomerular Disease**
- IgA nephropathy - Membranoproliferative nephritis - Postinfectious GN - Collapsing glomerulopathy - C3 GN	- Cryoglobulinemia - Goodpasture's syndrome - Lupus nephritis - Henoch-Schönlein purpura (HSP) - Vasculitis (e.g., granulomatosis with polyangiitis {formerly Wegener's granulomatosis}, ANCA vasculitis, polyarteritis nodosa) - HIV may cause collapsing glomerulopathy - Infective endocarditis or ventriculoatrial shunt nephritis - Light-chain GN with myeloma

ANCA, Antineutrophil cytoplasmic antibody; *GN*, glomerulonephritis; *IgA*, immunoglobulin A.

Pulmonary-Renal Syndromes[14]

Pulmonary-renal syndromes are a subset of diseases causing acute glomerulonephritis and diffuse alveolar hemorrhage. These should be differentiated from hemorrhagic pulmonary edema associated with renal failure from superimposed CHF or pulmonary emboli. The majority of pulmonary-renal syndrome cases are associated with positive antineutrophil cytoplasmic antibody (ANCA) levels.

- Microscopic polyangiitis, often associated with p-ANCA (proteinase 3 [PR3]-ANCA, anti-PR3) positivity
- Granulomatosis with polyangiitis (formerly Wegener's granulomatosis), often associated with c-ANCA (myeloperoxidase [MPO]-ANCA, anti-myeloperoxidase) positivity
- Churg-Strauss syndrome
- Systemic lupus erythematosus (SLE) with lung involvement
- Goodpasture's syndrome, associated with an anti–glomerular basement membrane (anti-GBM) antibody
- Behçet's disease
- Rheumatoid vasculitis

Acute Interstitial Nephritis[15]

Causes of Acute Interstitial Nephritis

- Infection
  - Bacterial (*Corynebacterium diphtheriae*, *Legionella* sp., staphylococci, streptococci, *Yersinia* sp.)
  - Viral (cytomegalovirus [CMV], Epstein-Barr virus [EBV], hantavirus, HIV, herpes simplex virus [HSV], hepatitis C, mumps, BK virus)
  - Other (*Leptospira* sp., mycobacterium, mycoplasma, *Rickettsia* sp., syphilis, toxoplasmosis)
- Immune diseases (SLE, sarcoid, Sjögren's syndrome, vasculitis, lymphoproliferative disorders)
- Acute rejection of kidney transplant
- Medications[16]
  - Antivirals
  - Antibiotics (penicillin, cephalosporins, rifampin, ciprofloxacin)
  - Sulfa-based drugs (trimethoprim/sulfamethoxazole [TMP/SMZ], hydrochlorothiazide [HCTZ], furosemide)
  - Proton pump inhibitors (PPIs) (the most common cause of acute interstitial nephritis [AIN])
  - NSAIDs, 5-aminosalicylic acid (5-ASA), others

Diagnosis of AIN

- Light proteinuria (<2 g/day), white blood cells (WBCs) in urinary sediment
- Eosinophiluria and/or eosinophilia
- Gallium scan positivity
- Kidney biopsy

Treatment of AIN

- Removing drug responsible for AIN
- Brief course of corticosteroids

Renal Toxicities of Medications and Anticancer Treatments[6,8,17–23]

It is well recognized that many medications can cause kidney dysfunction either as a direct effect of their action or as an undesirable side effect. This may occur by various mechanisms as will be outlined in the table below. This is particularly true of the new anticancer agents which can exhibit nephrotoxic properties, typically by inducing one or a combination of intrarenal vasoconstriction, direct tubular toxicity, intratubular obstruction, or thrombotic microangiopathy.

The reasons for this vulnerability of the kidney to toxic effects are as follows:
- Rich blood supply (20% of the cardiac output) causes high levels of potential toxicant delivery
- High tubular reabsorptive capacity results in increased tubule concentration causing high tubular intracellular concentrations
- Ability to concentrate toxins to high levels within the medullary interstitium
- Kidneys are an important site for xenobiotic metabolism, potential for transforming parent compounds into toxic metabolites
- Kidneys have high metabolic rate and the workload for oxidative energy requirements in renal cells causes increased sensitivity to toxins and high sensitivity to vasoactive agents
- Kidneys are a major elimination pathway for many antineoplastic drugs and their metabolites[23]

AKI Induced by Medications: Brief Summary

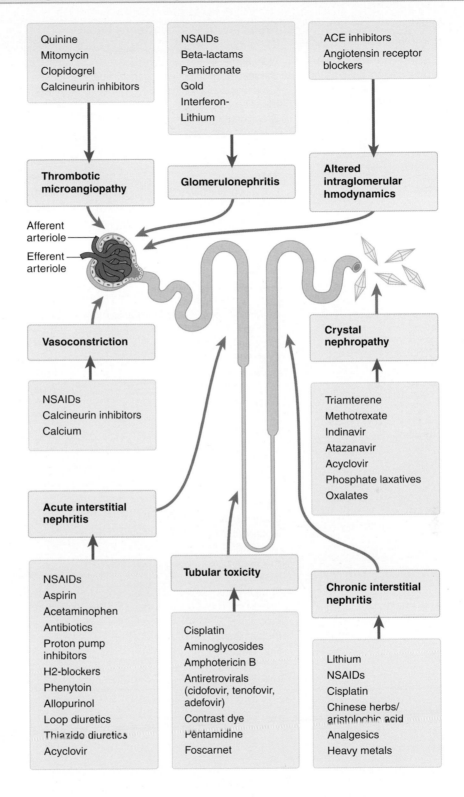

Quinine
Mitomycin
Clopidogrel
Calcineurin inhibitors

NSAIDs
Beta-lactams
Pamidronate
Gold
Interferon-
Lithium

ACE inhibitors
Angiotensin receptor blockers

Thrombotic microangiopathy

Glomerulonephritis

Altered intraglomerular hmodynamics

Afferent arteriole
Efferent arteriole

Vasoconstriction

NSAIDs
Calcineurin inhibitors
Calcium

Crystal nephropathy

Triamterene
Methotrexate
Indinavir
Atazanavir
Acyclovir
Phosphate laxatives
Oxalates

Acute interstitial nephritis

NSAIDs
Aspirin
Acetaminophen
Antibiotics
Proton pump inhibitors
H2-blockers
Phenytoin
Allopurinol
Loop diuretics
Thiazide diuretics
Acyclovir

Tubular toxicity

Cisplatin
Aminoglycosides
Amphotericin B
Antiretrovirals (cidofovir, tenofovir, adefovir)
Contrast dye
Pentamidine
Foscarnet

Chronic interstitial nephritis

Lithium
NSAIDs
Cisplatin
Chinese herbs/ aristolochic acid
Analgesics
Heavy metals

AKI Induced by Medications: Extended List

Site of Kidney Injury	Medications With Potential Renal Toxicity	Anticancer Medications
Vascular perfusion: Altered glomerular hemodynamics, afferent arteriole vasoconstriction, prerenal AKI, or thrombotic microangiopathy (TMA)	ACEI and ARB Calcineurin inhibitors (vasoconstriction) Cyclooxygenase inhibitors Diuretics Drugs causing hypercalcemia (vitamins D and A, high calcium intake) NSAID **TMA** Calcineurin inhibitors (CNI) Interferon Quinine Sirolimus Thienopyridines (clopidogrel)	Proteasome inhibitors (carfilzomib) **TMA** Anthracyclines (daunorubicin, doxorubicin) Anti-angiogenesis drugs Cellular TKIs/BCR-ABL (dasatinib) Cisplatin Gemcitabine Interferon Mitomycin Proteasome inhibitors (bortezomib, carfilzomib) VEGF/R antibodies (bevacizumab)
Glomerular lesions: hematuria, proteinuria ± AKI	Acebutolol Allopurinol Anabolic steroids Antiviral sofosbuvir in kidney transplant recipients Beta-lactam antibiotics Captopril Carbamazepine Carbimazole Chlorpromazine Cocaine adulterated with levamisole Febuxostat Gold therapy Hydralazine Interferon Isoniazid Lithium Methimazole Methyldopa Minocycline mTOR inhibitors (sirolimus, temsirolimus) NSAIDs Pamidronate Penicillamine and bucillamine Procainamide Propylthiouracil (PTU) Quinidine Sulfasalazine TNF-α inhibitors	Anthracyclines Anti-VEGF agents BRAF inhibitors (vemurafenib) Cellular TKIs/BCR-ABL (dasatinib) CTLA-4 antagonists (ipilimumab) EGFR inhibitors (gefitinib, cetuximab [monoclonal antibody]) Interferon Lenalidomide (immunomodulator) TKIs: receptor TKIs, VEGF family TKI (sunitinib, sorafenib), cellular TKIs/BCR-ABL (dasatinib)

Site of Kidney Injury	Medications With Potential Renal Toxicity	Anticancer Medications
Interstitial inflammation	**AIN** Antibiotics (penicillins, cephalosporins, macrolides, cyprofloxacin, vancomycin, rifampin, tetracyclines) NSAIDs Aspirin (ASA) Acetaminophen PPI (omeprazole, etc.) H2-blockers (cimetidine, ranitidine) Phenytoin Valproic acid Allopurinol Loop diuretics Thiazide diuretics Acyclovir **Chronic interstitial nephritis** Lithium NSAIDs Chinese herbs/aristolochic acid Analgesics Heavy metals, e.g., lead, cadmium, arsenic	**AIN** Lenalidomide (immunomodulator) Proteasome inhibitors (carfilzomib) BRAF inhibitors (vemurafenib, dabrafenib) Immune check point (PD-1, PD-L1) inhibitors (nivolumab, pembrolizumab) CTLA-4 antagonists (ipilimumab) TKIs, e.g., receptor TKIs VEGF family TKI (sunitinib, sorafenib) Anti–CTLA-4 **Chronic interstitial nephritis** Receptor TKIs VEGF family TKI (sunitinib, sorafenib)Cisplatin
AKI: tubular toxicity or ATN	Amphotericin B Antifungal drugs Antimicrobials, e.g., vancomycin, polymyxin, aminoglycosides Antiviral/antiretroviral drugs (cidofovir, tenofovir, adefovir) Calcineurin inhibitors Deferasirox Foscarnet IVIG containing sucrose mTOR inhibitors (sirolimus, temsirolimus) NSAIDs Pentamidine Radiocontrast media	ALK inhibitors Anti-KIR agents (lirilumab) BRAF inhibitors (vemurafenib) Cellular TKIs/BCR-ABL (imatinib, dasatinib) Cisplatin EGFR antagonists (cetuximab [monoclonal antibody], panitumumab [monoclonal antibody], erlotinib [anti-EGFR TKI], afatinib [anti-EGFR TKI], gefitinib [anti-EGFR TKI]) HER-2 antagonists MEK inhibitors (trametinib) Melphalan Pomalidomide (immunomodulator) SLAMF7 inhibitors (elotuzumab)

ALK, Anaplastic lymphoma kinase; *CTLA-4*, cytotoxic T-lymphocyte–associated protein 4; *EGFR*, epidermal growth factor receptor; *HER-2*, human epidermal growth factor receptor 2; *IVIG*, intravenous immunoglobulin; *KIR*, Killer cell immunoglobulin-like receptor; *mTOR*, mechanistic target of rapamycin; *PD-1*, programmed death-1; *PD-1L*, programmed cell death ligand 1; *SLAMF7*, signaling lymphocytic activation molecule F7; *TKIs*, tyrosine kinase inhibitors; *TNF-α*, tumor necrosis factor-α; *VEGF-R*, vascular endothelial growth factor receptor.

Medication-Related Kidney Damage: Renal Tubular Electrolyte and Acid-Base Disorders and Intratubular Crystal Formation

Site and Type of Disorder	Medications With Potential Renal Toxicity	Anticancer Medications
Tubular electrolyte disorders	**Hypokalemia** Loop and thiazide diuretics Insulin Amphotericin **Hyperkalemia** ACEI ARB Aldosterone antagonists (spironolactone, eplerenone) Potassium-sparing diuretics (amiloride, triamterene) Trimethoprim Pentamidine Cyclosporine, tacrolimus Succinylcholine (depolarizing anesthetic agents) Beta-blockers Heparin at high dose **Hypomagnesemia** Loop and thiazide diuretics Antibiotics (i.e., aminoglycosides, amphotericin, pentamidine, gentamicin, tobramycin, viomycin) Amphotericin B Cyclosporine, tacrolimus PPI medications (e.g., omeprazole) **Hyponatremia/SIADH** Multiple medications, including: Diuretics, mainly thiazides SSRIs Amphotericin Aripiprazole Atovaquone Amiodarone ACEI, ARB Bromocriptine Carbamazepine Carvedilol NSAIDs Desmopressin Sulfonylureas Trazodone Tolbutamide **Fanconi's syndrome** Tetracycline antibiotics Antiviral drugs Aminoglycosides Anticonvulsants **Hypophosphatemia** Diuretics Theophylline, bronchodilators Corticosteroids Mannitol Insulin treatment of acute diabetes **Hypocalcemia** Rifampin Antiseizure drugs (phenytoin, phenobarbital) Bisphosphonates Calcitonin Chloroquine Corticosteroids Plicamycin	**Hypokalemia** BRAF inhibitors (vemurafenib) Receptor TKIs VEGF family TKI (vandetanib) EGFR inhibitors (gefitinib, afatinib [anti-EGFR TKI], cetuximab [monoclonal antibody]), panitumumab [monoclonal antibody] [anti-EGFR TKI]) **Hyperkalemia** Anti–IL-6 agents (siltuximab) **Hypomagnesemia** Cisplatin EGFR inhibitors (erlotinib [anti-EGFR TKI], cetuximab, panitumumab [monoclonal antibody]) **Salt wasting/hyponatremia** Cisplatin, carboplatin Melphalan Cyclophosphamide Vincristine Basiliximab BRAF inhibitors (vemurafenib) MEK inhibitors (trametinib) Immune check point inhibitors (nivolumab, pembrolizumab) PD-1 inhibitors (nivolumab, pembrolizumab) CTLA-4 antagonists (ipilimumab) EGFR antagonists (cetuximab (monoclonal antibody), afatinib [anti-EGFR TKI]) **Fanconi's syndrome** Cisplatin Lenalidomide (immunomodulator) BRAF inhibitors (vemurafenib) Ifosfamide **Hypophosphatemia** BRAF inhibitors (dabrafenib) Anti-KIR agents (lirilumab) Akt inhibitors (perifosine) Receptor TKIs VEGF family TKI (sorafenib, regorafenib) Cellular TKIs/BCR-ABL (imatinib, bosutinib) EGFR inhibitors (erlotinib [anti-EGFR TKI]) Some anti-VEGF TKIs **Hypocalcemia** Receptor TKIs VEGF family TKI (regorafenib, vandetanib)

Site and Type of Disorder	Medications With Potential Renal Toxicity	Anticancer Medications
Renal tubular acidosis	**Type 1 ("distal")** Amphotericin Toluene a1 **Type 2 ("proximal")** Tenofovir, adefovir Didanosine, lamivudine, stavudine Valproic acid Aminoglycosides, expired tetracyclines Cidofovir Streptozocin **Type 4 ("hyperkalemic")** Potassium-sparing diuretics (amiloride, triamterene) Aldosterone antagonists (spironolactone, eplerenone) ACEIs Trimethoprim Pentamidine	**Type 2 ("proximal")** Ifosfamide Oxaplatin, cisplatin
Crystal nephropathy/intratubular obstruction	Phosphate laxatives Oxalate excess (starfruit, high-dose vitamin C) Acyclovir Amoxicillin Indinavir Atazanavir Ciprofloxacin Orlistat Sodium phosphate Sulfadiazine Triamterene Foscarnet	Methotrexate Pomalidomide (immunomodulator)

SIADH, Syndrome of inappropriate antidiuretic hormone secretion; *SSRIs,* selective serotonin reuptake inhibitors.

Types of Urine Crystals Associated With Specific Medications[19,24]

Acyclovir	Birefringent needle-shaped
Amoxicillin	Birefringent needle-shaped
Indinavir	Plate-like, fan-shaped, sun burst
Atazanavir	Needle-like crystals
Ciprofloxacin	Needles, sheaves, stars, birefringent
Methotrexate	Crystalline, birefringent compact or needle-shaped golden, arranged in annular structures. Positive on methenamine silver and negative von Kossa and alizarin red stains
Orlistat	Calcium oxalate (poorly birefringent, eight-faced bipyramid, "mail envelope")
Sodium phosphate	Calcium phosphate (amorphous, granular, white)
Sulfadiazine	Sheaves of wheat or shell-shaped rosettes
Triamterene	Birefringent colored spheres

Other Medication Side Effects With Potential Effect on Renal Function

Problem	Medications With Potential Renal Toxicity	Anticancer Medications
Hyperuricemia	Diuretics Salicylates Pyrazinamide Ethambutol Nicotinic acid Cyclosporine, tacrolimus (less so) 2-Ethylamino-1,3,4-thiadiazole	Anti–IL-6 agents (siltuximab) Cytotoxic agents
Hyperuricosuria	Atorvastatin Amlodipine Losartan (decreased serum urate)	
Osmotic nephrosis	Immunoglobulins Sucrose (intravenously) Hydroxyethyl starch Mannitol Contrast media	
Hemorrhagic cystitis	Rare: penicillins, danazol	Cyclophosphamide, ifosfamide Bacillus Calmette-Guérin (BCG) infusion in the bladder
Cyst formation		ALK inhibitor
Hypertension	Acetaminophen Alcohol Amphetamines, ecstasy (MDMA and derivatives), and cocaine Antidepressants (including venlafaxine, bupropion, and desipramine) Caffeine Corticosteroids Cyclosporine, tacrolimus Ephedra and many other herbal products Erythropoietin Estrogens Migraine medicines, e.g. ergotamine or triptans Nasal vasoconstrictor decongestants Nicotine NSAIDs	Anti-VEGF antibodies (bevacizumab, aflibercept) Cellular TKIs/BCR-ABL (nilotinib, ponatinib) MEK inhibitors (trametinib) Receptor TKIs VEGF family TKI (sunitinib, pazopanib, axitinib, sorafenib, regorafenib, vandetanib)
Rhabdomyolysis	Statins Anti-HIV medications Cyclosporine, tacrolimus Erythromycin Colchicine Cocaine (especially with heroin), amphetamines, ecstasy, LSD	Cellular TKIs/BCR-ABL (imatinib, dasatinib)

LSD, Lysergic acid diethylamide; *MDMA*, 3,4-methylenedioxymethamphetamine.

Treatment of AKI

- First look for reversible causative factors, e.g., infection, obstruction, nephrotoxins, circulatory failure, hypercalcemia, and so on
- Supportive care with careful fluid balance and electrolyte balance
- Pharmacologic manipulations (loop diuretics may increase urine output, dopamine for low cardiac output only, most drug trials ineffective)
- Phosphate binders for hyperphosphatemia ($CaCO_3$ if serum Ca is low, aluminum hydroxide or carbonate can be used for acute management without aluminum toxicity in short courses of <1 month)
- Renal replacement therapy (RRT)

Nutritional considerations in patients with AKI

- Energy requirements: 35 kcal/kg/day
- Protein requirements: 1.2 g protein/kg/day but >1.25 g/kg/day not beneficial and will increase rate of BUN rise
- Other nutrients: ratio between glucose and lipids 70/30 to provide calories
- Usually low-Na, low-K, low-phosphate diet is desirable to control fluid retention, hyperkalemia and hyperphosphatemia (see Chapter 4)

Renal Replacement Therapy

Indications for renal replacement therapy
Indications for initiating dialysis, either hemodialysis (HD), continuous veno-venous hemofiltration (CVVH), or peritoneal dialysis (PD) in acute or chronic renal failure are similar—to alleviate symptoms or signs of uremia, abnormalities of electrolyte or acid-base balance, or uncontrolled hypervolemia. Dialysis may be started in severe acute renal failure when no quick recovery is expected to avoid "impending uremia".

Acute Kidney Injury:
- Symptoms or signs of the uremic syndrome (pericarditis, neuropathy, encephalopathy, seizures, coagulopathy, enteropathy with GI symptoms)
- Refractory hypervolemia
- Severe uncontrolled electrolyte abnormalities (e.g., hyperkalemia)
- Severe uncontrolled acid-base disorder (e.g., metabolic acidosis)
- Rapidly rising BUN and creatinine with persistent oliguria
- Some poisonings, e.g., methanol, ethylene glycol

Chronic Kidney Disease (ESRD):
- Absolute indications:
  - Uncontrollable hyperkalemia (K^+ >6.5 mEq/L)
  - CHF, fluid overload, and pulmonary edema unresponsive to diuretics
  - Uremic symptoms (pericarditis, seizures, progressive neuropathy, encephalopathy, nausea, vomiting, weight loss)
  - Significant bleeding with uremic coagulopathy

- Relative indications:
  * Low GFR <10 mL/min/1.73m², or <15 mL/min/1.73m² In a diabetic patient, creatinine ≥10 mg/dL. However, estimated GFR should have minor role in determining the time of dialysis initiation
  * Intractable hypertension with diuretic unresponsiveness in severe CKD

- Relative Contraindications:
  * Severe irreversible dementia
  * Short estimated survival
  * Severe or debilitating co-morbid diseases compromising patient's quality of life (decision left up to patient or health care proxy)

Appropriateness of Dialysis Initiation

The appropriateness of starting dialysis in a particular patient should be based upon two considerations:
- Expected patient survival with or without dialysis
- Quality of life.[25]

Elderly patients (>80 years old) with end-stage renal disease (ESRD) and significant comorbidities might need to be informed that hemodialysis (HD) may extend life only 2 to 3 months more than conservative medical management without improving quality of life, although that should be decided individually on a case-by-case basis.

Timing of Dialysis Initiation

- AKI: In ARF there is a suggestion that early initiation of dialysis might be beneficial for survival, particularly in postoperative patients.[26–29] Consideration should be given to whether recovery of AKI may occur without the need for dialysis to avoid risks.
- CKD: Until recently, there was uncertainty about the timing of dialysis initiation (early versus. late start) in advancing CKD. The definition of early and late was based on the degree of renal dysfunction, measured by creatinine clearance or creatinine-based eGFR. But studies have found that there is no benefit to early initiation of dialysis[30] and in fact there is a suggested benefit of a late start[31] based on symptoms or signs of uremia.

Potential Negative Effect of Dialysis

- Decreased urine output caused by removal of volume and urea by dialysis
- Repeated episodes of hypotension with HD (less common with peritoneal dialysis [PD] and continuous veno-venous hemofiltration [CVVH]) may cause delayed recovery of AKI and/or myocardial stunning
- Complement activation (less severe with biocompatible dialysis membranes)
- Risks and complications associated with vascular access catheter placement for HD or CVVH or peritoneal catheter for PD

Dialyzers

Hemodialysis membranes are manufactured with cellulose, modified cellulose, or synthetic polymers. Dialyzer clearance is determined by the surface area (A) and mass transfer coefficient, which is a function of the membrane itself (Ko).[32]

Types of Dialyzers/Membranes

- Low-flux membranes (standard dialyzers with small pores)
- High-efficiency dialyzers (dialyzers with large surface area A)

- High-flux dialyzers (increased pore size and increased hydraulic permeability Ko for greater dialysis of "middle" molecules and greater ultrafiltration)
- Protein-leaking membranes (for plasmapheresis to remove large molecules such as immunoglobulins at the price of leaking out albumin)

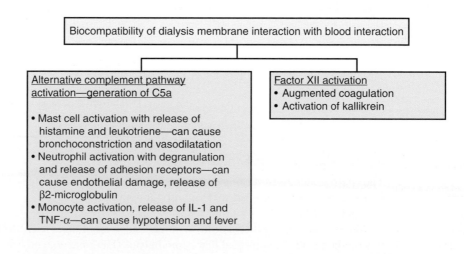

Vascular Access for Hemodialysis

There are three main types of vascular access for HD:
- Arterio-venous fistula (AVF),
- Arterio-venous graft (AVG), and
- Central venous catheter (CVC) (tunneled or not tunneled)

Hemodialysis access should be able to provide a blood flow of at least 300 mL/min.

Types of Vascular Access

AVF:

- AVF is the preferable dialysis access as it is associated with the best clinical outcomes.
- It has lower rates of infection and better long-term survival of the patient and of the access itself.
- However, it requires sufficient vasculature to create an adequate AVF that will mature and be useable to obtain satisfactory blood flow rates.
- It takes at least 1-2 months for an AVF to mature before being used, and often longer, with many fistulae never maturing adequately or requiring procedural interventions.

AVG:

- AVG is useful in patients where an AVF is not feasible due to poor veins.
- Provides good blood flow, and because it is internalized, it is less prone to infections than a CVC.

- AVG is considered to be inferior to AVF in terms of patient survival (except in elderly patients with comorbidities[35]).
- AVG does not require much time to mature and can often be used immediately or within days of placement.

CVC:

- CVC is considered to be the last choice for chronic dialysis access.
  - to be used only after AVF and AVG options are not feasible
  - if there is no time for AVF/AVG maturation
  - for patients likely to recover from AKI
  - for patients scheduled for renal transplantation but needing short-term dialysis
  - if patient survival is likely to be short
- Catheters are associated with poor patient survival, are often complicated by infection, generally have lower blood flow rates, and are more prone to clotting than AVF/AVG.
- The benefit of a CVC is that it can be used immediately after placement.

Acute Vascular Access: Dialysis Catheters

Acute HD or CVVH Access

- Double-lumen noncuffed dialysis catheters
  - semi-rigid at room temperature to facilitate insertion but soften at body temperature
  - proximal and distal lumens should be separated by at least 2 cm
  - maximum blood flow usually 350–400 mL/min

  - may be placed in internal jugular vein preferably, followed by femoral vein, or, less desirably, subclavian veins (due to high incidence of central vein stenoses)
  - also available with a third lumen for blood sampling or infusions
- Silastic, cuffed, tunneled dialysis catheters (either double-lumen or two single-lumen twin catheters usually placed in an internal jugular vein)

"Ideal" Dialysis Catheter

- Easy to insert and remove
- Inexpensive
- Low infection rate

- Does not clot or develop fibrin sheath
- Does not cause stenosis of central veins
- Delivers high flow (>400 mL/min) reliably
- Durable material to avoid kinking or leaks
- Comfortable and acceptable to the patient

Duration of Catheter Use

- Temporary (not tunneled) femoral catheters, inserted with sterile technique and meticulously cleaned daily in bed-bound patients, can usually be left in place safely for 3–7 days, occasionally longer, but are not suitable for ambulatory patients

- Subclavian and internal jugular temporary catheters (not tunneled) may be left in place for 2 to 4 weeks.
- Silastic/silicone cuffed catheters (tunneled) are suitable for long-term use

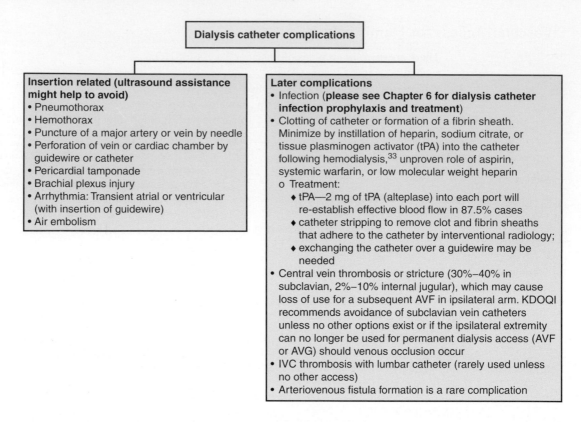

Approach to Central Venous Catheter Malfunction

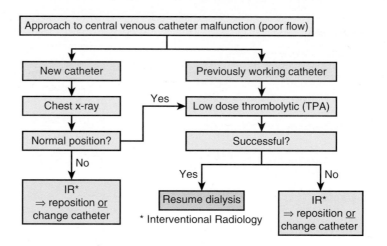

Anticoagulation in Hemodialysis

Anticoagulation is an important part of the HD or CVVH procedure though many dialyses can be performed without anticoagulation using frequent saline flushes in patients at high bleeding risk. Most common options for anticoagulation are unfractionated heparin (United States) and low-molecular-weight heparin (Western Europe),[34] and citrate, particularly for CVVH. Other agents are available when heparin is not an option (e.g., in heparin-induced thrombocytopenia).

Anticoagulants	Chemical Composition	Mechanism	Follow-Up Indicator	Heparin-Induced Thrombocytopenia
Unfractionated heparin	Mixture of glycosaminoglycan chains 5000–30,000 Da	Binds to antithrombin III ⇒ inhibits clotting factors IIa and Xa	PTT	1%–5% incidence
Low-molecular-weight heparin	Depolymerized fragments of larger heparins 4000–6500 Da	Binds to antithrombin III, inhibits clotting factor Xa (↓ incidence of bleeding)	Anti-Xa (therapeutic range 0.2–0.4 U/mL)	0%–3% incidence (90% cross-reactivity with HIT-IgG)
Citrate	Trisodium citrate solution, 3% (ACD-A sol'n) or citrate dialysate	Citrate binds to calcium and disrupts the coagulation cascade	Ionized calcium (therapeutic <0.4 mM/L in dialyzer) or an activated clotting time of 1.5–2.0 times baseline (180–250 seconds)	None
Other anticoagulants listed below are usually not used for HD barring unusual circumstances				
Heparinoids (danaparoid)	Sulfated glycosaminoglycans 4000–8000 Da	Binds to antithrombin III ⇒ inhibits clotting factor Xa (incidence of bleeding)	Anti-Xa (therapeutic range 0.2–04 U/mL)	0%–3% incidence (<10% cross-reactivity with HIT-IgG)
Argatroban	Arginine derivative	Thrombin inhibitor	aPTT 2.0–2.5; decrease dose with liver disease	None
Hirudin, lepirudin (recombinant hirudin)	Peptide of 65 amino acids—not currently available	Binds to thrombin	PTT	None
Iloprost	Analog of prostacyclin	Inhibits platelets aggregation	—	None
Ancrod	Extract from pit viper venom	Cleaves fibrinogen, prevents conversion into fibrin	—	None

ACD-A, Anticoagulant citrate dextrose solution, solution A; *aPTT,* activated partial thromboplastin time; *PTT,* partial thromboplastin time.

Hemodialysis Adequacy

Determining the adequate dose of dialysis for an individual patient remains uncertain. It is known that adding more dialysis clearance above a certain amount does not continue to provide additional survival benefit.[36,37] While goals for adequate dialysis dose might change as we learn more, it is important to know the tools to measure dialysis dose. Different approaches to measuring dialysis dose have one common component—the measurement is based on clearance of a particular chemical compound from the blood. Most often urea or creatinine is used as such compounds. Dialysis dose therefore may be expressed as percent reduction in plasma urea concentration (urea reduction ratio or URR). An alternate would be clearance of urea or creatinine in a given time period (Kt = clearance × time) and usually to individualize this indicator to patient size with this calculation based on the patient's total body water volume (V) and expressed as Kt/V. Urea Kt/V and URR are used most often as indicators of HD dose, while urea Kt/V and creatinine clearance are used as indicators of PD dose. The formulae below have been derived for chronic maintenance HD provided three times per week whereas HD adequacy for AKI is uncertain. HD for AKI should provide adequate clearance, electrolyte and acid-base balance, and volume control, often ~4 hours three times per week or less time more frequently, e.g., four to six times per week.

```
┌─────────────────────────────────────────┐
│           Hemodialysis Adequacy           │
└─────────────────────────────────────────┘
```

Urea Reduction Ratio (URR)
URR = *(BUN predialysis - BUN post dialysis) / BUN predialysis)* × 100%
Minimally adequate URR ≥65% for each treatment with three times per week dialysis, though target dose ≥70% is common in patients with little or no residual kidney function[38]

Kt/V (urea)
K - clearance of the dialyzer in mL/min, may be calculated from the URR or provided by the manufacturer (eg, at QB = 400, mL/min QD = 800 mL/min, and UF = 15 mL/min urea clearance of Fresenius Optiflux 160NR, Optiflux 200NR, and Gambro Polyflux 210H are approx. 0.28, 0.29, and 0.31 L/min)
t - time of dialysis (min)
V - volume of distribution of urea based on total body water (mL)
Kt - total volume of fluid cleared of urea (mL)
Kt/V - how many total body water volumes of distribution of urea cleared with each dialysis treatment.
It can be calculated from URR using empiric formulae or websites such as http://www.kt-v.net/. Minimally adequate Kt/V ≥1.2 with three times per week dialysis, though target dose Kt/V ≥1.4 is common, particularly in patients with little or no residual kidney function[38]

Dialysis Drug Clearance

Clearance of drugs and pharmacokinetics during HD is complex. It is important to estimate dialysis clearance of medications to adequately adjust the dose. That is especially true in drugs with relatively narrow therapeutic windows (e.g., chemotherapy, antibiotics).[39] The complexity of the process has to do with multiple factors affecting drug clearance in dialysis, specifically, the characteristics of the dialyzer, dialysis procedure, dialysate, and properties of the drug itself. Using these considerations, only very crude approximations of the clearance are possible in the absence of experimental data. Such experimental data are obtained for some but not all drugs (e.g., vancomycin).[40]

Drug Properties That Affect Dialytic Clearance

- Molecular size
  - <1000 Da—small molecules—diffusion-dependent transport
  - 1000–2000 Da—only convective transport
  - >2000 Da partially reflected by membrane even during UF
- Protein binding reduces clearance (heparin increases free fraction of many drugs)
- Volume of distribution (the greater the volume of distribution the less the dialyzability)
  - 1 L/kg BW distribution volume—likely removed by dialysis
  - 1–2 L/kg BW distribution volume—marginal clearance by dialysis
  - >2 L/kg BW—unlikely to be effectively removed by dialysis
  - multicompartmental distribution leads to dramatic rebound after dialysis
- Charge of drug molecule
- Water or lipid solubility: poor dialyzability of lipid-soluble compounds
- Dialyzer membrane binding increases clearance of the compound

BW, Body weight; *UF*, ultrafiltration.

Dialysis Properties That Affect Drug Clearance

- Dialyzer properties (pore size, surface area, type of membrane might affect binding)
- Dialysis procedure properties (blood flow rate, dialysate flow rate, ultrafiltration rate)
- Dialysate properties (solute concentration, pH, temperature)
- Time of dialysis treatment

Continuous Renal Replacement Therapy

Indications for continuous renal replacement therapy (CRRT): need for renal replacement therapy (fluid overload, uremia, uncorrectable acidosis, hyperkalemia, some intoxications), particularly in a hemodynamically unstable patient. CRRT clearance is based on diffusion (dialysis), convection (ultrafiltration), and adsorption by the membrane, similar to clearance by intermittent dialysis though usually less efficient on an hourly basis. Most CRRT is done by CVVH, rather than continuous arteriovenous hemofiltration (CAVH), without or with concomitant dialysis, called continuous veno-venous hemodiafiltration (CVVHD).

What Do You Need to Know to Write CRRT Orders?

Pumps
- Blood flow rate 120–250 (average 180) mL/min
- UF rate 1–2 L/h total but net UF depends on patient volume status and overall goals of treatment
- Clearance of volumes ≥25 mL/kg/h does not have improved outcomes[41]

Replacement Fluids
- If standard commercial replacement fluid is not available, normal saline and sodium bicarbonate, PD fluid, Ringer's lactate, or pharmacy-made solutions can be used

Dialysis Fluid
- The composition of dialysis fluid is selected based on the same principles as for intermittent HD; peritoneal dialysate solutions are often used, though calcium-free dialysate may be preferable for citrate anticoagulation

Anticoagulation
- Systemic heparin or regional citrate[42] anticoagulation
- Citrate anticoagulation
  - ○ ACD-A solution of 3% trisodium citrate infused at a rate of 150% (in mL/h) of the blood flow rate (QB) in mL/min, e.g., 225 mL/h for a QB of 150 mL/min
  - ○ Ca^{++} infusion rate is calculated based on the principle of giving about 1 mmol of Ca^{++} for each mmol of citrate, and then adjust infusion rate based on ionized calcium (iCa^{++}) level (e.g., calcium gluconate 20 g in 500 mL D5W at 30 mL/h with an increase for iCa^{++} <1.0 mmol/L or a decrease for iCa^{++} >1.2 mmol/L)

Parameters to Monitor
- Serum electrolytes, iCa^{++}, Mg^{++} Q 4–6 hours
- For citrate anticoagulation, iCa^{++} Q4h initially until stable, and then Q6h and total calcium Q12h to assess for citrate toxicity (by an increasing gap between total and ionized calcium levels)
- Activated clotting time measured at the post-filter maintained between 180 and 200 seconds with either heparin or citrate is usually adequate

D5W, Dextrose 5% in water.

Peritoneal Dialysis[43–45]

Peritoneal Dialysis Techniques[46,47]

Manual Technique
- CAPD—continuous ambulatory PD (continuous technique with about four 2–3-L exchanges per day, 4–6-hour dwell cycles)

Techniques Requiring a Cycler Machine or Automated PD (APD)
- CCPD—continuous cycling PD using a cycler machine usually during the night; with shorter dwell times than CAPD but more exchanges and commonly with increased total volume of dialysate and a long dwell, or even a PD exchange, during the day
- CCPD with abdomen dry during the day may be called intermittent PD (IPD) or nocturnal intermittent PD (NIPD) performed as frequent, short cycles during the night with no daytime dwell
- TPD—tidal PD (series of quick fills with incomplete drains, so that some residual volume [1/2 of usual dwell volume] remains in the peritoneal space; used infrequently as a peritoneal "conditioning" regimen)

Continuous Flow
- CFPD—continuous flow PD (requires double-lumen catheter or two separate catheters to support continuous flow of dialysate to increase efficiency, rarely used)

Peritoneal Dialysis Prescription

Adequate prescription of PD should provide adequate clearance, volume removal, and fit patient's lifestyle/schedule. PD prescription includes PD modality, number of exchanges, volume of exchange, and dialysate solution osmolarity ("strength" of PD dialysate to ultrafilter off fluid is usually determined by dextrose concentration, though icodextrin is available to enhance ultrafiltration over a longer dwell time.) The choice of the modality is based on transport characteristics of the peritoneal membrane that can be determined by the peritoneal equilibration test (PET). However, in the acute or ICU setting, it would be common to start empirically with CAPD using four or more 2- to 3-L exchanges per day (though initial smaller volumes would be utilized if a new catheter is placed to avoid peritoneal fluid leaks). Volume and number of exchanges are determined based on target clearance with the PD fluid dextrose concentration based on target ultrafiltration rate needed for fluid removal.

PD Adequacy

- Creatinine clearance >60 L/week/1.73 m^2 body surface area (best calculated using serum and dialysate creatinine measurements from a 24-hour collection of dialysate though in the acute setting target goals of fluid removal and serum chemistries are often used instead)
- Weekly Kt/V$_{urea}$ >1.7–2.0 (either just dialysis clearance or a combination of dialysis clearance and residual kidney function). Calculate from the website: http://www.kt-v.net/ using addition of residual renal function if urine output is >100 mL/day. To calculate weekly Kt/V for peritoneal dialysis:
  - K = clearance of urea (not creatinine)—measured by timed urine or dialysate collection
  - t = 10,080 minutes (per week)
  - V = 0.6 (for males) or 0.5 (for females) × body weight in kg

Complications of Peritoneal Dialysis

PD Peritonitis (See Chapter 6 for PD Peritonitis Management)

Acid-Base and Electrolyte Disturbances in Peritoneal Dialysis

ACID-BASE AND ELECTROLYTE DISTURBANCES IN PERITONEAL DIALYSIS		
	Mechanism	Correction
Hypernatremia	Hypertonic dialysate causes water to shift into peritoneal space (removing water in excess of Na)	Water orally or D5W IV or lower glucose or Na level in dialysate
Hyponatremia	Low Na intake, excessive thirst, renal or stool losses, inadequate UF	Salt intake must be proportional to the volume loss induced by dialysis,[48] increase hypertonic dialysate if water overload
Hyperkalemia	High K intake with low renal excretion and inadequate PD removal, extracellular shift of K may occur due to low insulin or drugs	Higher dialysis clearance, standard treatment for acute hyperkalemia (see Chapter 4)
Hypokalemia	Excessive K clearance by PD, occurs in 60% of ESRD patients on PD[49]	10%–30% of patients need K supplement
Lactic acidosis	Conversion of lactate to bicarbonate can be affected in sepsis or by metformin	Replace lactate buffer with bicarbonate in dialysate[50]

Hemoperitoneum

Causes of Hemoperitoneum	
Benign Causes	More Serious Causes
• Ovulation • Menstruation • Post-lithotripsy • Laparoscopic abdominal procedures, e.g., cholecystectomy • Shedding of ectopic endometrium	• Femoral hematoma leakage • Cyst rupture in PKD • Hematologic: low platelets, coagulopathy • Adenocarcinoma of the colon • Ischemic bowel • Splenic rupture • Pancreatitis • Sclerosing peritonitis
Treatment	
• Intraperitoneal heparin (does not change systemic coagulation, but prevents clotting of the catheter) • If benign—observe • If no obvious cause—investigate, e.g., PD fluid cytology, CT scan, etc.	

CT, Computed tomography; PKD, polycystic kidney disease.

Other Non-infectious Complications of PD

Conditions	Diagnosis	Treatment
Hernia (caused by ↑ intraabdominal pressure)	Clinical examination or CT scan	Surgical repair, corsets, dialysis with lower intraabdominal pressure (CAPD, eliminate daytime dwell or decrease volume)
Genital edema (<10% CAPD Pts): Tracking of PD fluid to scrotum/labia	Clinical exam, decreased PD fluid effluent return, Ultrasound/CT scan	Stop PD and use temporary HD, low volume CAPD at bed rest, further treatment depends on source of leak
Abdominal wall leak	Clinical exam, decreased PD fluid effluent return, Ultrasound/CT scan	Stop PD and use temporary HD, low volume CAPD at bed rest, consider catheter replacement or injecting fibrin glue (1 ml of a solution of fibrinogen and thrombin)[a]
Hydrothorax/Pleural effusion (incidence <5%)	Dyspnea, no improvement with hypertonic exchange, decreased PD fluid effluent return, diagnostic chest x-ray with pleural effusion, thoracentesis with pleural fluid analysis showing high glucose, scan with isotope in abdomen	Stop PD and use temporary HD, thoracentesis, low volume PD (after 2 weeks of HD may return to PD), pleurodesis (autologous blood, talc, tetracycline), surgical repair

Conditions	Diagnosis	Treatment
Sclerosing encapsulating peritonitis	Recurrent abdominal pain with fills, repeated peritonitis predisposes to it, may cause bowel obstruction, or hemoperitoneum, decreased solute and water transport, characteristic appearance with CT	Careful attention to nutrition and bowel function, laparoscopy[b], surgical intervention, anti-inflammatory or immunosuppressive meds (controversial), tamoxifen[c]

[a]From Herbrig K, Pistrosch F, Gross P, Palm C: Resumption of peritoneal dialysis after transcutaneaous treatment of a peritoneal leakage using fibrin glue, *Nephrol Dial Transplant* 21(7):2037-2038.
[b]From Kropp J, Sinaskul M, Butsch J, Rodby R: Laparoscopy in the Early Diagnosis and Management of Sclerosing Encapsulating Peritonitis, *Semin. Dial* 22(3):304–307.
[c]From Allaria PM, Giangrande A, Gandini E, Pisoni IB: Continuous ambulatory peritoneal dialysis and sclerosing encapsulating peritonitis: Tamoxifen as a new therapeutic agent?, *J. Nephrol* 12(6): 395–397

REFERENCES

1. Kellum JA, Lameire N, KDIGO AKI Guideline Work Group. Diagnosis, evaluation, and management of acute kidney injury: a KDIGO summary (Part 1). *Crit Care*. 2013;17(1):1–15.
2. Bellomo R, Ronco C, Kellum JA, Mehta RL, Palevsky P. Acute renal failure—definition, outcome measures, animal models, fluid therapy and information technology needs: the Second International Consensus Conference of the Acute Dialysis Quality Initiative (ADQI) Group. *Crit Care*. 2004;8(4):R204–R212.
3. Mehta RL, Kellum JA, Shah SV, et al. Acute Kidney Injury Network: report of an initiative to improve outcomes in acute kidney injury. *Crit Care*. 2007;11(2):R31.
4. Pavkov ME, Harding JL, Burrows NR. Trends in hospitalizations for acute kidney injury—United States, 2000–2014. *MMWR Morb Mortal Wkly Rep*. 2018;67(10):289–293.
5. Cartin-Ceba R, Kashiouris M, Plataki M, Kor DJ, Gajic O, Casey ET. Risk factors for development of acute kidney injury in critically ill patients: a systematic review and meta-analysis of observational studies. *Crit Care Res Pract*. 2012;2012:691013.
6. Mas-Font S, Ros-Martinez J, Pérez-Calvo C, Villa-Díaz P, Aldunate-Calvo S, Moreno-Clari E. Prevention of acute kidney injury in intensive care units. *Med Intensiva*. 2017;41(2):116–126.
7. Bonventre JV, Yang L. Cellular pathophysiology of ischemic acute kidney injury. *J Clin Invest*. 2011;121(11):4210–4221.
8. Gupta A, Biyani M, Khaira A. Vancomycin nephrotoxicity: myths and facts. *Neth J Med*. 2011;69(9):379–383.
9. Weisbord SD, Palevsky PM. Contrast-induced acute kidney injury: short- and long-term implications. *Semin Nephrol*. 2011;31(3):300–309.
10. Mosca L, Grundy SM, Judelson D, et al. AHA/ACC scientific statement: consensus panel statement. guide to preventive cardiology for women. American Heart Association/American College of Cardiology. *J Am Coll Cardiol*. 1999;33(6):1751–1755.
11. Morcos SK. Prevention of contrast media nephrotoxicity—the story so far. *Clin Radiol*. 2004;59(5):381–389.
12. Freeman RV, O'Donnell M, Share D, et al. Nephropathy requiring dialysis after percutaneous coronary intervention and the critical role of an adjusted contrast dose. *Am J Cardiol*. 2002;90(10):1068–1073.
13. Kellum JA, Lameire N, Aspelin P, et al. Kidney disease: improving global outcomes (KDIGO) acute kidney injury work group. KDIGO clinical practice guideline for acute kidney injury. *Kidney Int Suppl*. 2012;2(1):1–138.
14. Jara LJ, Vera-Lastra O, Calleja MC. Pulmonary-renal vasculitic disorders: differential diagnosis and management. *Curr Rheumatol Rep*. 2003;5(2):107–115.
15. Kodner CM, Kudrimoti A. Diagnosis and management of acute interstitial nephritis. *Am Fam Physician*. 2003;67(12):2527–2534. + 2539.
16. Rossert J. Drug-induced acute interstitial nephritis. *Kidney Int*. 2001;60(2):804–817.
17. Wanchoo R, Abudayyeh A, Doshi M, et al. Renal toxicities of novel agents used for treatment of multiple myeloma. *Clin J Am Soc Nephrol*. 2017;12(1):176–189.
18. Jhaveri KD, Wanchoo R, Sakhiya V, Ross DW, Fishbane S. Adverse renal effects of novel molecular oncologic targeted therapies: a narrative review. *Kidney Int Rep*. 2017;2(1):108–123.
19. Izzedine H, Perazella MA. Anticancer drug-induced acute kidney injury. *Kidney Int Rep*. 2017;81(4):504–514.
20. Naughton CA. Drug-induced nephrotoxicity. *Am Fam Physician*. 2008;78(6):743–750.
21. Awdishu L, Mehta RL. The 6R's of drug induced nephrotoxicity. *BMC Nephrol*. 2017;18(1):124.
22. Perazella MA. Pharmacology behind common drug nephrotoxicities. *Clin J Am Soc Nephrol*. 2018;13(12):1897–1908.
23. Lameire N. Nephrotoxicity of recent anti-cancer agents. *Clin Kidney J*. 2014;7(1):11–22.
24. Yarlagadda SG, Perazella MA. Drug-induced crystal nephropathy: an update. *Expert Opin Drug Saf*. 2008;7(2):147–158.
25. Moss AH. Ethical principles and processes guiding dialysis decision-making. *Clin J Am Soc Nephrol*. 2011;6(9):2313–2317.

26. Karvellas CJ, Farhat MR, Sajjad I, et al. A comparison of early versus late initiation of renal replacement therapy in critically ill patients with acute kidney injury: a systematic review and meta-analysis. *Crit Care.* 2011;15(1):R72.

27. do Nascimento GVR, Gabriel DP, Abrão JMG, Balbi AL. When is dialysis indicated in acute kidney injury? *Ren Fail.* 2010;32(3):396–400.

28. Shiao CC, Wu VC, Li WY, et al. Late initiation of renal replacement therapy is associated with worse outcomes in acute kidney injury after major abdominal surgery. *Crit Care.* 2009;13(5):R171.

29. Lameire N, Vanbiesen W, Vanholder R. When to start dialysis in patients with acute kidney injury? when semantics and logic become entangled with expectations and beliefs. *Crit Care.* 2011;15(4):171.

30. Cooper BA, Branley P, Bulfone L, et al. A randomized, controlled trial of early versus late initiation of dialysis. *N Engl J Med.* 2010;363(7):609–619.

31. Wright S, Klausner D, Baird B, et al. Timing of dialysis initiation and survival in ESRD. *Clin J Am Soc Nephrol.* 2010;5(10):1828–1835.

32. Ward RA, Ronco C. Dialyzer and machine technologies: application of recent advances to clinical practice. *Blood Purif.* 2005;24(1):6–10.

33. Daeihagh P, Jordan J, Chen GJ, Rocco M. Efficacy of tissue plasminogen activator administration on patency of hemodialysis access catheters. *Am J Kidney Dis.* 2000;36(1):75–79.

34. Cronin RE, Reilly RF. Unfractionated heparin for hemodialysis: still the best option. *Semin Dial.* 2010;23(5):510–515.

35. DeSilva RN, Sandhu GS, Garg J, Goldfarb-Rumyantzev AS. Association between initial type of hemodialysis access used in the elderly and mortality. *Hemodial Int.* 2012;16(2):233–241.

36. Eknoyan G, Beck GJ, Cheung AK, et al. Effect of dialysis dose and membrane flux in maintenance hemodialysis. *N Engl J Med.* 2002;347(25):2010–2019.

37. Paniagua R, Amato D, Vonesh E, et al. Effects of increased peritoneal clearances on mortality rates in peritoneal dialysis: ADEMEX, a prospective, randomized, controlled trial. *J Am Soc Nephrol.* 2002;13(5):1307–1320.

38. Hemodialysis Adequacy Peritoneal Dialysis Adequacy Vascular Access A Curriculum for CKD Risk Reduction and Care Kidney Learning System (KLS)™ 2006 Updates Clinical Practice Guidelines and Recommendations. www.kidney.org.

39. Pistolesi V, Morabito S, Di Mario F, Regolisti G, Cantarelli C, Fiaccadori E. A guide to understanding antimicrobial drug dosing in critically ill patients on renal replacement therapy. *Antimicrob Agents Chemother.* 2019;63(8):e00583-1.

40. Launay-Vacher V, Izzedine H, Mercadal L, Deray G. Clinical review: use of vancomycin in haemodialysis patients. *Crit Care.* 2002;6(4):313–316.

41. Prowle JR, Schneider A, Bellomo R. Clinical review: optimal dose of continuous renal replacement therapy in acute kidney injury. *Crit Care.* 2011;15(2):207.

42. Swartz R, Pasko D, O'Toole J, Starmann B. Improving the delivery of continuous renal replacement therapy using regional citrate anticoagulation. *Clin Nephrol.* 2004;61(02):134–143.

43. El Shamy O, Patel N, Abdelbaset MH, et al. Acute start peritoneal dialysis during the COVID-19 pandemic: outcomes and experiences. *J Am Soc Nephrol.* 2020;31(8):1680–1682.

44. Adapa S, Aeddula NR, Konala VM, et al. COVID-19 and renal failure: challenges in the delivery of renal replacement therapy. *J Clin Med Res.* 2020;12(5):276–285.

45. Vinsonneau C, Allain-Launay E, Blayau C, et al. Renal replacement therapy in adult and pediatric intensive care: recommendations by an expert panel from the French Intensive Care Society (SRLF) with the French Society of Anesthesia Intensive Care (SFAR) French Group for Pediatric Intensive Care Emergencies (GFRUP) the French Dialysis Society (SFD). *Ann Intensive Care.* 2015;5(1):58.

46. Liakopoulos V, Stefanidis I, Dombros NV. Peritoneal dialysis glossary 2009. *Int Urol Nephrol.* 2009;42(2):417–423.

47. Twardowski ZJ. Peritoneal dialysis glossary III. *Perit Dial Int.* 1990;10(2):173–175.

48. Uribarri J, Prabhakar S, Kahn T. Hyponatremia in peritoneal dialysis patients. *Clin Nephrol.* 2004;61(01):54–58.

49. Zanger R. Hyponatremia and hypokalemia in patients on peritoneal dialysis. *Semin Dial.* 2010;23(6):575–580.

50. Otte K, Gonzalez MT, Bajo MA, et al. Clinical experience with a new bicarbonate (25 mmol/L)/lactate (10 mmol/L) peritoneal dialysis solution. *Perit Dial Int.* 2003;23(2):138–145.

51. Herbrig K, Pistrosch F, Gross P, Palm C. Resumption of peritoneal dialysis after transcutaneous treatment of a peritoneal leakage using fibrin glue. *Nephrol Dial Transplant.* 2006;21(7):2037–2038.

52. Kropp J, Sinsakul M, Butsch J, Rodby R. Laparoscopy in the early diagnosis and management of sclerosing encapsulating peritonitis. *Semin Dial.* 2009;22(3):304–307.

53. Allaria PM, Giangrande A, Gandini E, Pisoni IB. Continuous ambulatory peritoneal dialysis and sclerosing encapsulating peritonitis: tamoxifen as a new therapeutic agent? *J Nephrol.* 1999;12(6):395–397.

CHAPTER 4

Water and Electrolyte Disorders

Robert Stephen Brown and Alexander Goldfarb-Rumyantzev

Water Distribution Between Body Compartments[1–7]

The diagram below illustrates water distribution between different body compartments: intracellular and extracellular, the latter including interstitial and intravascular spaces.

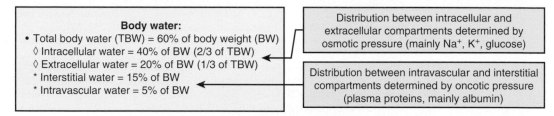

Body water:
- Total body water (TBW) = 60% of body weight (BW)
  ◊ Intracellular water = 40% of BW (2/3 of TBW)
  ◊ Extracellular water = 20% of BW (1/3 of TBW)
  * Interstitial water = 15% of BW
  * Intravascular water = 5% of BW

Distribution between intracellular and extracellular compartments determined by osmotic pressure (mainly Na^+, K^+, glucose)

Distribution between intravascular and interstitial compartments determined by oncotic pressure (plasma proteins, mainly albumin)

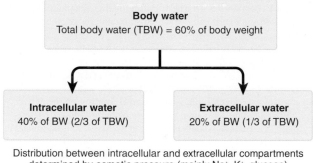

Body water
Total body water (TBW) = 60% of body weight

Intracellular water
40% of BW (2/3 of TBW)

Extracellular water
20% of BW (1/3 of TBW)

Distribution between intracellular and extracellular compartments
determined by osmotic pressure (mainly Na^+, K^+, glucose)

Interstitial water
15% of BW

Intravascular water
5% of BW

Distribution between both compartments determined by
oncotic pressure (plasma proteins, mainly albumin)

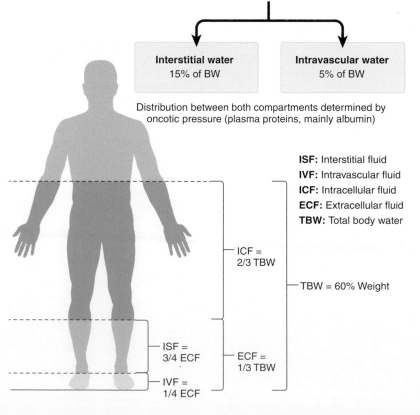

ISF: Interstitial fluid
IVF: Intravascular fluid
ICF: Intracellular fluid
ECF: Extracellular fluid
TBW: Total body water

ICF =
2/3 TBW

TBW = 60% Weight

ISF =
3/4 ECF

ECF =
1/3 TBW

IVF =
1/4 ECF

Sites of Important renal Tubular Electrolyte Reabsorption and Secretion

The simplified diagram below illustrates important sites of electrolyte reabsorption of sodium, chloride, bicarbonate, and secretion of potassium and hydrogen ions.[1-6,8] We discuss renal tubular reabsorption of calcium and magnesium below and targets of diuretic therapy in more detail at the end of this chapter.

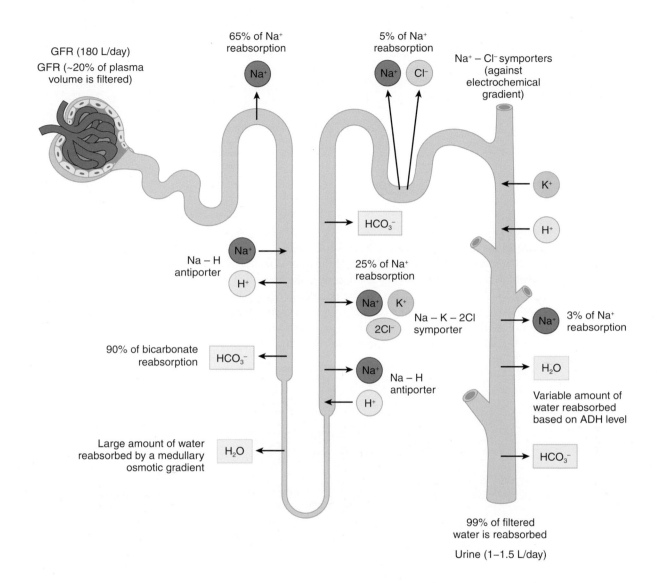

Sodium and Water Handling by the Kidney

Renal Water Reabsorption

Since some electrolyte disbalances are caused by water homeostasis problems (e.g., hyponatremia in the syndrome of inappropriate antidiuretic hormone secretion [SIADH]), it is helpful to have a general understanding of the physiology of water handling by the kidney. A simplified schema of the tubular water reabsorption mechanisms to reduce the urine volume to approximately 1% of the filtered fluid volume is depicted in the figure above.

- One mechanism is the passive water reabsorption in the proximal tubule, Loop of Henle, and distal tubule based on the iso-osmolar cortical and hyperosmolar medullary environments.
- The second is the ADH-dependent water reabsorption mainly in the collecting duct to determine the final urine concentration.

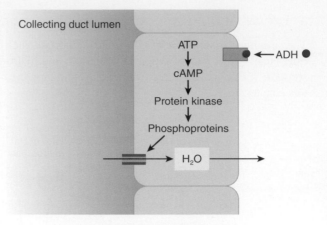

Urine osmolarity 50–1200 mOsm/L

ADH ↓ ⟹ ↓ water reabsorption and low
urine osmolarity

ADH increases water reabsorption
and urine osmolarity

Sodium

Sodium Reabsorption by the Kidney

Under common conditions, over 99% of the filtered sodium is reabsorbed, primarily with bicarbonate and chloride as "accompanying" anions, or in the collecting ducts in exchange for secretion of hydrogen and potassium cations. The reabsorption of sodium and water to maintain homeostasis of body volumes is largely under the control of the following factors: (1) glomerular filtration rate (GFR), (2) glomerulo-tubular balance to increase or decrease sodium reabsorption in parallel with the GFR, and (3) a number of regulatory hormones, the major ones of which are shown below.

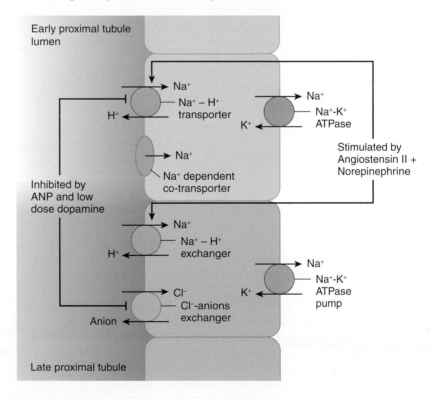

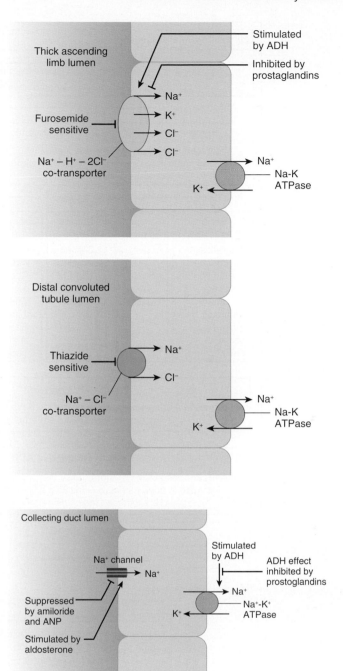

Hypernatremia[9]

Causes of hypernatremia are divided into three categories based on the patient's volume status. Hypernatremia in hospitalized patients is not very frequent (0.1% to 0.2% of hospitalized patients).[10] It is always associated with hypertonicity (hyperosmolality).

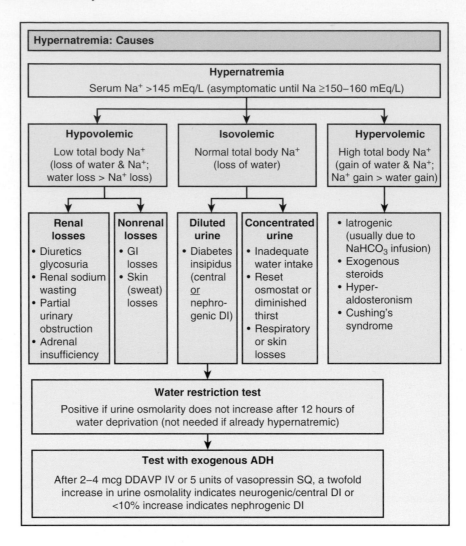

Hypernatremia: Causes

Hypernatremia
Serum Na⁺ >145 mEq/L (asymptomatic until Na ≥150–160 mEq/L)

Hypovolemic	**Isovolemic**	**Hypervolemic**
Low total body Na⁺ (loss of water & Na⁺; water loss > Na⁺ loss)	Normal total body Na⁺ (loss of water)	High total body Na⁺ (gain of water & Na⁺; Na⁺ gain > water gain)

Renal losses
- Diuretics glycosuria
- Renal sodium wasting
- Partial urinary obstruction
- Adrenal insufficiency

Nonrenal losses
- GI losses
- Skin (sweat) losses

Diluted urine
- Diabetes insipidus (central or nephrogenic DI)

Concentrated urine
- Inadequate water intake
- Reset osmostat or diminished thirst
- Respiratory or skin losses

- Iatrogenic (usually due to NaHCO₃ infusion)
- Exogenous steroids
- Hyper-aldosteronism
- Cushing's syndrome

Water restriction test
Positive if urine osmolarity does not increase after 12 hours of water deprivation (not needed if already hypernatremic)

Test with exogenous ADH
After 2–4 mcg DDAVP IV or 5 units of vasopressin SQ, a twofold increase in urine osmolality indicates neurogenic/central DI or <10% increase indicates nephrogenic DI

Hypernatremia Clinical Manifestations

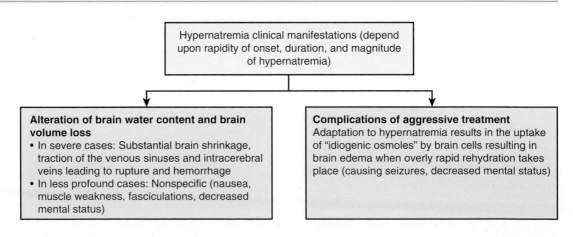

Hypernatremia clinical manifestations (depend upon rapidity of onset, duration, and magnitude of hypernatremia)

Alteration of brain water content and brain volume loss
- In severe cases: Substantial brain shrinkage, traction of the venous sinuses and intracerebral veins leading to rupture and hemorrhage
- In less profound cases: Nonspecific (nausea, muscle weakness, fasciculations, decreased mental status)

Complications of aggressive treatment
Adaptation to hypernatremia results in the uptake of "idiogenic osmoles" by brain cells resulting in brain edema when overly rapid rehydration takes place (causing seizures, decreased mental status)

Treatment of Hypernatremia

For practical purposes one can imagine that the body maintains the homeostasis of the basic components in the following order of priority:
1) Circulatory volume
2) Osmotic equilibrium
3) Electrolyte concentration

Similarly, in the treatment of electrolyte disorders, the therapeutic measures should be directed at the same aspects in the same order (e.g., attempts to correct the circulatory volume should take priority and precede correction of sodium concentration and osmolality).

Helpful Points in Treating Hypernatremia

- In patients with hypovolemia—start with volume expansion with isotonic saline or Ringer's lactate, then correct water deficit
- In patients with hypervolemia—water + loop diuretic to avoid pulmonary or cerebral edema
- Replace calculated water deficit plus ongoing losses (urinary, GI) plus insensible losses (no more than half of calculated water deficit in the first 24 hours to prevent cerebral edema)
- Reduce Na+ concentration by ≤1 mmol/L/h if symptomatic but <12 mmol/L/day
- When symptoms are resolved, replace the remaining water deficit in 24–48 hours
- Worsening neurologic status after initial improvement suggests brain edema—discontinue water replacement
- Central DI—treat with desmopressin (DDAVP)
- Nephrogenic DI—treat with thiazides that inhibit urinary diluting capacity and cause mild intravascular volume depletion which decreases water delivery to the collecting duct that will decrease polyuria for symptomatic benefit
- Amiloride for lithium-induced DI: like thiazides, amiloride decreases polyuria, but spares K+ wasting and may diminish lithium toxicity (by blocking lithium entry into collecting duct cells in exchange for Na+)

DI, Diabetes insipidus; *GI*, gastrointestinal.

Water deficit formula to correct hypernatremia (assuming distribution volume of Na^+ to be 0.6 of the body mass):

$$\text{Water deficit (L)} = \frac{\text{Serum Na (mEq/L)} - 140}{140} \cdot 0.6 \cdot \text{body mass (kg)}$$

Hyponatremia[9]

Hyponatremia is relatively common (1%–2% of hospitalized patients).[10] Unlike hypernatremia (which is always associated with hypertonicity), hyponatremia can be associated with hypotonicity, isotonicity, or hypertonicity.

To identify the cause of hyponatremia, one has to collect the following information:
- Plasma osmolality
- Patient volume status
- Urine sodium concentration
- Urine osmolality (latter reflects ADH secretion)[11]

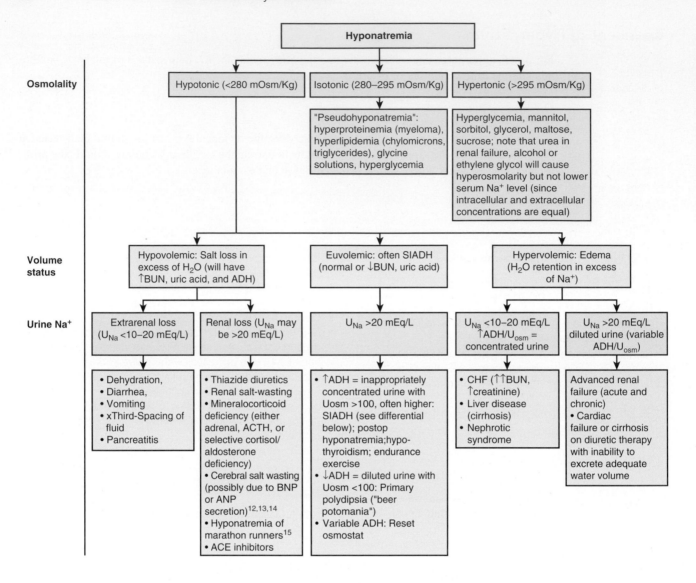

Other Helpful Points

- Low ADH level results in diluted urine, so that U_{Osm} <100 (e.g., in primary polydipsia or "beer potomania").
- SIADH is the most common cause of euvolemic hyponatremia.
- SIADH is hard to distinguish from cerebral salt wasting as volume status might be difficult to estimate, but cerebral salt wasting is usually due to intracranial hemorrhage. It does not have strict diagnostic criteria, though hypotension is common, or laboratory tests associated with it, though management is often similar to SIADH.[13,14]
- Diagnostic criteria for SIADH:
    - hypoosmolarity (serum osmolarity < 280 mOsm/kg)
    - hyponatremia (Na ≤ 134 mEq/L)
    - clinical euvolemia, urinary Na > 40 mEq/L
    - inappropriately concentrated urine (U_{Osm} > 100 mOsm/kg)
    - normal adrenal, thyroid, cardiac, renal, and hepatic function, frequently with hypouricemia[10,11]

Causes of SIADH

SIADH is the most frequent cause of hyponatremia in a hospitalized patient.[11] It is important to identify the underlying cause of SIADH, as it may be due to serious or even urgent medical conditions or may recur.

1. Malignant neoplasia
   - Carcinoma (bronchogenic, duodenal, pancreatic, ureteral, prostatic, bladder)
   - Lymphoma and leukemia
   - Thymoma, mesothelioma, and Ewing's sarcoma
2. CNS disorders
   - Trauma, subarachnoid hemorrhage, subdural hematoma
   - Infection (encephalitis, meningitis, brain abscess)
   - Tumors
   - Porphyria
   - Stroke
   - Vasculitis
3. Pulmonary disorders
   - Tuberculosis
   - Pneumonia
   - Vasculitis
   - Mechanical ventilators with positive pressure
   - Lung abscess
4. Drugs
   - Desmopressin
   - Vasopressin
   - Chlorpropamide
   - Thiazide diuretics
   - Oxytocin
   - Haloperidol
   - Phenothiazines
   - Tricyclic and other antidepressants
   - High-dose cyclophosphamide
   - Vincristine
   - Vinblastine
   - Nicotine
5. Others
   - "Idiopathic" SIADH
   - Hypothyroidism
   - HIV
   - Guillain-Barre syndrome
   - Multiple sclerosis
   - Nephrogenic SIADH[16]

Clinical Manifestations of Hyponatremia

Symptoms of hyponatremia depend on degree and rapidity of onset, underlying central nervous system (CNS) status, and other metabolic factors, such as hypoxia, acidosis, hypercalcemia, or hypercapnia. The underlying mechanism causing symptoms is hypoosmolar encephalopathy (brain edema from water shift).

- Mild symptoms: headache, nausea
- More severe symptoms (usually with Na <125): confusion, obtundation, focal neurological deficits, seizures

Treatment of Hyponatremia

As in the case of hypernatremia, the therapeutic measures aimed to correct hyponatremia should be directed at correcting the circulatory volume first and only then at correcting the sodium concentration. If the hyponatremia developed rapidly (<24 hours), it should be corrected rapidly; if it developed slowly, it should be corrected slowly to decrease the risk of a CNS demyelinating syndrome.

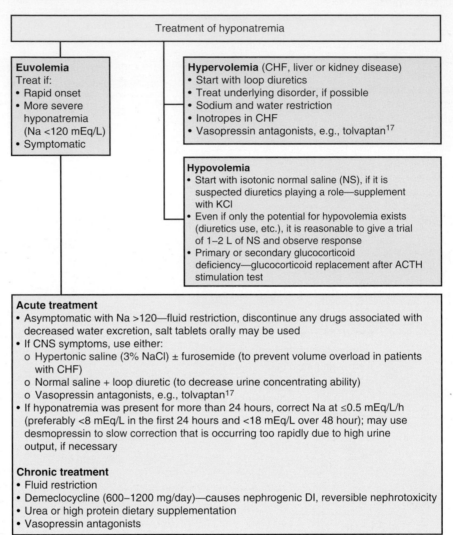

Additional Considerations for Using 3% NaCl

- Stop 3% NaCl infusion if symptoms are abolished, or serum Na has risen to ≥125 mEq/L
- Correct serum Na at 0.5 mEq/L/h (max 1 mOsm/kg/h), raising Na not more than 8 mEq/L over the first 24 hours unless hyponatremia developed acutely in <24 hr
- Overly rapid or overcorrection can occur with vasopressin antagonists, such as tolvaptan, as well[18,19]
- Rapid osmolality correction can cause the demyelination syndrome and pontine and extrapontine myelinolysis, with substantial neurological morbidity and mortality

Calculations to Establish the Rate of 3% NaCl Infusion

Calculations are based on the following assumptions: Although NaCl is distributed mainly in the extracellular space, the distribution volume of NaCl is total body water, or therefore, roughly $0.6 \times$ body mass (in kg). The calculations below are crude approximations since they do not account for the rate of Na and water excretion or potassium losses.

Amount of Na (mEq) to give per hour = Body mass $\cdot$ 0.6 $\cdot$ rate of correction (e.g., 0.5 mEq/L/h)

For example, considering that 1 L of 3% NaCl has 512 mEq/L of Na, the rate of infusion (mL/h) is:

$$\text{Rate of infusion} = \frac{\text{Body mass} \times 0.6 \times \text{rate of correction} \times 1000 \text{ mL}}{512}$$
$$= \text{Body mass} \times \text{rate of correction} \times 1.17$$

Therefore if the rate of serum Na correction is to be 0.5 mEq/L/h for a 70-kg individual:
Rate of 3% NaCl infusion = 70 × 0.5 × 1.17 (or body mass in kg × 0.585) = 41 mL/h

Calculation of Total Na Deficit to Fully Correct Hyponatremia

Calculated Na Deficit (mEq) = 0.6 (body mass in kg) × (140 − serum Na in mEq/L)

This would correct the hyponatremia to a serum Na of 140 mEq/L.

If volume depletion is also present, replace estimated volume deficit in liters with normal saline in addition.

Risk vs. Benefit in Treatment of Hyponatremia

	Risk of Uncorrected Hyponatremia	Risk of Demyelination
Rapid onset, symptoms, Na <120	Higher	Lower
Slow onset, asymptomatic	Lower	Higher

Potassium

Overview of Potassium Physiology[20]
Regulation of potassium distribution
Total body stores of potassium amount to about 3000 mEq, most of which is intracellular, as in muscle cells, and in bone, while only about 60 mEq or 2% of potassium is in the extracellular fluid. Since maintenance of the potassium electrical gradient across heart muscle cell membranes is so important, precise regulation of potassium distribution between the intracellular and extracellular fluid compartments is essential.

The major factors increasing cellular uptake of potassium are:
- Insulin
- Beta-sympathetic catecholamines (epinephrine) which stimulate Na-K ATPase
- Alkalosis with low intracellular H^+ ion and increased intracellular K^+ that will lower serum K^+
- Increased K^+ in the diet or high serum K^+ causes adaptation that increases intracellular uptake of K^+ by muscle cells

The opposite process wherein low insulin, low beta—or high alpha-sympathetic catecholamines, acidosis, or low K^+ diet will decrease cellular K^+ uptake to raise serum K^+ as shown below.

Total body potassium regulation
The ultimate regulation of total body potassium depends upon renal excretion of the approximately 60 to 100 mEq/day of potassium ingested in the diet to maintain proper potassium balance.
- Tubular reabsorption: About 90% of the roughly 700 mEq/day of potassium filtered by the glomeruli is reabsorbed in the proximal and distal nephron to conserve potassium
- Urinary excretion: Potassium is secreted into the collecting duct to excrete potassium to maintain balance
- The major factors affecting potassium excretion are aldosterone, distal tubular Na^+ delivery, urine flow rate, and acid-base status as shown below
- Increased K^+ in the diet or high serum K^+ causes increased renal K^+ excretion to protect against worsening hyperkalemia (with the opposite conservation of K^+ in cases of low K^+ diets and low serum K^+ levels to protect against hypokalemia)

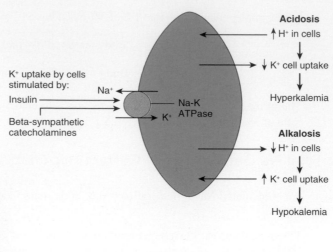

Acidosis

↑ H⁺ in cells

↓ K⁺ cell uptake

Hyperkalemia

K⁺ uptake by cells
stimulated by:

Insulin

Beta-sympathetic
catecholamines

Na⁺

Na-K
ATPase

K⁺

Alkalosis

↓ H⁺ in cells

↑ K⁺ cell uptake

Hypokalemia

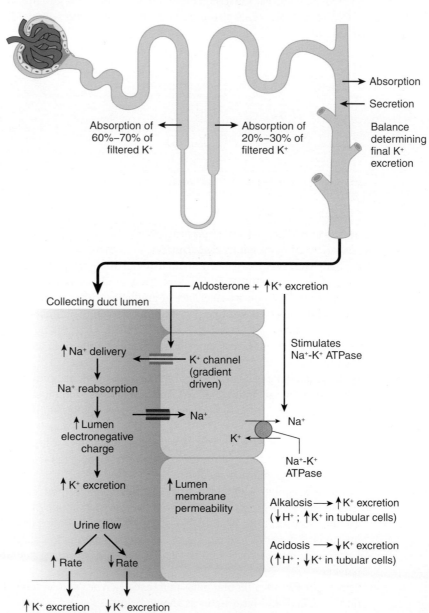

Absorption

Secretion

Balance
determining
final K⁺
excretion

Absorption of
60%–70% of
filtered K⁺

Absorption of
20%–30% of
filtered K⁺

Aldosterone + ↑K⁺ excretion

Collecting duct lumen

↑ Na⁺ delivery

K⁺ channel
(gradient
driven)

Stimulates
Na⁺-K⁺ ATPase

Na⁺ reabsorption

Na⁺

↑ Lumen
electronegative
charge

Na⁺

K⁺

↑ K⁺ excretion

↑ Lumen
membrane
permeability

Na⁺-K⁺
ATPase

Urine flow

Alkalosis ⟶ ↑K⁺ excretion
(↓H⁺ ; ↑K⁺ in tubular cells)

↑ Rate   ↓ Rate

Acidosis ⟶ ↓K⁺ excretion
(↑H⁺ ; ↓K⁺ in tubular cells)

↑ K⁺ excretion   ↓ K⁺ excretion

Hypokalemia

Similar to other electrolytes, hypokalemia can be explained either by lower intake, higher excretion, or intracellular redistribution of potassium. To identify the cause of hypokalemia, the following tests are very helpful: urine potassium, and for concentrated urines (U_{Osm} >300 mOsm/kg), the transtubular potassium gradient (TTKG described below), urine chloride, and plasma bicarbonate.[21]

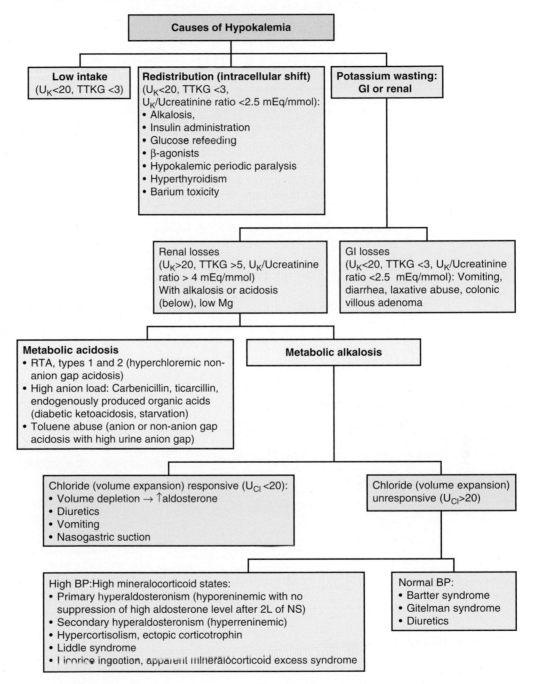

Causes of Hypokalemia

Low intake
(U_K<20, TTKG <3)

Redistribution (intracellular shift)
(U_K<20, TTKG <3,
U_K/Ucreatinine ratio <2.5 mEq/mmol):
• Alkalosis,
• Insulin administration
• Glucose refeeding
• β-agonists
• Hypokalemic periodic paralysis
• Hyperthyroidism
• Barium toxicity

Potassium wasting:
GI or renal

Renal losses
(U_K>20, TTKG >5, U_K/Ucreatinine ratio > 4 mEq/mmol)
With alkalosis or acidosis (below), low Mg

GI losses
(U_K<20, TTKG <3, U_K/Ucreatinine ratio <2.5 mEq/mmol): Vomiting, diarrhea, laxative abuse, colonic villous adenoma

Metabolic acidosis
• RTA, types 1 and 2 (hyperchloremic non-anion gap acidosis)
• High anion load: Carbenicillin, ticarcillin, endogenously produced organic acids (diabetic ketoacidosis, starvation)
• Toluene abuse (anion or non-anion gap acidosis with high urine anion gap)

Metabolic alkalosis

Chloride (volume expansion) responsive (U_{Cl} <20):
• Volume depletion → ↑aldosterone
• Diuretics
• Vomiting
• Nasogastric suction

Chloride (volume expansion) unresponsive (U_{Cl}>20)

High BP:High mineralocorticoid states:
• Primary hyperaldosteronism (hyporeninemic with no suppression of high aldosterone level after 2L of NS)
• Secondary hyperaldosteronism (hyperreninemic)
• Hypercortisolism, ectopic corticotrophin
• Liddle syndrome
• Licorice ingestion, apparent mineralocorticoid excess syndrome

Normal BP:
• Bartter syndrome
• Gitelman syndrome
• Diuretics

Transtubular K Gradient[21–23]

The concept of TTKG helps to identify renal wasting of potassium (high TTKG), as opposed to gastrointestinal (GI) losses or intracellular shift (low TTKG). TTKG compensates for a high urinary concentration above 300 mOsm/kg which raises the U_K concentration by removing tubular fluid from the final urine, but without excreting more potassium.

Note that this formula is valid only when U_{Osm} >300 mOsm/kg and U_{Na} >25 mEq/L and should not be used to "correct" for dilute urines.

$$TTKG = \frac{Urine_K}{Plasma_k} \div \frac{Urine_{osm}}{Plasma_{osm}}$$

$$= \frac{U_K \times P_{Osm}}{P_K \times U_{Osm}}$$

TTKG <3—GI loss, intracellular redistribution with renal K conservation when hypokalemic

TTKG >5—renal K wasting when hypokalemic

TTKG ≥6–8—denotes appropriate renal and aldosterone effect when hyperkalemic

TTKG <6—denotes inadequate renal tubular K excretion when hyperkalemic

An alternative is to use the urine potassium-to-urine creatinine ratio[24]:

$U_K/U_{creatinine}$ **<2.5 mEq/mmol**—GI loss, intracellular redistribution with renal K conservation when hypokalemic

$U_K/U_{creatinine}$ **>4 mEq/mmol**—renal K wasting when hypokalemic

$U_K/U_{creatinine}$ **>15–20 mEq/mmol**—denotes appropriate renal and aldosterone effect when hyperkalemic

$U_K/U_{creatinine}$ **<15 mEq/mmol**—denotes inadequate renal tubular K excretion when hyperkalemic

---

Clinical Manifestations of Hypokalemia

- ECG changes (prominent U-wave, T-wave flattening, ST depression, arrhythmias)
- Skeletal muscle weakness to the point of paralysis
- Respiratory arrest with severe hypokalemia
- Decreased motility of the smooth muscle: ileus, urinary retention
- Rhabdomyolysis
- Nephrogenic DI (hypokalemia interferes with concentrating mechanism in the distal nephron)

Treatment of Hypokalemia

- Oral or IV K (oral is safer)
- IV (for K < 3.0 mEq/L) not more than 10 mmol/h, recheck K every 2–3 hours
- Magnitude of K replacement cannot be calculated from serum K but is often over 200 mEq when serum K <3.0 mEq/L

Hyperkalemia

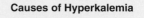

```
                    ┌─────────────────────────┐
                    │ Causes of Hyperkalemia  │
                    └─────────────────────────┘
```

Increased intake (TTKG >6–8, U_K/Ucreatinine ratio >15–20 mEq/mmol)	Redistribution from cells (TTKG >6–8, U_K/Ucreatinine ratio >15–20 mEq/mmol)	Inadequate excretion
• Use of salt substitutes or K^+ supplements (usually is in the setting of CKD)	• Shift of K^+ out of cells due to acidosis, depolarizing paralytic agents (e.g., succinylcholine), or decreased functioning of Na-K-ATPase related to hypoxia, insulin deficiency, beta blockade, or severe digitalis toxicity • Cell destruction—crush injuries, tumor lysis syndrome, rhabdomyolysis, burns or hemolysis • Receiving old or improperly administered blood or massive blood transfusion[25]	• Renal failure, oliguria • Inadequate renal tubular secretion (TTKG <6, U_K/Ucreatinine ratio <15 mEq/mmol): • Hypoaldosteronism • Renal tubular defects: Type 4 RTA, interstitial renal diseases • Medications: aliskiren, ACEI, ARB[26], aldosterone receptor antagonists[27], amiloride, trimethoprim, calcineurin inhibitors • Pseudohypoaldosteronism

Clinical Manifestations of Hyperkalemia

- Skeletal muscle weakness to the point of paralysis and respiratory failure
- ECG changes
  - Peaking of T wave
  - First-degree AV block
  - Widening of QRS
  - ST depression
  - Shallow P waves → atrial standstill
  - Biphasic waves → ventricular standstill

AV, Atrioventricular.

Acute Rx of Hyperkalemia

1. Stabilize the myocardium if there is widening of the QRS by ECG (IV calcium chloride 1 g over 1 minute or calcium gluconate 3 g over 2–3 minutes, repeat once in 5 minutes if no ECG improvement)
2. Shift K to the intracellular space
   - Insulin at doses of 10 units IV (K decreases in 15–30 minutes) with glucose (to avoid hypoglycemia)
   - Beta-agonists (K decreases in 30 minutes): are as effective as insulin for lowering serum potassium and have a longer duration of action but may promote arrhythmia[28]
   - Sodium bicarbonate 50–150 mEq IV (K decreases in 1–4 hours): supported only by studies with weak or equivocal results but useful when acidotic[28]
3. Remove potassium from the body
   - Diuresis
   - Sodium polystyrene sulfonate (Kayexalate) 15 g orally (preferably without sorbitol to protect against GI toxicity with possible GI perforation) and repeat in 1–2 hours up to 60 g/day; or 30–50 g rectally and repeat in 6 hours[29]
   - Patiromer (Veltassa) 8.4–25.2 g/day orally in water in nonacute hyperkalemia due to delayed onset of action[30]
   - Sodium zirconium cyclosilicate (Lokelma) 10 g suspension 3 times per day for up to 48 hours orally in nonacute hyperkalemia due to delayed onset of action[31]
   - Dialysis

Calcium

Regulation of Calcium and Phosphate[32–35]

Calcium and phosphate regulation is described together since they are tightly interconnected and are regulated by the same factors (i.e., parathyroid hormone [PTH], vitamin D, fibroblast growth factor 23 [FGF23]). The following figures show the main effects of these three factors which play the dominant role in controlling homeostasis of calcium and phosphate:

- PTH increases serum calcium by releasing calcium from bone, increasing kidney tubular reabsorption of filtered calcium, and activating vitamin D to 1,25-dihydroxycholecalciferol and decreases serum phosphate by inhibiting kidney tubular reabsorption of phosphate.
- Vitamin D, once activated, increases calcium mainly by augmenting GI small intestinal uptake of calcium and also increasing kidney reabsorption of calcium.
- FGF23 regulates serum phosphate levels by decreasing kidney tubular reabsorption of phosphate and decreases the kidney activation of vitamin D to decrease GI calcium and phosphate absorption.[36]

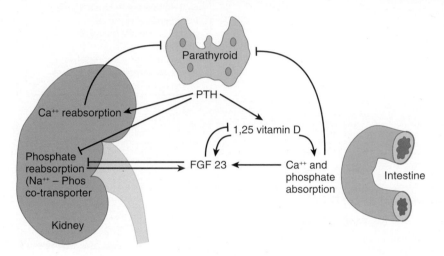

Renal Handling of Calcium

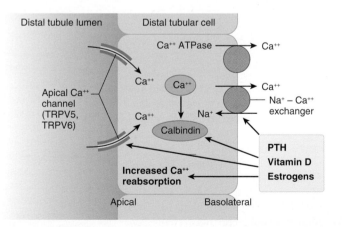

Since calcium is partially bound to albumin, about 6 mg/dL of calcium is filtered, amounting to about 10,800 mg/day in the 180 L/day of glomerular filtrate. With the net intestinal absorption of about 200 mg of calcium per day, and therefore renal excretion amounting to about 200 mg/day to maintain balance in a non-growing adult, 98% of the filtered calcium is reabsorbed by the tubules.

- In the proximal tubule and the Loop of Henle, about 80% of the calcium is reabsorbed, largely paralleling sodium reabsorption.
- In the distal tubule where about 15% of the calcium is reabsorbed, hormonal regulation controls calcium reabsorption to achieve body balance by the mechanisms described above.

Hypercalcemia

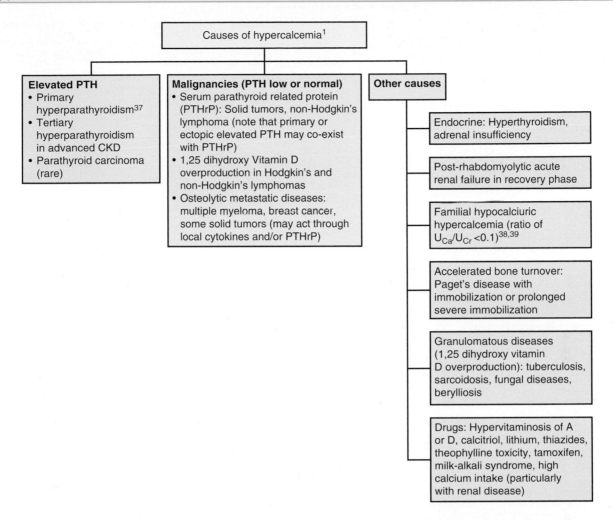

Calcium, Phosphate and PTH in Hyperparathyroidism, Malignancy, and Vitamin D Excess			
	Ca⁺⁺	Phosphate	PTH
Primary hyperparathyroidism: adenoma (85%), hyperplasia (15%), or carcinoma (<1%) of the parathyroid glands	↑	↓	↑
Malignancy	↑	↓	↓
1,25-Dihydroxyvitamin D overproduction (e.g., sarcoidosis)	↑	↑	↓

Hyperparathyroidism Mechanisms	
Type of Hyperparathyroidism	Mechanism
Primary	Primary elevated PTH production
Secondary	Elevated PTH secondary to other factors (low Ca⁺⁺ levels, vitamin D deficiency, renal failure) causing ↑PTH
Tertiary	After long-standing secondary hyperparathyroidism, presents with elevated Ca⁺⁺ (due to prolonged overstimulation of parathyroid glands—with hypertrophy/hyperplasia and sometimes develop adenoma)
Pseudohypoparathyroidism	Elevated PTH with resistance in end-organs' response which presents with low serum calcium and high phosphate causing ↑PTH

Linglart A, Levine MA, Jüppner H. Pseudohypoparathyroidism. *Endocrinol Metab Clin North Am.* 2018;47(4):865–888. http://dx.doi.org/10.1016/j.ecl.2018.07.011.

Clinical Manifestations of Hypercalcemia

- Cardiovascular:
  - dysrhythmia/arrhythmia
  - ECG changes (short corrected QT interval, broad T waves, first-degree AV block)
  - digoxin sensitivity
  - hypertension
- Gastrointestinal:
  - anorexia
  - nausea/vomiting
  - constipation
  - abdominal pain
  - pancreatitis
- Genitourinary:
  - polyuria
  - polydipsia
  - nephrolithiasis
- Neurologic:
  - insomnia
  - delirium
  - dementia
  - psychosis
  - lethargy
  - somnolence
  - coma
- Musculoskeletal:
  - muscle weakness
  - hyporeflexia
  - bone pain
  - fractures

Treatment of Hypercalcemia

Treat aggressively if Ca >14 or altered mental status/ECG changes:

- Saline 2.5–4 L/day + furosemide 10–40 mg IV every 6 hrs
- Calcitonin
- Bisphosphonates (pamidronate, zoledronic acid, etidronate)
- Calcimimetics in those with high PTH (cinacalcet)[40]
- Gallium nitrate (Ganite) for cancer-associated hypercalcemia[41]
- Glucocorticoids (especially in hematologic malignancies, sarcoid, vitamin D toxicity)[42]
- Estrogens, raloxifene
- Chloroquine/hydroxychloroquine for sarcoid
- Ethylenediaminetetraacetic acid (EDTA) chelates calcium for rare emergency use
- Dialysis

Criteria for parathyroidectomy in patients with hyperparathyroidism

In patients with asymptomatic primary hyperparathyroidism[42]

- Serum calcium >1–2 mg/dL (0.25 mmol/L) above the upper limit of the local reference range
- Creatinine clearance less than 60 mL/min attributed to calcemic nephropathy
- Age <50 years
- BMD T-score ≤2.5 determined by DXA scan at any site (forearm, lumbar spine, hip)

In secondary/tertiary hyperparathyroidism in ESRD[43]

- Marked hypercalcemia resistant to medical or dialysis treatment
- High total alkaline phosphatase accompanied by specific radiologic and/or histomorphologic changes of renal osteopathy
- Hyperphosphatemia with extraskeletal soft tissue calcifications resistant to treatment
- Calciphylaxis
- Symptomatic disease: severe pruritus, myopathy
- Marked hyperparathyroidism (PTH level >10 times upper normal limit) resistant to calcimimetic treatment, i.e., cinacalcet, etelcalcetide[44]

Hypocalcemia[45–47]

Causes of Hypocalcemia

- Renal failure, particularly with hyperphosphatemia
- Magnesium deficiency with severe hypomagnesemia
- Pancreatitis, rhabdomyolysis
- Vitamin D deficiency or Vitamin D receptor defects, malabsorption syndrome, osteomalacia
- Drugs (bisphosphonates, calcimimetics, denosumab, calcitonin, imatinib, citrate overload with anticoagulation for renal replacement therapy, or multiple blood transfusions)
- Calcium-sensing receptor (CaSR) activating mutations
- Hypoparathyroidism: neck radiation, thyroidectomy, parathyroidectomy, genetic diseases, autoimmune polyendocrine syndrome type 1 (APS1), idiopathic, or infiltrative
- Pseudohypocalcemia (hypoalbuminemia with normal ionic Ca^{++}, gadolinium-contrast agents interfering with lab measurement)
- Osteoblastic metastases

Signs and Symptoms of Hypocalcemia

- Muscle spasms, cramps, tremors (tetany)
- Hyperactive reflexes
- Diarrhea
- Tingling paresthesias of the fingers, toes, lips, face
- Tetany
- Positive Trousseau's sign—carpopedal spasm (hand spasm when BP cuff inflated above arterial pressure for 3–4 minutes)
- Positive Chvostek's sign (the twitching of the circumoral muscles with tapping lightly over the facial nerve)
- Seizures
- ECG changes/arrhythmia

Treatment of Hypocalcemia

- Monitor lab for other disturbances such as hypokalemia, hyperphosphatemia, hypomagnesemia, alkalosis
- Cardiac ECG monitor
- Seizure precautions and quiet room to decrease external stimuli
- Administer oral calcium supplements and/or vitamin D plus calcium supplements for mild to moderate hypocalcemia
- Give oral calcium between meals to increase intestinal absorption
- Administer IV calcium gluconate for severe hypocalcemia via slow IV bolus followed by slow IV drip or IV calcium chloride with severe cardiac indications
- Watch for infiltration with IV administration, calcium chloride extravasation can cause necrosis and tissue sloughing (Never give calcium intramuscularly or subcutaneously; check Chvostek's sign every hour when giving IV calcium)
- Teach patient about foods and fluids high in calcium

Phosphate

Regulation of phosphate is tightly connected with regulation of calcium level and is depicted in the diagram below. We added to the diagram the effect of chronic kidney disease (CKD) and anemia, as these factors are a frequent cause of abnormal phosphate levels.

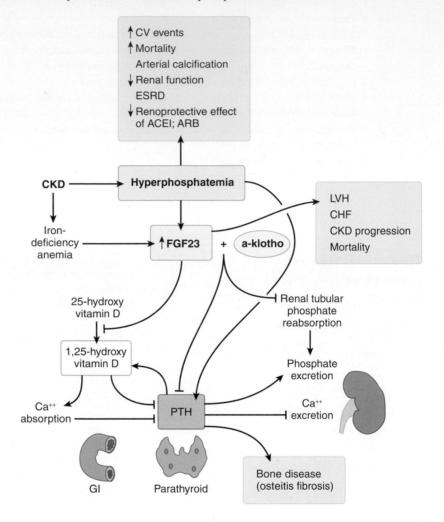

Kidney Handling of Phosphate

Phosphate is filtered at the glomerulus and is reabsorbed mainly in the proximal tubule with a urinary fractional excretion of about 15% to 20% commonly, but which is quite variable depending upon dietary phosphate intake. Tubular reabsorption of phosphate is under the regulation of the hormones PTH and FGF23, both of which exert a phosphaturic action by blocking phosphate reabsorption as shown below.

In the kidney, about 70% of phosphate is reabsorbed in the proximal tubule with sodium and about 10% to 20% in the distal tubule under the influence of PTH and FGF23 which inhibit reabsorption to increase phosphate excretion (presented in the figure below).

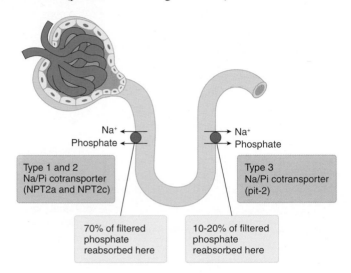

The figure below represents the role of proximal tubular cell in phosphate excretion and reabsorption.

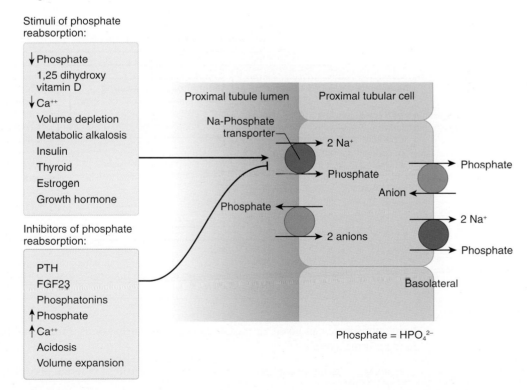

Hyperphosphatemia[48,49]

Causes

- Excessive phosphate load
  - o Tumor lysis syndrome, rhabdomyolysis, severe hemolysis
  - o Exogenous phosphate (ingestion of large amounts of phosphate-containing laxatives)
  - o Vitamin D intoxication
- Decreased renal excretion
  - o Late stages of CKD
  - o Hypoparathyroidism and pseudohypoparathyroidism
- Transcellular shifting
  - o Lactic acidosis
  - o Diabetic ketoacidosis
- Acromegaly
- Familial tumoral calcinosis

Treatment—Generally Reserved for Serum Phosphate >5.5 mg/dL

- Acute hyperphosphatemia with preserved renal function: extracellular volume expansion by saline infusion and diuretics
- Chronic hyperphosphatemia
  - o Dietary phosphate restriction
  - o Phosphate binders
    - ▪ Calcium-based binders
    - ▪ Aluminum hydroxide or carbonate for short-term use is effective
    - ▪ Sevelamer
    - ▪ Lanthanum carbonate
    - ▪ Ferric citrate
    - ▪ Sucroferric oxyhydroxide
    - ▪ Magnesium carbonate
  - o Drugs targeting intestinal phosphate transporters to decrease absorption
    - ▪ Nicotinic acid and nicotinamide[50]
    - ▪ Tenapanor[51]
  - o Renal replacement therapies
  - o Management of secondary hyperparathyroidism in end-stage kidney disease

Hypophosphatemia

Urine phosphate can be either measured in 24-hour urine or as a fractional phosphate excretion in a random urine sample:

$$FEPO4 = (\text{urine phosphate} \times \text{serum creatinine} \times 100\%) / (\text{serum phosphate} \times \text{urine creatinine})$$

$FEPO_4$ usually varies between 5% and 20% but should increase with hyperphosphatemia and decrease with hypophosphatemia when hormonal control is normal.[52]

Magnesium[53–56]

Renal Handling of Magnesium

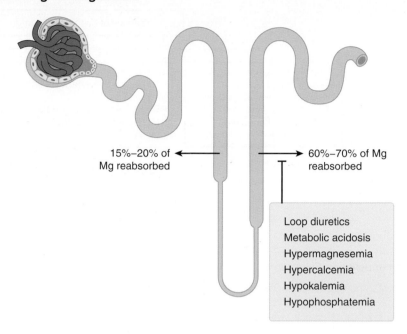

15%–20% of Mg reabsorbed

60%–70% of Mg reabsorbed

Loop diuretics
Metabolic acidosis
Hypermagnesemia
Hypercalcemia
Hypokalemia
Hypophosphatemia

Magnesium Effects in the Body

Magnesium is the fourth most common cation in the body, and the second most common intracellular cation. It has numerous effects among which are the following:

- Vasodilatation by direct action on blood vessels (Mg acts as a calcium antagonist) and exerts antisympathetic activity
- Negative inotropic effect
- Bronchodilation
- Tocolytic effect to suppress premature labor
- Renal vasodilation and diuresis
- Cofactor for many intracellular enzymes
- Responsible for the maintenance of transmembrane gradients of sodium and potassium

Hypermagnesemia[57]

Causes of Hypermagnesemia

- Iatrogenic: parenteral magnesium administration (usually for preeclampsia treatment)
- Excessive use of magnesium-containing laxatives and antacids

Effects of Hypermagnesemia/Symptoms

- Depressed CNS, muscle weakness, areflexia (usually with serum Mg >6 mg/dL)
- Depressed cardiac conduction, widened QRS complexes, prolonged P-QRS intervals

Treatment of Hypermagnesemia

- Forced diuresis
- Dialysis
- Intravenous calcium

Hypomagnesemia[58,59]

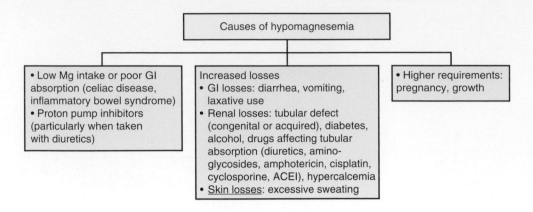

Effects of Hypomagnesemia/Symptoms

- Neurological: nystagmus, convulsions, numbness
- Fatigue
- Muscle spasms, cramps, or muscle weakness
- Cardiac arrhythmias
- Hypocalcemia, hypokalemia from renal wasting
- In severe cases, cardiac arrest or respiratory arrest

The diagnosis of GI vs. renal losses of Mg in hypomagnesemic patients can be made by calculating the fractional excretion of magnesium (FEMg) as follows:

$$FE_{Mg} = \frac{U_{Mg} \times P_{Cr}}{(0.7^* \times P_{Mg}) \times U_{Cr}} \times 100\%$$

—————

*Factoring the plasma or serum Mg level by 0.7 is because of the protein-bound Mg of about 30% which is not filtered by the kidney.

In hypomagnesemic patients, FE_{Mg} >4% indicates renal magnesium wasting whereas FE_{Mg} <2% indicates a GI loss or low Mg intake.[60]

Therapeutic Use of Magnesium

- Preeclampsia and eclampsia
- Cardiac arrhythmias (torsades de pointes, digoxin toxicity, any serious ventricular or atrial arrhythmias especially with hypokalemia)
- Asthma or chronic obstructive pulmonary disease (COPD) exacerbation
- Refractory hypokalemia or hypocalcemia in the context of hypomagnesemia
- Tocolytic agent to suppress premature labor

Polyuria Workup[61,62]

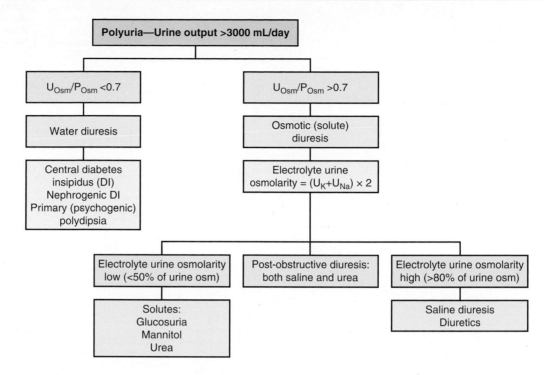

Diuretic Therapy[63–74]

The three major classes of diuretics used for enhancing sodium excretion are:
- Thiazide diuretics, e.g., hydrochlorothiazide
- Loop diuretics, e.g., furosemide
- Potassium-sparing diuretics (either aldosterone antagonists, e.g., spironolactone, or collecting duct sodium channel blockers, e.g., amiloride)

  Other drugs have diuretic action, but are used for more specific purposes, such as:
- Carbonic anhydrase inhibitors (to cause bicarbonaturia or alkalinize the urine to correct metabolic alkalosis)
- Osmotic diuretics (to enhance urinary excretion of poisons or for CNS edema)
- Low-dose dopamine (for congestive heart failure [CHF] and acute kidney injury [AKI], but probably no longer indicated for AKI treatment)
- ADH antagonists (to induce a water diuresis to correct hyponatremia)

Diuretic Sites of Action

Their sites of action in the renal tubule are shown in the diagram below.

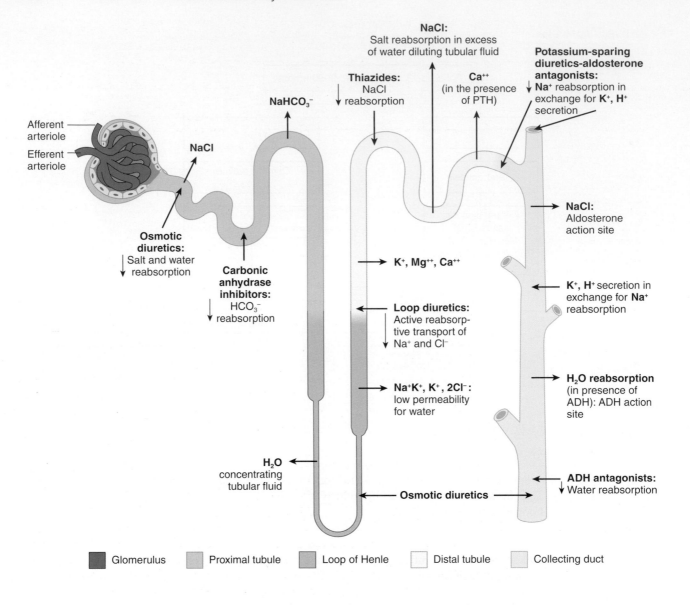

	Loop Diuretics	Thiazides	K+-Sparing Diuretics: Amiloride/Triamterene
Mechanism	Block Na+-K+-Cl− transporter in the Loop of Henle	Block electroneutral Na+-Cl− transporter in the distal tubule	Block apical Na+ channels
Water and Na+	Impair urinary concentration ability: water is excreted in excess of sodium	Impair the ability to dilute urine (decreased ability to excrete a water load while diuresing sodium may cause hyponatremia)	
Other electrolytes	Loss of K+ and Mg++, increase urinary Ca++ excretion	Loss of K+ and Mg++, urinary Ca++ retention	Impair the excretion of K+ and H+ in exchange for collecting duct Na+ absorption

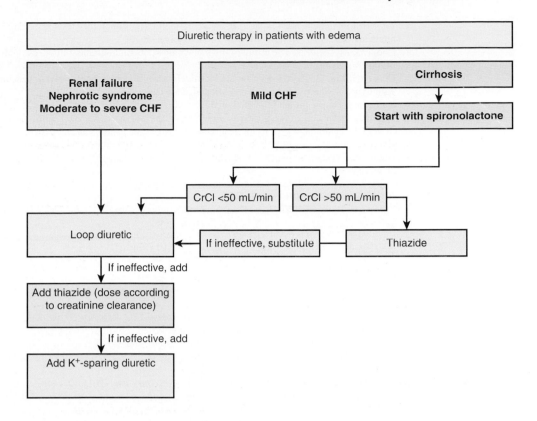

REFERENCES

1. Danziger J, Zeidel M, Parker MJ. *Renal Physiology: A Clinical Approach*. Philadelphia: Lippincott Williams & Wilkins; 2012.
2. Rose BD, Post TW. *Clinical Physiology of Acid-Base and Electrolyte Disorders*. New York: McGraw-Hill; 2001.
3. Schrier RW. *Renal and Electrolyte Disorders*. 7th ed. Philadelphia: Lippincott Williams & Wilkins; 2010.
4. Rennke B, Denker HG. *Renal Pathophysiology: The Essentials*. 3rd ed. Philadelphia: Lippincott Williams & Wilkins; 2009.
5. Eaton J, Pooler D. *Vander's Renal Physiology*. 8th ed. New York: McGraw-Hill; 2013.
6. Jameson J, Loscalzo J. *Harrison's Nephrology and Acid-Base Disorders*. New York: McGraw-Hill; 2010.
7. Goldfarb-Rumyantzev AS, Brown RS. *Nephrology Pocket. El Segundo*. Borm Bruckmeier Publishing; 2014.
8. Eladari D, Chambrey R, Peti-Peterdi J. A new look at electrolyte transport in the distal tubule. *Annu Rev Physiol*. 2012;74(1):325–349.
9. Seay NW, Lehrich RW, Greenberg A. Diagnosis and management of disorders of body tonicity—hyponatremia and hypernatremia: core curriculum 2020. *Am J Kidney Dis*. 2020;75(2):272–286.
10. Offenstadt G, Das V. Hyponatremia, hypernatremia: a physiological approach. *Minerva Anestesiol*. 2006;72(6):353–356.
11. Hannon MJ, Thompson CJ. The syndrome of inappropriate antidiuretic hormone: prevalence, causes and consequences. *Eur J Endocrinol*. 2010;162(suppl 1):S5–S12.
12. Sterns RH, Silver SM. Cerebral salt wasting versus SIADH: what difference? *J Am Soc Nephrol*. 2008;19(2):194–196.
13. Cui H, He G, Yang S, et al. Inappropriate antidiuretic hormone secretion and cerebral salt-wasting syndromes in neurological patients. *Front Neurosci*. 2019;13:1170.
14. Kalita J, Singh RK, Misra UK. Cerebral salt wasting is the most common cause of hyponatremia in stroke. *J Stroke Cerebrovasc Dis*. 2017;26(5):1026–1032.
15. Noakes TD. Overconsumption of fluids by athletes. *BMJ*. 2003;327(7407):113–114.
16. Feldman BJ, Rosenthal SM, Vargas GA, et al. Nephrogenic syndrome of inappropriate antidiuresis. *N Engl J Med*. 2005;352(18):1884–1890.
17. Schrier RW, Gross P, Gheorghiade M, et al. Tolvaptan, a selective oral vasopressin V2-receptor antagonist, for hyponatremia. *N Engl J Med*. 2006;355(20):2099–2112.
18. Kim Y, Lee N, Lee KE, Gwak HS. Risk factors for sodium overcorrection in non-hypovolemic hyponatremia patients treated with tolvaptan. *Eur J Clin Pharmacol*. 2020;76(5):723–729.
19. Morris JH, Bohm NM, Nemecek BD, et al. Rapidity of correction of hyponatremia due to syndrome of inappropriate secretion of antidiuretic hormone following tolvaptan. *Am J Kidney Dis*. 2018;71(6):772–782.
20. Palmer BF, Clegg DJ. Physiology and pathophysiology of potassium homeostasis: core curriculum 2019. *Am J Kidney Dis*. 2019;74(5):682–695.

21. Lin SH, Lin YF, Chen DT, Chu P, Hsu CW, Halperin ML. Laboratory tests to determine the cause of hypokalemia and paralysis. *Arch Intern Med*. 2004;164(14):1561.

22. Choi MJ, Ziyadeh FN. The utility of the transtubular potassium gradient in the evaluation of hyperkalemia. *JASN (J Am Soc Nephrol)*. 2008;19(3):424–426.

23. Ethier JH, Kamel KS, Magner PO, Lemann J, Halperin ML. The transtubular potassium concentration in patients with hypokalemia and hyperkalemia. *Am J Kidney Dis*. 1990;15(4):309–315.

24. Kamel KS, Halperin ML. Intrarenal urea recycling leads to a higher rate of renal excretion of potassium: an hypothesis with clinical implications. *Curr Opin Nephrol Hypertens*. 2011;20(5):547–554.

25. Sihler KC, Napolitano LM. Complications of massive transfusion. *Chest*. 2010;137(1):209–220.

26. Harel Z, Gilbert C, Wald R, et al. The effect of combination treatment with aliskiren and blockers of the renin-angiotensin system on hyperkalaemia and acute kidney injury: systematic review and meta-analysis. *BMJ*. 2012;344:e42.

27. Nappi JM, Sieg A. Aldosterone and aldosterone receptor antagonists in patients with chronic heart failure. *Vasc Health Risk Manag*. 2011;7:353–363.

28. Elliott MJ, Ronksley PE, Clase CM, Ahmed SB, Hemmelgarn BR. Management of patients with acute hyperkalemia. *Can Med Assoc J*. 2010;182(15):1631–1635.

29. Kayexalate® SODIUM POLYSTYRENE SULFONATE, USP Cation-Exchange Resin. https://www.rxlist.com/kayexalate-drug.htm#description. Accessed August 17, 2021.

30. Desai NR, Rowan CG, Alvarez PJ, Fogli J, Toto R. Hyperkalemia treatment modalities: a descriptive observational study focused on medication and healthcare resource utilization. *PloS One*. 2020;15(1).

31. Packham DK, Rasmussen HS, Lavin PT, et al. Sodium zirconium cyclosilicate in hyperkalemia. *N Engl J Med*. 2015;372(3):222–231.

32. Peacock M. Calcium metabolism in health and disease. *Clin J Am Soc Nephrol*. 2010;5(suppl 1):S23–S30.

33. Lambers TT, Bindels RJM, Hoenderop JGJ. Coordinated control of renal Ca2+ handling. *Kidney Int*. 2006;69(4):650–654.

34. Goltzman D, Mannstadt M, Marcocci C. Physiology of the calcium-parathyroid hormone-vitamin D axis. *Front Horm Res*. 2018;50:1–13.

35. Song L. Calcium and bone metabolism indices. *Adv Clin Chem*. 2017;82:1–46.

36. Richter B, Faul C. FGF23 actions on target tissues-with and without Klotho. *Front Endocrinol*. 2018;9:189.

37. Masi L. Primary hyperparathyroidism. *Front Horm Res*. 2018;51:1–12.

38. Varghese J, Rich T, Jimenez C. Benign familial hypocalciuric hypercalcemia. *Endocr Pract*. 2011;17(suppl 1):13–17.

39. Lee JY, Shoback DM. Familial hypocalciuric hypercalcemia and related disorders. *Best Pract Res Clin Endocrinol Metab*. 2018;32(5):609–619.

40. Makras P, Papapoulos S. Medical treatment of hypercalcaemia. *Hormones (Basel)*. 2009;8(2):83–95.

41. Chitambar CR. Medical applications and toxicities of gallium compounds. *Int J Environ Res Public Health*. 2010;7(5):2337–2361.

42. Khan A, Grey A, Shoback D. Medical management of asymptomatic primary hyperparathyroidism: proceedings of the third international workshop. *J Clin Endocrinol Metab*. 2009;94(2):373–381.

43. Schlosser K, Zielke A, Rothmund M. Medical and surgical treatment for secondary and tertiary hyperparathyroidism. *Scand J Surg*. 2004;93(4):288–297.

44. Eidman KE, Wetmore JB. Treatment of secondary hyperparathyroidism: how do cinacalcet and etelcalcetide differ? *Semin Dial*. 2018;31(5):440–444.

45. Shoback D. Hypoparathyroidism. *N Engl J Med*. 2008;359(4):391–403.

46. Mannstadt M, Bilezikian JP, Thakker RV, et al. Hypoparathyroidism. *Nat Rev Dis Prim*. 2017;3:17055.

47. Bilezikian JP, Brandi ML, Cusano NE, et al. Management of hypoparathyroidism: present and future. *J Clin Endocrinol Metab*. 2016;101(6):2313–2324.

48. Goyal R, Jialal I. Hyperphosphatemia. In: *StatPearls—NCBI Bookshelf [Online]*. Treasure Island: StatPearls Publishing; 2020. https://www.ncbi.nlm.nih.gov/books/NBK551586/.

49. Lee R, Weber TJ. Disorders of phosphorus homeostasis. *Curr Opin Endocrinol Diabetes Obes*. 2010;17(6):561–567.

50. Müller D, Mehling H, Otto B, et al. Niacin lowers serum phosphate and increases HDL cholesterol in dialysis patients. *Clin J Am Soc Nephrol*. 2007;2(6):1249–1254.

51. Ketteler M, Liangos O, Biggar PH. Treating hyperphosphatemia—current and advancing drugs. *Expert Opin Pharmacother*. 2016;17(14):1873–1879.

52. Assadi F. Hypophosphatemia an evidence-based problem-solving approach to clinical cases. *Iran J Kidney Dis*. 2010;4(3):195–201.

53. Byrd RP, Roy TM. Magnesium: its proven and potential clinical significance. *South Med J*. 2003;96(1):104.

54. Fawcett WJ, Haxby EJ, Male DA. Magnesium: physiology and pharmacology. *Br J Anaesth*. 1999;83(2):302–320.

55. Quamme GA. Renal magnesium handling: new insights in understanding old problems. *Kidney Int*. 1997;52(5):1180–1195.

56. Saris NEL, Mervaala E, Karppanen H, Khawaja JA, Lewenstam A. Magnesium: an update on physiological, clinical and analytical aspects. *Clin Chim Acta*. 2000;294(1–2):1–26.

57. Van Laecke S. Hypomagnesemia and hypermagnesemia. *Acta Clin Belg*. 2019;74(1):41–47.

58. Gröber U. Magnesium and drugs. *Int J Mol Sci*. 2019;20(9):2094.

59. Ahmed F, Mohammed A. Magnesium: the forgotten electrolyte—a review on hypomagnesemia. *Med Sci*. 2019;7(4):56.

60. Elisaf M, Panteli K, Theodorou J, Siamopoulos KC. Fractional excretion of magnesium in normal subjects and in patients with hypomagnesemia. *Magnes Res*. 1997;10(4):315–320.

61. Fenske W, Refardt J, Chifu I, et al. A copeptin-based approach in the diagnosis of diabetes insipidus. *N Engl J Med*. 2018;379(5):428–439.
62. Ranieri M, Di Mise A, Tamma G, Valenti G. Vasopressin–aquaporin-2 pathway: recent advances in understanding water balance disorders [version 1; referees: 3 approved]. *F1000Res*. 2019;8:F1000. Faculty Rev-149.
63. Kennelly P, Sapkota R, Azhar M, Cheema FH, Conway C, Hameed A. Diuretic therapy in congestive heart failure. *Acta Cardiol*. 2021;3:1–8.
64. Bernstein PL, Ellison DH. Diuretics and salt transport along the nephron. *Semin Nephrol*. 2011;31(6):475–482.
65. Brater DC. Update in diuretic therapy: clinical pharmacology. *Semin Nephrol*. 2011;31(6):483–494.
66. Palmer BF. Metabolic complications associated with use of diuretics. *Semin Nephrol*. 2011;31(6):542–552.
67. Sarafidis PA, Georgianos PI, Lasaridis AN. Diuretics in clinical practice. Part I: mechanisms of action, pharmacological effects and clinical indications of diuretic compounds. *Expert Opin Drug Saf*. 2010;9(2):243–257.
68. Sarafidis PA, Georgianos PI, Lasaridis AN. Diuretics in clinical practice. Part II: electrolyte and acid-base disorders complicating diuretic therapy. *Expert Opin Drug Saf*. 2010;9(2):259–273.
69. Ernst ME, Gordon JA. Diuretic therapy: key aspects in hypertension and renal disease. *J Nephrol*. 2010;23(5):487–493.
70. Maaskant JM, De Boer JP, Dalesio O, Holtkamp MJ, Lucas C. The effectiveness of chlorhexidine-silver sulfadiazine impregnated central venous catheters in patients receiving high-dose chemotherapy followed by peripheral stem cell transplantation. *Eur J Cancer Care (Engl)*. 2009;18(5):477–482.
71. Wile D. Diuretics: a review. *Ann Clin Biochem*. 2012;49(5):419–431.
72. Kassamali R, Sica DA. Acetazolamide: a forgotten diuretic agent. *Cardiol Rev*. 2011;19(6):276–278.
73. Sica DA, Carter B, Cushman W, Hamm L. Thiazide and loop diuretics. *J Clin Hypertens*. 2011;13(9):639–643.
74. Epstein M, Calhoun DA. Aldosterone blockers (mineralocorticoid receptor antagonism) and potassium-sparing diuretics. *J Clin Hypertens*. 2011;13(9):644–648.

CHAPTER 5

Acid-Base Disorders

Alexander Goldfarb-Rumyantzev and Robert Stephen Brown

This chapter will discuss the interpretation of arterial or venous blood gas results and routine serum electrolytes to identify, diagnose and treat the acid-base disorder.[1–3]

The figure below depicts a brief summary of the main metabolic pathways involved in the metabolism of glucose, amino acids, and lipids. A general understanding of these processes is helpful to get a better insight into acid-base physiology.

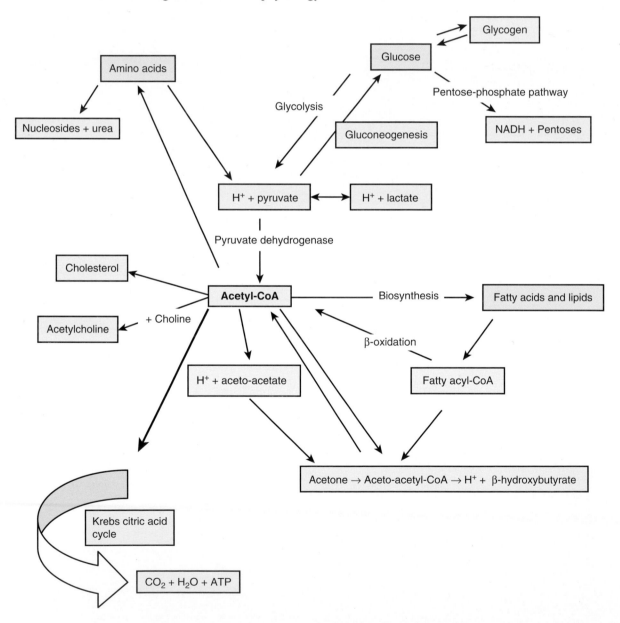

When oxidative metabolism in the Krebs cycle is inhibited by hypoxia or shock or when acetyl-CoA is generated from fat rather than glucose as in diabetic ketoacidosis, the metabolic pathway shows the un-metabolized hydrogen ion as lactic acid or ketoacids, respectively, resulting in metabolic acidosis.

Henderson-Hasselbalch Equation

Interpretations of blood gas findings start with the Henderson-Hasselbalch equation:

$$pH = pKa + \log \frac{[Base]}{[Acid]}$$

where pKa is the negative log of the acid dissociation constant.

The blood buffering system uses bicarbonate as the base and carbonic acid as the acid; therefore this equation can be rewritten as follows:

$$pH = pKa + \log \frac{[HCO_3^-]}{[H_2CO_3]}$$

Using a pKa value of 6.1 for carbonic acid, and a conversion factor of 0.03 to express the acid concentration in terms of partial arterial pressure of CO_2 (paCO_2), which is measured in arterial blood gases (ABGs), this is finally rewritten as follows:

$$pH = 6.1 + \log \frac{[HCO_3^-]}{0.3 \, paCO_2}$$

Since this final expression includes a logarithm, which is difficult for quick bedside calculation, several simple approximations may be used, as discussed on the pages that follow.

Note that a normal pH of 7.4, the concentration of the base [HCO_3] of about 25 mEq/L is 20 times that of carbonic acid with a concentration of 1.2 mEq/L (or a pCO_2 of 40 mm Hg).

Acid-Base Regulation by the Kidney[4–9]

General view of kidney handling of bicarbonate reabsorption and H^+ excretion is represented in the diagram below summarizing renal tubular physiology relevant to acid-base balance.

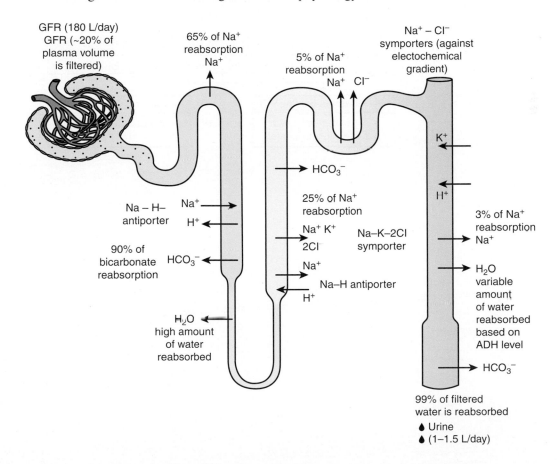

To maintain normal blood pH, the kidney must first reabsorb the filtered bicarbonate. This takes place mainly in the proximal tubule in a process largely coupled to sodium reabsorption and hydrogen ion (H$^+$) secretion which is dependent upon carbonic anhydrase by the mechanisms shown below.

Bicarbonate reabsorption

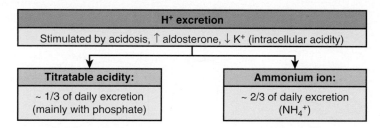

Since most human diets produce metabolic acids to excrete, after reabsorption of bicarbonate takes place, additional hydrogen ions are secreted into the urine to be excreted as "titratable" acid at urine pH levels that can be reduced below 5 and by ammonium ions.

H$^+$ excretion	
Stimulated by acidosis, ↑ aldosterone, ↓ K$^+$ (intracellular acidity)	
Titratable acidity:	**Ammonium ion:**
~ 1/3 of daily excretion (mainly with phosphate)	~ 2/3 of daily excretion (NH$_4^+$)

Proximal tubule

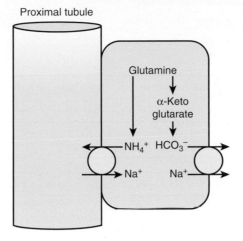

Distal tubule and collecting duct

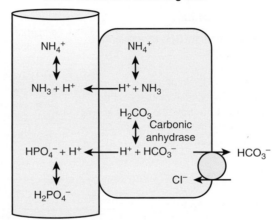

Alkalinization of the urine by bicarbonate secretion, though also shown below, can take place but is usually unnecessary unless there is an alkali load, e.g., sodium bicarbonate ingestion or metabolic alkalosis.

Bicarbonate secretion

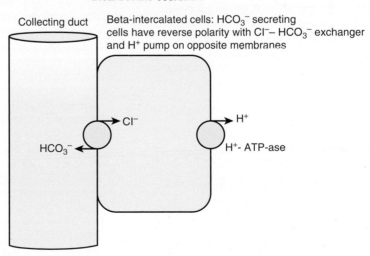

Potassium and Acid-Base Balance Interrelation

The diagram below illustrates the association between alkalosis and hypokalemia and between acidosis and hyperkalemia.

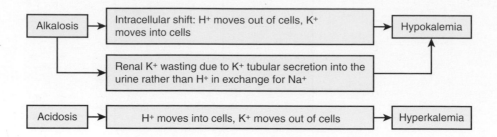

Acid-Base Disorder Diagnostic Algorithm

This algorithm provides an interpretation of ABGs in conjunction with plasma chemistry.

To use this algorithm:
- First examine the pH and identify acidemia or alkalemia
- Then, using the bicarbonate (HCO_3^-) concentration obtained from serum electrolytes and the $paCO_2$ from the ABG, identify whether the primary cause of the disorder is metabolic or respiratory (see ABG algorithm below)

- Then perform a calculation to examine whether a primary respiratory disorder has appropriate metabolic compensation, or a primary metabolic disorder has appropriate respiratory compensation (refer to the "Evaluation for Appropriate Compensation" table on the next pages)
- If not, there is a second "primary" disorder, considered to be a "complex" (meaning more than just one) acid-base disorder, rather than a "simple" (meaning a single) acid-base disorder underlying the observed changes

"Complex" (Double or Triple) Acid-Base Disorders

A single patient may have two or even three primary acid-base disorders. It is possible to have a primary metabolic acidosis, e.g., diabetic ketoacidosis, and a simultaneous primary metabolic alkalosis, e.g., vomiting with HCl loss. This can be diagnosed using the anion gap. In an increased anion-gap metabolic acidosis, a "hidden" metabolic alkalosis can be discovered with the "delta/delta" concept. It is based on the assumption that for a given increase in the anion gap (ΔAG), there is a concomitant decrease in bicarbonate concentration (ΔHCO_3) from the added unmeasured acid titrating away the bicarbonate.

The delta/delta calculation is as follows:

$$\Delta AG = \text{Measured AG} - \text{Normal AG (12mEq/L)}$$
$$= \text{Unmeasured anions}$$

$$\Delta HCO_3 = \text{Normal } HCO_3 \text{ (24mEq/L)} -$$
$$\text{Measured } HCO_3 = \text{Decrease in } HCO_3$$

If $\Delta AG/\Delta HCO_3 >2$ it suggests a concomitant metabolic alkalosis.

Looked at another way, if the unmeasured anions in the large anion gap were rapidly metabolized to HCO_3, the patient would have a high serum bicarbonate level and become alkalotic. This would indicate the concomitance of both a metabolic acidosis and alkalosis. Were such a patient to also overbreathe or underbreathe, the added primary respiratory disorder would give rise to a triple acid-base disturbance.

It is important to note that because there are other buffers besides serum bicarbonate, the AG often increases somewhat more than the serum bicarbonate falls, so the $\Delta AG/\Delta HCO_3$ is usually more than 1, between 1 and 2 is usual in a simple increased anion-gap metabolic acidosis.

However, if the AG is significantly less than the fall in serum bicarbonate, it suggests that there may be a concomitant primary non–anion-gap metabolic acidosis from loss of HCO_3, e.g., from diarrhea, present.

This can be calculated as follows:
$$\Delta AG/\Delta HCO_3 <1 \text{ suggests a combined normal and high anion-gap metabolic acidosis.}$$

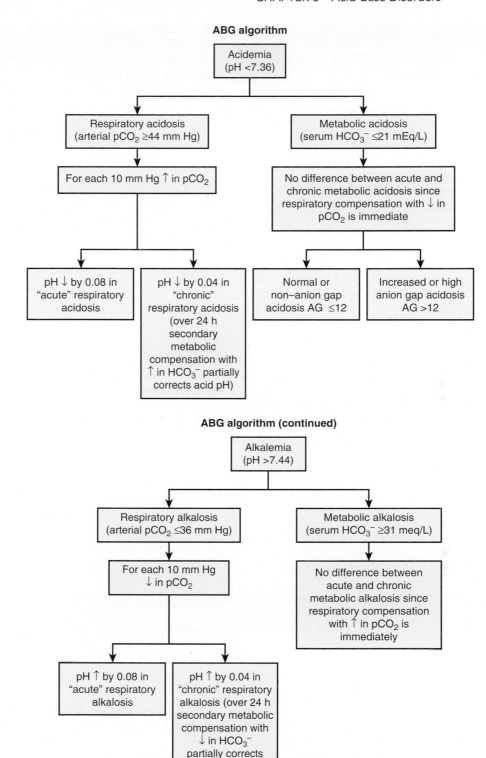

ABG algorithm

Acidemia
(pH <7.36)

Respiratory acidosis
(arterial pCO₂ ≥44 mm Hg)

Metabolic acidosis
(serum HCO₃⁻ ≤21 mEq/L)

For each 10 mm Hg ↑ in pCO₂

No difference between acute and chronic metabolic acidosis since respiratory compensation with ↓ in pCO₂ is immediate

pH ↓ by 0.08 in "acute" respiratory acidosis

pH ↓ by 0.04 in "chronic" respiratory acidosis (over 24 h secondary metabolic compensation with ↑ in HCO₃⁻ partially corrects acid pH)

Normal or non–anion gap acidosis AG ≤12

Increased or high anion gap acidosis AG >12

ABG algorithm (continued)

Alkalemia
(pH >7.44)

Respiratory alkalosis
(arterial pCO₂ ≤36 mm Hg)

Metabolic alkalosis
(serum HCO₃⁻ ≥31 meq/L)

For each 10 mm Hg ↓ in pCO₂

No difference between acute and chronic metabolic alkalosis since respiratory compensation with ↑ in pCO₂ is immediately

pH ↑ by 0.08 in "acute" respiratory alkalosis

pH ↑ by 0.04 in "chronic" respiratory alkalosis (over 24 h secondary metabolic compensation with ↓ in HCO₃⁻ partially corrects alkaline pH)

Evaluation for appropriate compensation

Compensation for Respiratory Alkalosis	Compensation for Respiratory Acidosis
Acute	**Acute**
Expect serum HCO₃ to fall about 2 mEq/L for each 10-mm Hg decrease in pCO₂ for normal metabolic compensation	Expect serum HCO₃ to rise about 1 mEq/L for each 10-mm Hg increase in pCO₂ for normal metabolic compensation

cont'd	
Compensation for Respiratory Alkalosis	**Compensation for Respiratory Acidosis**
Chronic (over 24 hours)	**Chronic (over 24 hours)**
Expect serum HCO_3 to fall about 5 mEq/L for each 10-mm Hg decrease in pCO_2 for normal metabolic compensation	Expect serum HCO_3 to rise about 3.5 mEq/L for each 10-mmHg increase in pCO_2 for normal metabolic compensation

Compensation for Metabolic Alkalosis	**Compensation for Metabolic Acidosis**
There are three common ways to evaluate for normal respiratory compensation response (±2 mm Hg): • Expect pCO_2 to rise 0.7 mm Hg for each 1-mEq/L rise in serum HCO_3^- for normal respiratory compensation • pCO_2 should be equal to serum HCO_3 + 15 mm Hg up to a pCO_2 of about 60 when the pCO_2 rises no further • The easy way: pCO_2 should be equal to the last two digits of the pH up to pH 7.60	There are three common ways to evaluate for normal respiratory compensation response (±2 mm Hg): • Expect pCO_2 to decrease 1.2 mm Hg for each 1-mEq/L fall in HCO_3 • pCO_2 should be equal to 1.5 (HCO_3) + 8 • The easy way: pCO_2 should be equal to the last two digits of the pH down to pH 7.10

Useful Tips

1. Acid-base disorders do not compensate completely, so if the pH is acidic, assume acidosis; if it is alkaline, assume alkalosis.
2. In interpreting serum bicarbonate level:
   • If HCO_3 is ↑, there is either a primary metabolic alkalosis or compensation for a respiratory acidosis.
   • If HCO_3 is ↓, there is either a primary metabolic acidosis or compensation for a respiratory alkalosis.[10]
   • If HCO_3 is normal, there is either a normal acid-base state or a complex (double or triple) disorder may be present.
3. An ↑ anion gap almost always indicates a metabolic acidosis.
4. Serum K^+ concentration may be helpful: If K^+ is ↓, there is usually an alkalosis; if K^+ is ↑, there is usually an acidosis.
5. When blood urea nitrogen (BUN) and creatinine levels are ↑, renal failure may be associated with a metabolic acidosis that often has a normal anion gap when mild, and an increased anion gap when renal failure is more severe.
6. Liver failure is usually associated with metabolic acidosis.

Metabolic Acidosis[11]

Causes of Metabolic Acidosis

• Once the diagnosis of metabolic acidosis is established, the next step is to identify the cause.
• The first step is to assess whether the metabolic acidosis is associated with a normal anion gap or an abnormally high anion gap.
• An increased anion gap indicates the presence of unmeasured acids which may be endogenous, e.g., lactic acid, or exogenous, e.g., oxalic acid from ethylene glycol poisoning.
• Metabolic acidosis with a normal anion gap is caused by either loss of bicarbonate (from the gastrointestinal [GI] tract or in the urine) or failure to excrete acid (H+) by the kidneys.

Serum Osmolar Gap

Using the serum or plasma osmolar gap will help to differentiate between a non-osmolar gap (usually endogenous) and a high osmolar gap (exogenous toxin) acidosis.

The osmolar gap is determined by comparing the measured serum or plasma osmolality to the calculated serum osmolality.

Serum Osmolality

Calculated serum osmolality (to compare with measured S_{osm} for assessment of an osmolar gap):

$$S_{osm} = 2\,(Na^+) + \frac{Glucose\ (mg/dL)}{18} + \frac{BUN\ (mg/dL)}{2.8}$$

An osmolar gap greater than 10 mOsm/kg indicates the presence of abnormal, unmeasured osmotically active molecules[12] such as an alcohol or ethylene glycol.

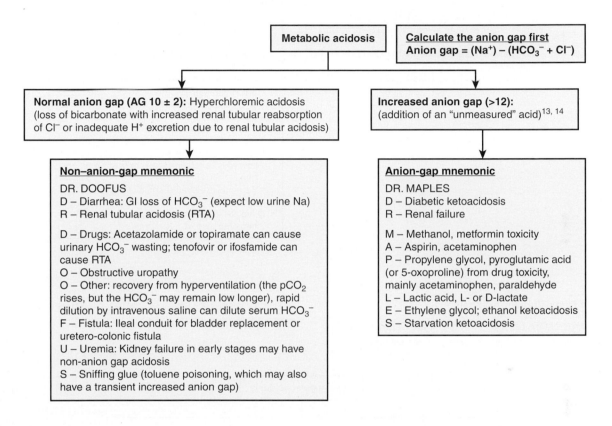

Metabolic acidosis

Calculate the anion gap first
Anion gap = $(Na^+) - (HCO_3^- + Cl^-)$

Normal anion gap (AG 10 ± 2): Hyperchloremic acidosis (loss of bicarbonate with increased renal tubular reabsorption of Cl^- or inadequate H^+ excretion due to renal tubular acidosis)

Increased anion gap (>12): (addition of an "unmeasured" acid)[13, 14]

Non–anion-gap mnemonic

DR. DOOFUS
D – Diarrhea: GI loss of HCO_3^- (expect low urine Na)
R – Renal tubular acidosis (RTA)

D – Drugs: Acetazolamide or topiramate can cause urinary HCO_3^- wasting; tenofovir or ifosfamide can cause RTA
O – Obstructive uropathy
O – Other: recovery from hyperventilation (the pCO_2 rises, but the HCO_3^- may remain low longer), rapid dilution by intravenous saline can dilute serum HCO_3^-
F – Fistula: Ileal conduit for bladder replacement or uretero-colonic fistula
U – Uremia: Kidney failure in early stages may have non-anion gap acidosis
S – Sniffing glue (toluene poisoning, which may also have a transient increased anion gap)

Anion-gap mnemonic

DR. MAPLES
D – Diabetic ketoacidosis
R – Renal failure

M – Methanol, metformin toxicity
A – Aspirin, acetaminophen
P – Propylene glycol, pyroglutamic acid (or 5-oxoproline) from drug toxicity, mainly acetaminophen, paraldehyde
L – Lactic acid, L- or D-lactate
E – Ethylene glycol; ethanol ketoacidosis
S – Starvation ketoacidosis

Non–Anion-Gap Metabolic Acidosis

Renal Tubular Acidosis (RTA) vs. GI Losses

In metabolic acidosis associated with a normal anion gap, the low serum bicarbonate level is either due to loss of bicarbonate from the GI tract from diarrhea, or from failure of the kidneys to conserve bicarbonate or to regenerate bicarbonate by excreting acid.

The differential diagnosis between these two conditions is based on showing a normal renal response to acidemia in GI losses.

- First, with normal renal response to GI loss of bicarbonate, the urine pH should be acidic.
- Second, the urine anion gap (urine $Na^+ + K^+ - Cl^-$) should be negative, indicating the presence of the unmeasured positively charged urinary cation, NH_4^+, which provides additional acid excretion. If renal tubular NH_4^+ secretion is impaired, the urinary anion gap remains positive or around zero. Remember that calculating a urine anion gap has no role in an increased anion gap metabolic acidosis because there is an unmeasured anion in the urine that obscures the quantity of the unmeasured NH_4^+ cation.[23]

Differential diagnosis between RTA and GI loss of bicarbonate

Measure urine pH
Measure urine anion gap = $Na^+ + K^+ - Cl^-$

GI loss of bicarbonate

- Urine is acidic: pH <5.5
- Appropriately increased urinary NH_4^+ excretion leads to negative urine anion gap ($Na^+ + K^+ - Cl^- = -20$ to -50)
- Also, hypovolemia associated with diarrhea leads to low urine Na^+

RTA (see below for more detailed discussion)

- Urine pH >5.5: Type 1 "distal" or "classic" RTA
  - Will have low serum K^+ and bicarbonate may be <10
- Urine pH <5.5: Type 2 "proximal" RTA
  - Low NH_4^+ excretion leads to positive urine anion gap. Waste urinary HCO_3^- when given alkali therapy and then urine pH will be >5.5. Serum K^+ may be low and bicarbonate usually 14–20
  - May have full blown Fanconi's syndrome
- Urine pH <5.5: Type 4 RTA
  - Low NH_4^+ excretion leads to positive anion gap
  - Serum K is elevated and bicarbonate usually >15
- Urine Na^+ is not low in RTA unless volume depleted also

Types of Renal Tubular Acidosis

The patterns of RTA of types 1, 2, and 4 are described below. Type 3 RTA (a mixture of types 1 and 2) was associated with renal insufficiency and is no longer recognized as a diagnostic entity. Localization of the defect in the nephron is illustrated below.

Renal tubular acidosis

Distal (type 1)

Mechanism:
- Defect in H^+-ATP-ase pump—defect in kidney tubular H^+ secretion into the urine
- Defect in Na^+-H^+ exchanger—decreased Na reabsorption leads to secondary hyperaldosteronism and hypokalemia
- Increase in membrane permeability leading to back-diffusion of H^+ and urinary K^+ wasting (hypokalemia)
- Downregulation of H^+-K^+ pump (leads to hypokalemia)

Features:
- Selective deficit of H^+ secretion in the distal nephron with increased K^+ secretion → alkalotic urine (pH >5.5) with hyperchloremia and hypokalemia, bicarbonate <10.
- May often be associated with secondary hypercalciuria, hypocitraturia and nephrolithiasis

Etiology:
- Familial (hereditary), toluene toxicity, Sjögren's syndrome, rheumatoid arthritis, active cirrhosis
- Obstructive uropathy and SLE may cause Type I RTA with hyperkalemia

Proximal (type 2)

Mechanism:
- Defect in Na^+-H^+ exchanger leads to decreased Na reabsorption which results in decreased luminal negative charge and decreased K^+ excretion (due to the decreased electric gradient). While this mechanism can lead to hyperkalema, the secondary hyperaldosteronism (from the decreased Na reabsorption) can cause hypokalemia (so serum K^+ is often only slightly low but will decrease if $NaHCO_3$ is given to correct acidosis)
- Defect in basolateral Na-K-ATP-ase
- Defect in carbonic anhydrase
- All three mechanisms lead to Na wasting, increased Na and water delivery to distal tubule and hypokalemia

Features:
- Inability to reabsorb filtered HCO_3^- with bicarbonate wasting (e.g. carbonic anhydrase inhibitors) → hyperchloremia, normal or low serum K^+, acidic urine: pH < 5.5 (once serum bicarbonate is low), bicarbonate usually between 14 and 20
- Not associated with nephrolithiasis except when carbonic anhydrase inhibitors cause proximal tubular HCO_3^- wasting

Etiology:
- Multiple myeloma with light chain nephropathy, heavy metals, tenofovir, ifosfamide, hereditary in children

Hyperkalemic (type 4)

Mechanism:
- Decreased aldosterone effect → decreased Na^+ reabsorption, decreased K^+ excretion → downregulation of Na^+-H^+ pump (which is also under control of aldosterone)
- Less commonly, tubulointerstitial disease can cause unresponsiveness to aldosterone

Features:
- Also called hyporeninemic hypoaldosteronism (though often renin level is not low).
- ↓ Aldosterone → impaired renal tubular Na^+ reabsorption leading to impaired K^+ and H^+ secretion with impaired ability to generate NH_3 → NH_4^+ excretion → hyperchloremia, hyperkalemia, acidic urine
- Hyperkalemia, urine pH <5.5, bicarbonate >15

Etiology:
- Diabetic or hypertensive nephropathy (usually with hypoaldosteronism), tubulointerstitial diseases, e.g., lupus nephritis, potassium-sparing diuretics, ACE inhibitors and trimethoprim

Illustration of Renal Tubular Acidosis Types

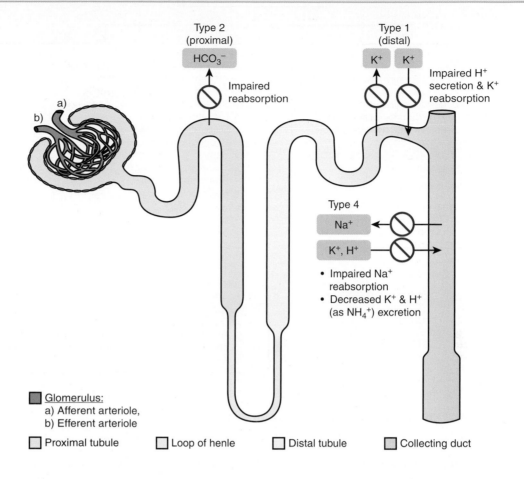

Lactic Acidosis

Types of Lactic Acidosis

Lactic acidosis is one of the most common types of metabolic acidosis associated with an increased anion gap. The diagram below illustrates underlying causes of lactic acidosis of type A (caused by tissue hypoxia) and type B (associated with other causes of increased lactate generation or decreased excretion).

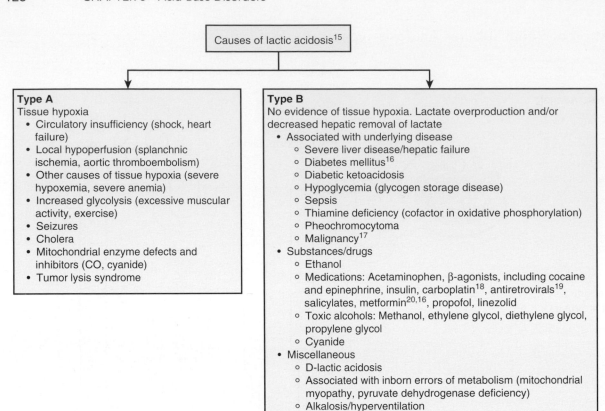

Causes of lactic acidosis[15]

Type A
Tissue hypoxia
- Circulatory insufficiency (shock, heart failure)
- Local hypoperfusion (splanchnic ischemia, aortic thromboembolism)
- Other causes of tissue hypoxia (severe hypoxemia, severe anemia)
- Increased glycolysis (excessive muscular activity, exercise)
- Seizures
- Cholera
- Mitochondrial enzyme defects and inhibitors (CO, cyanide)
- Tumor lysis syndrome

Type B
No evidence of tissue hypoxia. Lactate overproduction and/or decreased hepatic removal of lactate
- Associated with underlying disease
  - Severe liver disease/hepatic failure
  - Diabetes mellitus[16]
  - Diabetic ketoacidosis
  - Hypoglycemia (glycogen storage disease)
  - Sepsis
  - Thiamine deficiency (cofactor in oxidative phosphorylation)
  - Pheochromocytoma
  - Malignancy[17]
- Substances/drugs
  - Ethanol
  - Medications: Acetaminophen, β-agonists, including cocaine and epinephrine, insulin, carboplatin[18], antiretrovirals[19], salicylates, metformin[20,16], propofol, linezolid
  - Toxic alcohols: Methanol, ethylene glycol, diethylene glycol, propylene glycol
  - Cyanide
- Miscellaneous
  - D-lactic acidosis
  - Associated with inborn errors of metabolism (mitochondrial myopathy, pyruvate dehydrogenase deficiency)
  - Alkalosis/hyperventilation

Treatment of Other Metabolic Acidosis Disorders

Treatment of Lactic Acidosis[21]
- Treat underlying condition (e.g., restore tissue perfusion)
- Avoid vasoconstrictors but need caution to avoid fluid overload from volume expansion
- Bicarbonate therapy for pH <7.1 (be aware that bicarbonate stimulates phosphofructokinase ⇒ leading to enhanced lactate production, can increase pCO_2, and cause overshoot alkalosis after lactate eventually converts to bicarbonate)

First treat the underlying cause of the acidosis, e.g., insulin for diabetic ketoacidosis, glucose for alcoholic ketoacidosis, dialysis for severe toxicity from dialyzable toxins such as aspirin, methanol, or ethylene glycol (with fomepizole or ethanol for the latter two poisonings), restoration of circulatory insufficiency, and so on. Thereafter the consideration of alkalinizing therapy with bicarbonate has been controversial. The authors are in favor of alkali in cases of acidosis with pH levels <7.1 unless treatment is likely to quickly correct the condition such as insulin for diabetic ketoacidosis or antiseizure medication for status epilepticus.

Alkalinizing Therapy

Alkalinizing therapy, of which sodium bicarbonate is the most commonly used agent, should be considered in non–anion-gap metabolic acidosis and when pH is <7.1. The chart below describes the administration of sodium bicarbonate, complications of therapy, and alternative alkalinizing agents.

Sodium Bicarbonate Therapy

Bicarbonate Administration Guidelines

- Goal—return pH to 7.2 and serum bicarbonate to >8–10 mEq/L (goal is pH 7.45–7.5 in case of salicylate poisoning to enhance urinary excretion)
- Calculate bicarbonate deficit initially using a distribution volume of bicarbonate estimated at $0.5 \times$ body weight in kg

(this is an approximation due to the need to alkalinize both HCO_3^- and other buffers)
- Administer sodium bicarbonate as infusion rather than boluses which can be used in severe acidemia
- Check bicarbonate level ≥30 minutes after infusion is completed

---

Metabolic Alkalosis

Acute Conditions in Which Sodium Bicarbonate Therapy May Not Improve Outcomes[22]

- Diabetic ketoacidosis
- Lactic acidosis
- Septic shock
- Cardiac arrest
- Intraoperative metabolic acidosis

Potential Complications of Bicarbonate Therapy[22]

- Fluid overload
- Metabolic alkalosis occurring post recovery or as "overshoot" metabolic alkalosis (e.g., in lactic acidosis, when lactate is converted to bicarbonate)
- Electrolyte problems: hypernatremia, increase in urinary sodium excretion, hypokalemia, ionized hypocalcemia
- May promote precipitation of Ca phosphate, potential progression of vascular calcification
- Hyperosmolality
- May increase pCO_2 with paradoxical worsening of intracellular acidosis, paradoxical cerebrospinal fluid acidosis, impairment of tissue oxygenation
- Prolongation of the QTc interval
- Hypercapnia
- Slight blood pressure reduction, hemodynamic instability during hemodialysis
- Increased lactate production

Alternative Alkalinizing Agents to NaHCO$_3$

Carbicarb—Na bicarbonate + Na carbonate[21]
- Limits generation of CO_2
- Minimal ↑ in pCO_2

THAM: 0.3 N tromethamine—buffers metabolic and respiratory acids 1
Reactions take place as follows: $THAM + H^+ \rightarrow THAM^+$

$$TIIAM + H_2CO_3 \rightarrow THAM^+ + HCO_3^-$$

- Limits CO_2 generation
- Side effects: hyperkalemia, hypoglycemia, ventilatory depression, local injury in cases of extravasation, hepatic necrosis in neonates

---

Causes of Metabolic Alkalosis

Metabolic alkalosis is caused by H^+ and Cl^- loss, or bicarbonate accumulation

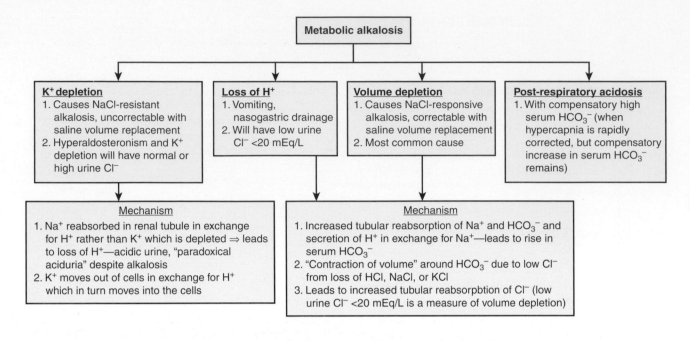

Diagnostic Workup

Diagnostic workup into causes of metabolic alkalosis is based on the following tests: urine chloride and potassium concentrations and arterial blood pressure. The figure below will provide an algorithm into the workup process.

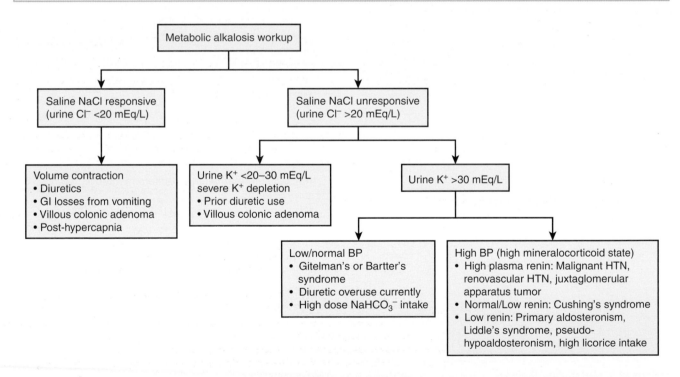

Treatment of Metabolic Alkalosis

- Saline for NaCl-responsive metabolic alkalosis due to volume depletion or GI losses
- Potassium chloride for K⁺ and Cl⁻ depletion saline-resistant metabolic alkalosis

- Acetazolamide (250–500-mg doses as needed) to lower high serum bicarbonate post-hypercapnia or when patient is hypervolemic to preclude saline volume expansion
- HCl 0.3 N rarely used (needs central intravenous catheter infusion)

REFERENCES

1. Narins RG, Emmett M. Simple and mixed acid-base disorders. *Medicine (Baltimore)*. 1980;59(3):161–182.
2. Adrogué HJ, Madias NE. Secondary responses to altered acid-base status: the rules of engagement. *J Am Soc Nephrol*. 2010;21(6):920–923.
3. Romero MF, Rossano AJ. Acid-base basics. *Semin Nephrol*. 2019;39(4):316–327.
4. Danziger J, Zeidel M, Parker MJ. *Renal Physiology: A Clinical Approach*. Philadelphia: Lippincott Williams & Wilkins; 2012.
5. Rose BD, Post TW. *Clinical Physiology of Acid-Base and Electrolyte Disorders*. New York: McGraw-Hill, Medical Pub. Division; 2001.
6. Schrier RW. *Renal and Electrolyte Disorders*. 7th ed. Philadelphia: Lippincott Williams & Wilkins; 2010.
7. Rennke B, Denker HG. *Renal Pathophysiology: The Essentials*. 3rd ed. Philadelphia: Lippincott Williams & Wilkins; 2009.
8. Eaton J, Pooler D. *Vander's Renal Physiology*. 8th ed. New York: McGraw-Hill; 2013.
9. Jameson J, Loscalzo J. *Harrison's Nephrology and Acid-Base Disorders*. New York: McGraw-Hill; 2010.
10. Krapf R, Beeler I, Hertner D, Hulter HN. Chronic respiratory alkalosis. *N Engl J Med*. 1991;324(20):1394–1401.
11. Bushinsky DA, Coe FL, Katzenberg C, Szidon JP, Parks JH. Arterial PCO_2 in chronic metabolic acidosis. *Kidney Int*. 1982;22(3):311–314.
12. Marts LT, Hsu DJ, Clardy PF. Case conferences: The clinical physiologist: Mind the gap. *Ann Am Thorac Soc*. 2014;11(4):671–674.
13. Emmett M, Narins RG. Clinical use of the anion gap. *Medicine (Baltimore)*. 1977;56(1):38–54.
14. Yan MT, Chau T, Cheng CJ, Lin SH. Hunting down a double gap metabolic acidosis. *Ann Clin Biochem*. 2010;47(3):267–270.
15. Seheult J, Fitzpatrick G, Boran G. Lactic acidosis: an update. *Clin Chem Lab Med*. 2017;55(3):322–333.
16. Scale T, Harvey JN. Diabetes, metformin and lactic acidosis. *Clin Endocrinol (Oxf)*. 2011;74(2):191–196.
17. Ruiz JP, Singh A, Hart P. Type B lactic acidosis secondary to malignancy: case report, review of published cases, insights into pathogenesis, and prospects for therapy. *Sci World J*. 2011;11:1316–1324.
18. Brivet FG, Slama A, Prat D, Jacobs FM. Carboplatin: a new cause of severe type B lactic acidosis secondary to mitochondrial DNA damage. *Am J Emerg Med*. 2011;29(7):842.e5–842.e7.
19. Goldfarb-Rumyantzev AS, Jeyakumar A, Gumpeni R, Rubin D. Lactic acidosis associated with nucleoside analog therapy in an HIV-positive patient. *AIDS Patient Care Stds*. 2000;14(7):339–342.
20. Lalau JD, Lacroix C, Compagnon P, et al. Role of metformin accumulation in metformin-associated lactic acidosis. *Diabetes Care*. 1995;18(6):779–784.
21. Kraut JA, Madias NE. Lactic acidosis: current treatments and future directions. *Am J Kidney Dis*. 2016;68(3):473–482.
22. Adeva-Andany MM, Fernández-Fernández C, Mouriño-Bayolo D, Castro-Quintela E, Domínguez-Montero A. Sodium bicarbonate therapy in patients with metabolic acidosis. *Sci World J*. 2014;2014:627673.
23. Palmer BF, Clegg DJ. The use of selected urine chemistries in the diagnosis of kidney disorders. *Clin J Am Soc Nephrol*. 2019;14(2):306–316.

CHAPTER 6

Infectious Disease in Critical Care Practice

Alexander Goldfarb-Rumyantzev

Severe Sepsis and Septic Shock

Sepsis represents a systemic inflammatory reaction to infection with life-threatening consequences triggered by inflammatory mediators released into systemic circulation. Septic shock is defined as hypotension and end-organ hypoperfusion as a result of severe inflammatory response. It is very important to recognize and treat sepsis early prior to end-organ damage.

Septic shock mechanisms[1]:
- Vasoplegic or distributive shock (excessive vasodilatation, abnormal distribution of the capillary blood flow)
- Myocardial depression
- Altered microvascular flow
- Diffuse endothelial injury

Organ dysfunction in sepsis[2]
- Respiratory: Acute respiratory distress syndrome (ARDS)
- Cardiovascular: Hypotension and elevated lactate
- Central nervous system (CNS): Obtundation, delirium
- Renal: Acute kidney injury, Acute tubular necrosis (ATN)
- Gastrointestinal (GI): Paralytic ileus, elevated liver enzymes
- Heme: Disseminated intravascular coagulation (DIC), thrombocytopenia
- Endo: Adrenal dysfunction, euthyroid sick syndrome

Symptoms of severe sepsis[1,2]:
- Chills and rigors
- Heart rate (HR) >120/min
- Systolic Blood pressure (BP) <90 mm Hg
- Respiratory rate: >20/min
- Temperature >38.5° or <36° C
- Confusion
- Lactate >2 mmol/L
- Procalcitonin >0.5 ng/mL
- White blood cell (WBC) count >12,000 or <4000 cells/μL
- Band count >5% of WBCs
- Lymphocytopenia <500/μL
- Thrombocytopenia <150,000/μL
- Oliguria
- Blood cultures are positive in only ~1/3 of cases

Treatment of Sepsis and Septic Shock

The treatment of sepsis (which is a systemic inflammatory response) targets several goals, in particular: infection control, accomplishing hemodynamic stability and end-organ perfusion, and addressing acid-base and electrolyte abnormalities.

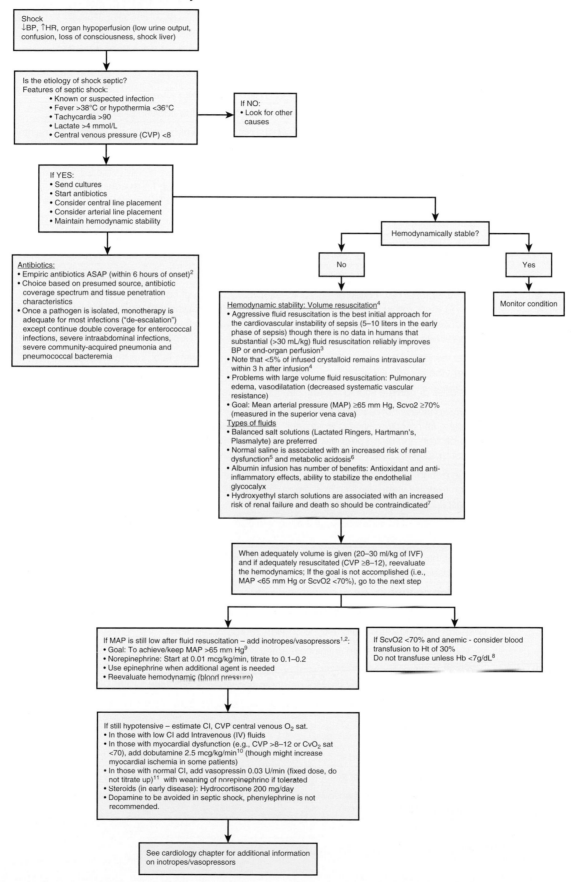

Guidelines for the Treatment of Severe Sepsis and Septic Shock From the Surviving Sepsis Campaign (Surviving sepsis campaign: international guidelines for management of severe sepsis and septic shock: 2012)[2,12]

For all grades, the number indicates the strength of the recommendation (1, recommended; 2, suggested), and the letter indicates the level of evidence, from high (A) to low (D), with UG indicating ungraded.

Element of Care	Grade
Resuscitation	
Begin goal-directed resuscitation during the first 6 hours after recognition	1C
Begin initial fluid resuscitation with crystalloid and consider the addition of albumin	1B
Consider the addition of albumin when substantial amounts of crystalloid are required to maintain adequate arterial pressure	2C
Avoid hetastarch formulations	1C
Begin initial fluid challenge in patients with tissue hypoperfusion and suspected hypovolemia, to achieve ≥30 mL of crystalloids per kilogram of body weight. The guidelines recommend completing the initial fluid resuscitation within 3 hours (UG)	1C
Continue fluid challenge technique as long as there is hemodynamic improvement	UG
Use norepinephrine as the first-choice vasopressor to maintain a MAP of ≥65 mm Hg	1B
Use epinephrine when an additional agent is needed to maintain adequate blood pressure	2B
Add vasopressin (at a dose of 0.03 units/min) with weaning of norepinephrine, if tolerated. Low-dose vasopressin is not recommended as the single initial vasopressor for treatment of sepsis-induced hypotension and vasopressin doses higher than 0.03–0.04 units/min should be reserved for salvage therapy (failure to achieve adequate MAP with other vasopressor agents)	UG
Avoid the use of dopamine except in carefully selected patients (e.g., patients with a low risk of arrhythmias and either known marked left ventricular systolic dysfunction or low heart rate)	2C
Low-dose dopamine should not be used for renal protection	1A
Phenylephrine is not recommended in the treatment of septic shock except in circumstances where (a) norepinephrine is associated with serious arrhythmias, (b) cardiac output is known to be high and blood pressure persistently low, or (c) as salvage therapy when combined inotrope/vasopressor drugs and low-dose vasopressin have failed to achieve MAP target	1C
Infuse dobutamine or add it to vasopressor therapy in the presence of myocardial dysfunction (e.g., elevated cardiac filling pressures or low cardiac output) or ongoing hypoperfusion despite adequate intravascular volume and MAP	1C
Avoid the use of IV hydrocortisone if adequate fluid resuscitation and vasopressor therapy restore hemodynamic stability; if hydrocortisone is used, administer at a dose of 200 mg/day	2C
Target a hemoglobin level of 7–9 g/dL in patients without hypoperfusion, critical coronary artery disease or myocardial ischemia, or acute hemorrhage	1B
Infection control	
Obtain blood cultures before antibiotic therapy is administered	1C
Perform imaging studies promptly to confirm source of infection	UG
Administer broad-spectrum antibiotic therapy within 1 hour after diagnosis of either severe sepsis or septic shock	1B/1C
Reassess antibiotic therapy daily for de-escalation when appropriate	1B
Perform source control with attention to risks and benefits of the chosen method within 12 hours after diagnosis	1C
Respiratory support	
Use a low tidal volume and limitation of inspiratory-plateau-pressure strategy for ARDS	1A/1B
Apply a minimal amount of positive end-expiratory pressure in ARDS	1B
Administer higher rather than lower positive end-expiratory pressure for patients with sepsis-induced ARDS	2C

continued

Element of Care	Grade
Use recruitment maneuvers in patients with severe refractory hypoxemia due to ARDS	2C
Use prone positioning in patients with sepsis-induced ARDS and a ratio of the partial pressure of arterial oxygen (mm Hg) to the fraction of inspired oxygen of <100, in facilities that have experience with such practice	2C
Elevate the head of the bed in patients undergoing mechanical ventilation, unless contraindicated	1B
Use a conservative fluid strategy for established acute lung injury or ARDS with no evidence of tissue hypoperfusion	1C
Use weaning protocols	1A
Central nervous system (CNS) support	
Use sedation protocols, targeting specific dose-escalation end points	1B
Avoid neuromuscular blockers if possible in patients without ARDS	1C
Administer a short course of a neuromuscular blocker (<48 hours) for patients with early, severe ARDS	2C
General supportive care	
Use a protocol-specified approach to blood glucose management, with the initiation of insulin after two consecutive blood glucose levels of >180 mg/dL (10 mmol/L), targeting a blood glucose level of <180 mg/dL	1A
Use the equivalent of continuous veno-venous hemofiltration or intermittent hemodialysis as needed for renal failure or fluid overload	2B
Administer prophylaxis for deep-vein thrombosis	1B
Administer stress-ulcer prophylaxis to prevent upper gastrointestinal bleeding	1B
Administer oral or enteral feedings, as tolerated, rather than either complete fasting or provision of only IV glucose within the first 48 hours after a diagnosis of severe sepsis or septic shock	2C
Address goals of care, including treatment plans and end-of-life planning as appropriate	1B

ARDS, Acute respiratory distress syndrome.

Recommendations that are specific to pediatric severe sepsis include:

Therapy with face-mask oxygen, high-flow nasal cannula oxygen, or nasopharyngeal continuous positive end-expiratory pressure in the presence of respiratory distress and hypoxemia	2C
Use of physical examination therapeutic end points, such as capillary refill	2C
Administration of a bolus of 20 mL of crystalloids (or albumin equivalent) per kilogram of body weight during a period of 5–10 minutes for hypovolemia	2C
Increased use of inotropes and vasodilators in septic shock with low cardiac output associated with elevated systemic vascular resistance	2C
Use of hydrocortisone only in children with suspected or proven absolute adrenal insufficiency	2C

Determination of the Quality of Evidence[12]

A (high): Randomized controlled trials (RCTs)
B (moderate): Downgraded RCTs or upgraded observational studies
C (low): Well-done observational studies with control RCTs
D (very low): Downgraded controlled studies or expert opinion based on other evidence

Specific Infections

Major Classes of Bacteria

The next diagram represents types of bacteria important in clinical practice. Most of the time selection of appropriate empiric antibiotic therapy can be based on the type of microorganism.

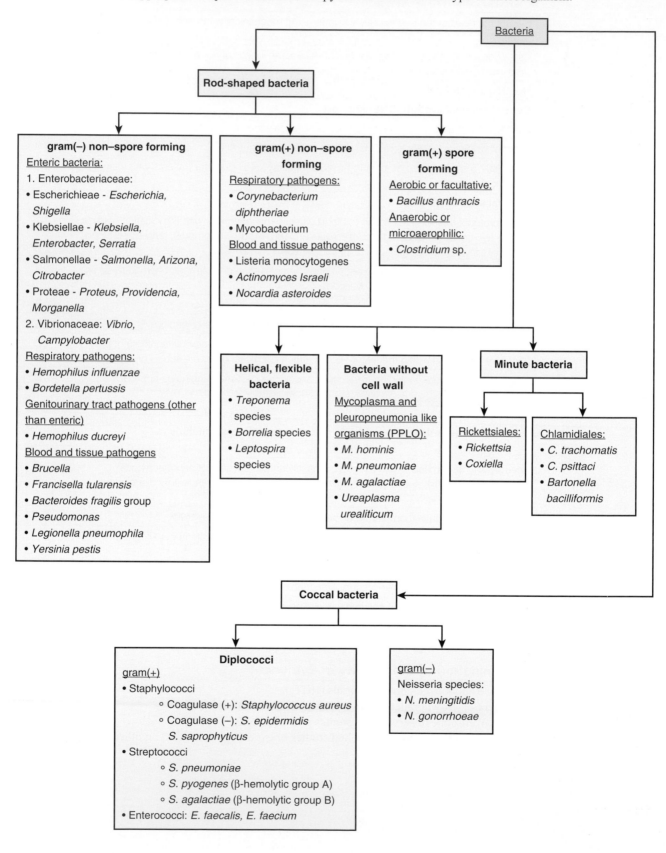

Major Classes of Antibiotics

Most important classes of antibiotics are based on the mechanism of action in the microorganism. In complex cases when combination therapy is used, antibiotics of different classes (affecting different elements of the bacterial cell) are preferable to use together.

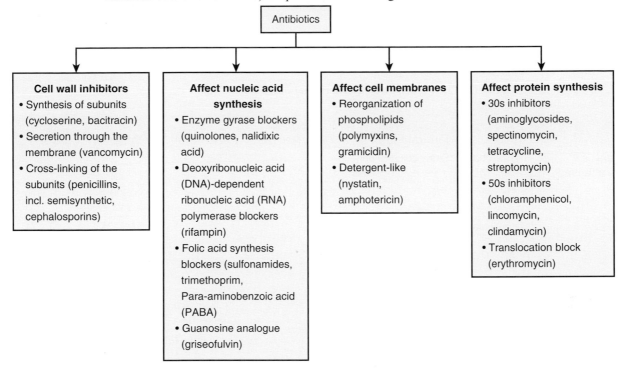

Quick Reference to Empiric Use of Antibiotics

Initiation of antibiotic therapy is frequently done with uncertainty of the exact nature of the pathogen, but most of the time cannot be delayed until microorganism identification. Below is a quick reference to guide initial use of antibiotics. More details on this subject are presented in the sections dealing with specific infections (e.g., pneumonia, urinary tract infection [UTI], endocarditis, meningitis).

	Most Common Microorganism	Empiric ABx
Common cold	Caused by rhinoviruses	No antibiotics
Sinusitis	75%—pneumococcus and *Haemophilus influenzae* Recent dental infection/foul smelling—anaerobes *Moraxella catarrhalis*—4% in adults, often in children *Staphylococcus*—very sick patient	Bactrim 3–7 days Ampicillin Amoxicillin
Meningitis	Pneumococci *H. influenzae*	Ceftriaxone ± ampicillin Vancomycin, rifampin for high-level resistance
Respiratory tract infection	*Pneumococcus, Chlamydia, Mycoplasma* *Haemophilus*	Erythromycin, clarithromycin, azithromycin Augmentin
Acute Strep pharyngitis	*Streptococcus*	Penicillin or erythromycin
Acute bronchitis		No benefits from the use of antibiotics
Exacerbation of chronic bronchitis		Very little benefit of antibiotics
Pneumonia	Multiple potential organisms	Third-generation cephalosporin + azithromycin
Infected implanted devices	Coagulase-negative *Staphylococcus*	Vancomycin + gentamicin
Sepsis with unknown pathogen		Aminoglycoside + ticarcillin-clavulanate or imipenem or third-generation cephalosporin Vancomycin + fluoroquinolones

	Most Common Microorganism	Empiric ABx
Sepsis in neutropenic patient		Aminoglycoside + antipseudomonal penicillin (ticarcillin-clavulanate or imipenem or third-generation cephalosporin or piperacillin or mezlocillin) If failed to respond add vancomycin after 48 hours, amphotericin after another 3–7 days

Diagnostic Tests

Diagnosis of infectious etiology based on body fluid analysis

		Pleural Fluid[13]	Peritoneal Fluid/Ascites[13]	Pericardial[13]	Synovial[14]	CSF[15]
Transudate (noninflammatory)	Physical characteristics	Straw colored, non-viscous, odorless				
	Leukocytes	<1000	<100		<1000 (normal <75)	0–5/mm³
	Predominate	Mononuclear			15%–25% Polymorphonuclear leukocytes (PMN)	
	Protein	<3 g/dL		<3, fluid/serum ratio <0.5		<40 mg/dL
	Glucose	>60 mg/dL		Fluid/serum ratio >1		40–70
	Other biochemistry	Lactate dehydrogenase (LDH) <200 IU, pH 7.45–7.55	High albumin gradient	Fluid/serum LDH ratio <0.6		
General exudate characteristics (inflammatory)	Leukocytes	>1000/µL, frequently 25,000–100,000	>100		<200–2000	>1000
	Predominate	PMN neutrophils	PMN neutrophils			PMN neutrophils
	Protein	>3 g/dL, pleural-to-serum ratio >0.5	Fluid/serum ratio ≥0.5	>3, fluid/serum ratio >0.5		>150 mg/dL (high)
	Glucose	<60 mg/dL		Fluid/serum ratio <1		<30 mg/dL (low)
	Other biochemistry	pH <7.3, elevated LDH (>200 IU, pleural-to-serum LDH >0.6), elevated cholesterol, C-reactive protein (CRP)	Elevated LDH (>400 IU, pleural-to-serum LDH >0.6), low albumin gradient, amylase >2000 U/L in pancreatic ascites, Blood urea nitrogen (BUN) and creatinine same or greater than serum in urine leak, high cholesterol, triglycerides in chylous ascites	Elevated LDH (>200 IU, fluid/serum LDH >0.6), fluid/serum cholesterol >0.3		

continued

		Pleural Fluid[13]	Peritoneal Fluid/Ascites[13]	Pericardial[13]	Synovial[14]	CSF[15]
Bacterial	Leukocytes	>1000/μL, frequently 25,000–100,000	>100	Exudate/inflammatory	>50,000	100–1000 or >1000
	Predominate	PMN neutrophils	PMN neutrophils		PMN (>75%)	PMN neutrophils
	Protein	>3 g/dL, pleural-to-serum ratio >0.5	Fluid/serum ratio ≥0.5			>150 mg/dL (high)
	Glucose	<60 mg/dL				<30 mg/dL (low)
	Other characteristics	pH < 7.3, elevated LDH (>200 IU, pleural-to-serum LDH >0.6), elevated cholesterol, CRP	Elevated LDH (>400 IU, pleural-to-serum LDH > 0.6), low albumin gradient			Opening pressure elevated (>20 cm), elevated lactate
TB	Leukocytes	5000–10,000	Exudate/inflammatory	Exudate/inflammatory	25,000	Usually <100
	Predominate	Mononuclear			PMN (50%)	Lymphocytes
	Protein					High or normal
	Glucose	Equal to serum level				low
	Other biochemistry	Adenosine deaminase >40 U/L	Adenosine deaminase >40	Adenosine deaminase >40		
Viral	Leukocytes	Transudate/noninflammatory	Transudate/noninflammatory	Transudate/noninflammatory	2000–20,000	10–1000, usually <100
	Predominate				Variable	Lymphocytes
	Protein					Elevated or normal
	Glucose					Normal
	Other biochemistry					Opening pressure normal or slightly elevated (20 cm)
Cancer	Leukocytes	1000–100,000	Exudate/inflammatory	Exudate/inflammatory		
	Predominate	Mononuclear				
	Protein	>3 g/dL, pleural-to-serum ratio > 0.5				
	Glucose	<60 mg/dL				
	Other biochemistry	Elevated LDH (>200 IU, pleural-to-serum LDH >0.6)				

		Pleural Fluid[13]	Peritoneal Fluid/Ascites[13]	Pericardial[13]	Synovial[14]	CSF[15]
Rheumatoid/ autoimmune	Leukocytes	1000–20,000	Exudate/inflam-matory	Exudate/inflam-matory	>2000–50,000	Normal (<15)
	Predominate	M or PMN				
	Protein					Elevated
	Glucose	<40 mg/dL				Normal
	Other bio-chemistry					

CRP, C-reactive protein.

Pneumonia

Pneumonia represents probably the most common infection among patients admitted to the Intensive care unit (ICU). Cases of severe pneumonia, frequently with respiratory failure, require ICU admission; however, some patients are admitted to medical floor and are transferred to ICU in a few days when their conditions deteriorate. Mortality among these cases has been reported to be higher.[16,17] Criteria for ICU admission listed below may be used as a guideline for patient triage.

Diagnostic Criteria for Pneumonia

- Constellation of suggestive clinical features
- Demonstrable infiltrate by chest radiograph is required for diagnosis of pneumonia
- Consider blood and sputum (or endotracheal aspirate) culture
- Urinary antigen tests for *Legionella pneumophila* and *Streptococcus pneumoniae*

Criteria for ICU Admission[16]

- Septic shock requiring vasopressors
- Acute respiratory failure requiring intubation and mechanical ventilation
- Three of the minor criteria for severe CAP:
  - Respiratory rate ≥30 breaths/min
  - PaO_2/FiO_2 ratio ≤250
- Multilobar infiltrates
- Confusion/disorientation
- Uremia (BUN level ≥20 mg/dL)
- Leukopenia (WBC count <4000 cells/mm^3)
- Thrombocytopenia (platelet count <100,000 cells/mm^3)
- Hypothermia (core temperature <36°C)
- Hypotension requiring aggressive fluid resuscitation

BUN, Blood urea nitrogen; *CAP*, community-acquired pneumonia; *WBC*, white blood cells.

Potential etiology of pneumonia

Typical: clinical features equated with *S. Pneumoniae* pneumonia: Onset of productive cough with green/yellow sputum, fever, chills, pleuritic chest pain, leukocytosis, lobar consolidation on chest x-ray (CXR)

Atypical: Gradual onset of irritating, non-productive cough, occasional scanty sputum, myalgias, arthralgias, upper respiratory tract symptoms, lack of consolidation on CXR

Streptococcus pneumoniae
Treatment: Cephalosporines, macrolides, quinolones

Hemophilus influenzae
Associated with: Chronic obstructive pulmonary disease (COPD), alcoholism, smoking, Human immunodeficiency virus (HIV)(+), elderly (Gram stain)
Treatment: Bactrim, ampicillin/sulbactam

Moraxella (Branhamella) catarrhalis
Associated with: Chronic lung disease, >50 age, immunocompromised
Treatment: Ampicillin/sulbactam, 3rd generation cephalosporines, macrolides

Klebsiella
Associated with: Diabetes mellitus (DM), alcoholism, COPD
Treatment: Ampicillin/sulbactam, piperacillin/tazobactam, ticarcillin/clavulanate, third-generation cephalosporines, quinolones, meropenem, ertapenem

Other: Fungi (e.g., *Coccidioides, Histoplasma*), Tuberculosis (TB)

In HIV/cellular immune dysfunction:
TB, *Coccidioides, Histoplasma, Aspergillus, Cryptococcus, Pneumocistis carinii*

Mycoplasma pneumoniae: 15%–35%
Associated with: Healthy young group, confined in closed quarters
Diagnosis: Rise in complement fixation antibody titer - for retrospective confirmation, serum cold agglutinins titer 1:64 or higher
Treatment: Macrolides

Legionella species*:* 1%–15%
Older patient, Hx of smoking, COPD
Diagnosis: Leg. pneum. antigen in the urine, direct fluorescent antibody in sputum, rise in antibody titer - for retrospective diagnosis
Treatment: Macrolides, quinolones, rifampin

Chlamydia pneumoniae: 6%–12% (rise in Ig M or G against Chlamydia)
Treatment: Doxycycline, macrolides

Viruses: Varicella-zoster, adenovirus, influenza A and B, Cytomegalovirus (CMV), Respiratory syncytial virus (RSV)
Treatment: Antiviral (oseltamivir, zanamivir)

HCAP (health–care associated)*:* Enteric organisms - gram(−): Klebsiella, *Pseudomonas*
NAP (nursing home–assoc. pneum): *Pseudomonas, E. coli, Enterobacter*
VAP (ventilator associated): Early onset - *Staphylococcus, Pseudomonas*, late onset - *Stenotrophomonas*

Community-Acquired Pneumonia

For the sake of completeness, we present the spectrum of severity of community-acquired pneumonia (CAP), though cases of less severe course of the disease are of less interest to critical care practitioners.

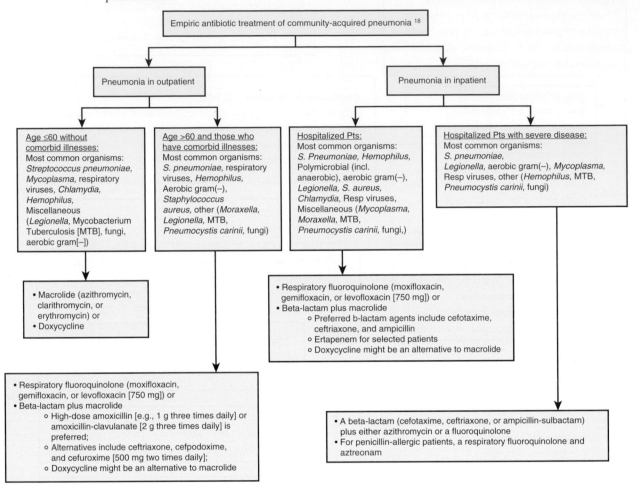

- Note: Early treatment (within 48 hours of the onset of symptoms) with oseltamivir or zanamivir is recommended for influenza. However, use of oseltamivir and zanamivir is not recommended for patients with uncomplicated influenza with symptoms for >48 hours.

Special Cases of CAP

CAP with septic shock or hypotension:
- fluid resuscitation
- treat per septic shock algorithm (see earlier in this chapter)
- consider drotrecogin alfa treatment patients who are at high risk of death
- screen for occult adrenal insufficiency

CAP with respiratory distress:
- try noninvasive ventilation
- intubate if severe hypoxemia (PaO_2/FiO_2 ratio <150) and bilateral alveolar infiltrates
- use low-tidal-volume ventilation (6 cm^3/kg of ideal body weight) if diffuse bilateral pneumonia or ARDS

Specific treatment and de-escalation of antibiotic therapy (change to antimicrobial Rx specific to etiology) is based on results of microbiology studies, once the potential pathogen is identified. Change from intravenous (IV) to oral antibiotics and duration of antibiotic therapy are discussed below.

Duration of ABx:

Switch from IV to oral prescription when hemodynamically stable, improving clinically, able to ingest medications, and have a normally functioning gastrointestinal tract.

Patients with CAP:

- treat for a minimum of 5 days
- should be afebrile for 48–72 hours

- should have no more than one CAP-associated sign of clinical instability before discontinuation of Rx (see criteria of clinical stability below)

Signs of Clinical Instability

- Temperature >37.8°C
- Heart rate >100 beats/min
- Respiratory rate >24 breaths/min

- Systolic blood pressure <90 mm Hg
- Arterial oxygen saturation <90% or pO$_2$ <60 mm Hg on room air
- Inability to maintain oral intake
- Altered mental status

Hospital-Acquired and Ventilator-Associated Pneumonia

Hospital-acquired (HAP) and ventilator-associated (VAP) pneumonia represent very common (~22%) of hospital-acquired infections. VAP is common in patients requiring mechanical ventilation, about 10% of the latter are diagnosed with VAP, which is associated with much higher mortality risk.[19] Risk factors for HAP/VAP include mechanical ventilation for longer than 20 days, male sex, the cause of ICU admission (specifically: multiple trauma, sepsis, Central nervous system [CNS] disease, and endocrine system and respiratory disease). Other important risk factors are invasive respiratory procedures, e.g., reintubation, tracheostomy, and bronchoscopy.[20]

Additional issues with Hospital-acquired pneumonia (HAP) and Ventilator-associated pneumonia (VAP)[19]

- HAP develops in hospitalised patients after 48 hours of admission.
- VAP occurs in ICU patients who have received mechanical ventilation for at least 48 hours.

- Recommended to obtain samples of respiratory secretions to identify the causative agent of nosocomial pneumonia before commencing antibiotic treatment.
- If samples are obtained within 48 hours of the start of antibiotic treatment the result may be altered or emerge as negative.

Diagnostic Points

- Noninvasive sampling (endotracheal aspiration) is preferred rather than invasive sampling: bronchoscopic

- Techniques (i.e., bronchoalveolar lavage [BAL], protected specimen brush [PSB]) and blind bronchial sampling)
- Diagnostic threshold for VAP (PSB with < 10^3 colony-forming units [CFU]/mL, BAL with < 10^4 CFU/mL)— if invasive sampling and quantitative cultures are preformed

Initial treatment of HAP/VAP should be based on antibiogram of the specific institution, which would help to reduce the development of resistant infection, minimize antibiotic use, specifically avoid the unnecessary use of methicillin-resistant *Staphylococcus aureus* (MRSA) coverage, use short courses of antibiotics and use a de-escalation strategy once the organism is identified.[19] Empiric treatment of HAP/VAP is discussed below. Decision to treat is based on clinical criteria.

General Principle of Antibiotics Therapy

- Initiation of Antibiotics (ABx) based on clinical criteria, while biomarkers (procalcitonin, sTREM-1, CRP) are not helpful
- Optimal choice of antibiotics based on each hospital antibiogram

- Minimize exposure to unnecessary antibiotics and reduce the development of antibiotic resistance
  - Use antibiogram data to decrease the unnecessary use of dual Gram-negative and empiric MRSA coverage
  - Short-course antibiotic therapy for most patients with HAP or VAP independent of microbial etiology
  - Antibiotic de-escalation

Below we list some of the antibiotics available for treatment of HAP/VAP. This is followed by the algorithm to select empiric antibiotic therapy based on local antibiogram, suspected infection, and patient's mortality risk.

Antibiotics Used in Treatment of HAP/VAP

Gram-positive antibiotics with MRSA activity:
- Vancomycin 15 mg/kg IV q8–12h (consider a loading dose of 25–30 mg/kg × 1 for severe illness)
- Linezolid 600 mg IV q12h

Gram-negative antibiotics with antipseudomonal activity: beta-lactam–based agents
- Piperacillin-tazobactam 4.5 g IV q6h
- Cefepime 2 g IV q8h
- Ceftazidime 2 g IV q8h
- Imipenem 500 mg IV q6h
- Meropenem 1 g IV q8h
- Aztreonam 2 g IV q8h

Gram-negative antibiotics with antipseudomonal activity: non–beta-lactam–based agents
- Ciprofloxacin 400 mg IV q8h
- Levofloxacin 750 mg IV q24h
- Amikacin 15–20 mg/kg IV q24h
- Gentamicin 5–7 mg/kg IV q24h
- Tobramycin 5–7 mg/kg IV q24h
- Colistin 5 mg/kg IV × 1 (loading dose) followed by 2.5 mg × (1.5 × CrCl + 30) IV q12h (maintenance dose)
- Polymyxin B 2.5–3.0 mg/kg/day divided into two daily IV doses

Empiric therapy for HAP

Initial choice of antibiotics is based upon
• Local antibiogram and local distribution of pathogens associated with VAP
• HAP patients Rx needs to include coverage for *Staphylococcus aureus,* and in addition in those with suspected VAP also for *Pseudomonas aeruginosa,* and other gram-negative bacilli in all empiric regimens

S. aureus coverage
• Cover for MRSA (vancomycin or linezolid) only if risk factor for MRSA infection are present:
  ◦ Risk for antimicrobial resistance (see below)
  ◦ Units with high prevalence (>10% of *S. aureus* are MRSA) or unknown prevalence
  ◦ High risk of mortality
• If no risk factors of MRSA (see above) and not a high risk for mortality – ABx with MSSA activity (piperacillin-tazobactam, cefepime, levofloxacin, imipenem, or meropenem) should be used

Pseudomonas and other gram-negative coverage:
• Avoid aminoglycosides and colistin if alternative agents are available
• Aminoglycoside should not be used as the sole antipseudomonal agent
• If two agents are to be used – avoid two beta-lactam ABx
• Two antipseudomonal antibiotics from different classes for the empiric treatment of suspected VAP <u>only</u> in patients with any of the following:
  ◦ Units where >10% of gram-negative isolates are resistant to an agent being considered for monotherapy or local antimicrobial susceptibility rates are not available
  ◦ Risk factor for antimicrobial resistance (see below)

Risk factors for multidrug-resistant pathogens in HAP and VAP
• In HAP (including VAP): Prior intravenous antibiotic use within 90 days
• In addition, risk factors for MDR in VAP:
  ◦ Septic shock at time of VAP
  ◦ ARDS preceding VAP
  ◦ Five or more days of hospitalization prior to the occurrence of VAP
  ◦ Acute renal replacement therapy prior to VAP onset

In summary suggested empiric treatment for HAP
• For patients not at high risk of mortality and no factors increasing the likelihood of MRSA: <u>One ABx from the right (not aminoglycoside and not colistin).</u> If VAP is suspected—same approach, but always use the ABx with *Pseudomonas* coverage
• For those patients not at high risk of mortality but with factors increasing the likelihood of MRSA: <u>One ABx from the left plus one from the right</u>
• For patients with high risk of mortality or receipt of intravenous antibiotics during the prior 90 days: <u>Two Abx from the right (avoid two beta-lactam) plus one from the left</u>

• Vancomycin 15 mg/kg IV q8–12h with goal to target 15–20 mg/mL trough level (consider a loading dose of 25–30 mg/kg IV × 1 for severe illness)
• Linezolid 600 mg IV q12h

• Piperacillin-tazobactam 4.5 g IV q6h
• Cefepime 2 g IV q8h
• Levofloxacin 750 mg IV daily
• Imipenem 500 mg IV q6h
• Meropenem 1 g IV q8h
• Amikacin 15–20 mg/kg IV daily
• Gentamicin 5–7 mg/kg IV daily
• Tobramycin 5–7 mg/kg IV daily
• Aztreonam 2 g IV q8h

Antibiotic De-Escalation in HAP

Once culture results are back and pathogen is established, antibiotic regimen is de-escalated and narrowed to specific microorganism, as discussed below.

Duration, De-Escalation, Discontinuation of Rx

- VAP or HAP: 7-day course
- De-escalate ABx, which means change empiric broad-spectrum antibiotic regimen to a narrower mono-

therapy antibiotic regimen by changing the antimicrobial agent
- Use procalcitonin and clinical criteria to guide the discontinuation of antibiotic therapy

---

Principles of pathogen-specific therapy

- MRSA: Vancomycin or linezolid
- *P. aeruginosa:*
  - Rx should be used upon the results of antimicrobial susceptibility testing
  - Recommendations are against aminoglycoside monotherapy
  - Monotherapy (other than aminoglycoside) using an antibiotic to which the isolate is susceptible is recommended (unless in septic shock or high risk of death)
  - If in septic shock or high risk of death: Combination therapy using two antibiotics to which the isolate is susceptible
    - An antipneumococcal, antipseudomonal b-lactam (piperacillin-tazobactam, cefepime, imipenem, or meropenem) plus either ciprofloxacin or levofloxacin (750 mg dose) OR
    - The above b-lactam plus an aminoglycoside and azithromycin OR
    - The above b-lactam plus an aminoglycoside and an antipneumococcal fluoroquinolone (for penicillin-allergic patients, substitute aztreonam for the above b-lactam)
- Extended-Spectrum β-Lactamase (ESBL)–producing Gram-negative bacilli: Based upon the results of antimicrobial susceptibility testing and patient-specific factors (i.e., allergies and comorbidities)
- *Acinetobacter* species
  - Either a carbapenem or ampicillin/sulbactam if the isolate is susceptible
  - If sensitive only to polymyxins → IV polymyxin (colistin or polymyxin B) plus adjunctive inhaled colistin
  - If sensitive only to colistin, do not use adjunctive rifampicin (potential adverse effects)
  - Recommendations are against the use of tigecycline
- Carbapenem-resistant pathogens
  - If sensitive only to polymyxins, then use intravenous polymyxins (colistin or polymyxin B)
  - Inhaled colistin may have potential pharmacokinetic advantages compared to inhaled polymyxin B

MRSA-Related Pneumonia[21]

Since MRSA infection is common, we specifically discuss the treatment of pneumonia with suspected (based on the severity) or demonstrated MRSA as a causative organism.

Is It Severe Pneumonia?

Pneumonia considered severe if:
- a requirement for ICU admission

- necrotizing or cavitary infiltrates
- empyema

For Severe Pneumonia

Empirical therapy for MRSA is recommended pending sputum and/or blood culture results

Once cultures are back and MRSA pneumonia is demonstrated	• Linezolid 600 mg PO/IV twice daily or clindamycin 600 mg PO/IV three times daily, if the strain is susceptible for 7–21 days, depending on the extent of infection
• IV vancomycin or	• If empyema—needs to be drained in addition to ABx

Nonresolving Pneumonia

Despite adequate therapy some cases of pneumonia either deteriorate or fail to improve. In general, this has to do with the high severity at presentation, inappropriate coverage, misdiagnosis, or complication (infectious or noninfectious) of the original disease.

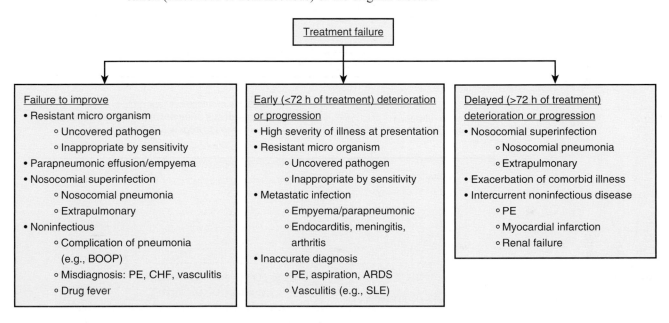

Meningitis

Etiology of Meningitis[22]	• Viral
• Bacterial	• Fungal

Most Common Bacterial Pathogens in the United States	• *Neisseria meningitidis* (meningococcus) (14%)
• *S. pneumoniae* (pneumococcus) (58%)	• *H. influenzae* (7%)
• Group B *Streptococcus* (18%)	• *Listeria monocytogenes* (3%)

Fungi Causing Meningitis

- *Cryptococcus neoformans*
- *Coccidioides immitis*

- *Aspergillus*
- *Candida*
- Mucormycosis (more common in DM; direct extension of sinus infection)

DM, Diabetes mellitus.

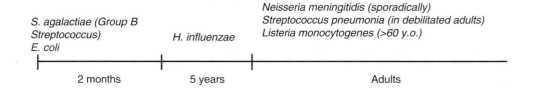

Etiology of meningitis[22]
- Bacterial
- Viral
- Fungal

Most common bacterial pathogens in the US
Streptococcus pneumonia (*Pneumococcus*) (58%)
group B *Streptococcus* (18%)
Neisseria meningitides (*Meningococcus*) (14%)
H-emophilus influenzae (7%)
Listeria monocytogenes (3%)

Fungi causing meningitis
- *Cryptococcus neoformans*
- *Coccidioides immitis*
- *Aspergillus*
- *Candida*
- Mucormycosis (more common in DM; direct extension of sinus infection)

Bacterial meningitis: Likely etiology in age groups

S. agalactiae (Group B Streptococcus)
E. coli
— 2 months —
H. influenzae
— 5 years —
Neisseria meningitidis (sporadically)
Streptococcus pneumonia (in debilitated adults)
Listeria monocytogenes (>60 y.o.)
Adults

Diagnosis

- Definitive diagnosis is based on the analysis of cerebrospinal fluid (CSF)
- CT is recommended prior to lumbar puncture (LP) in some patients (concern for herniation caused by LP, although incidence is <5%[23])
- Delay LP and perform CT if signs of impending herniation:
  - Glasgow Coma Scale (GCS) less than 11
  - Lethargy
  - Altered mental status
  - New-onset seizures
  - Focal neurologic deficit

- Lumbar puncture and CSF analysis
  - Pleiocytosis (>100 cells/mm^3)
  - Predominance of polynuclear neutrophils (>80%)
  - CSF/serum glucose <0.4
  - CSF protein >2 g/L
- Clinical biomarkers[23]
  - CSF lactate >3.5 mmol/mL
  - Serum procalcitonin level >0.3 ng/mL
  - High CRP
- Multiplex PCR for presence of bacterial genome in CSF

CT, Computed tomography; *PCR,* polymerase chain reaction.

Suspected meningitis needs to be treated immediately. Empiric choice of antibiotics is based primarily on patient's age.

> **Empiric antimicrobial treatment**
> Suitable treatment should be instituted within 60 minutes of admitting the patient

Neonates
- Ampicillin 100 mg/kg IV (or 50 mg/kg if >1 month old)
- Cefotaxime 75 mg/kg IV or Gentamicin 2.5 mg/kg IV if ≤1 month old or Ceftriaxone if >1 month old
- Acyclovir IV 40 mg/kg

Adults
- Ceftriaxone 2 g IV
- Vancomycin 20 mg/kg IV
- Add Ampicillin 2 g IV if >50 years old

Other special cases of meningitis

Meningitis associated with foreign body (post-procedure, penetrating trauma)
- Cefepime 2 g IV or Ceftazidime 2 g IV or Meropenem 2 g IV and
- Vancomycin 20 mg/kg IV

Meningitis with severe penicillin allergy
- Chloramphenicol 1 g IV and
- Vancomycin 20 mg/kg IV

Fungal (Cryptococcal) meningitis
- Amphotericin B 1 mg/kg IV and
- Flucytosine 25 mg/kg by mouth

Other Treatment Considerations

Steroids
- Dexamethasone 10 mg IV before or with the first dose of antibiotics
- No dexamethasone if the patient has already received antibiotics
- Oral glycerol is an alternative instead of IV dexamethasone[24]

To reduce intracranial pressure, if patient is symptomatic:
- Elevating the head of the bed to 30 degrees
- Inducing mild hyperventilation in the intubated patient
- Osmotic diuretics such as 25% mannitol or 3% saline

CNS Infection Caused by MRSA[21]

ABx
- IV vancomycin ± rifampin 600 mg daily or 300–450 mg twice daily
- Alternatively: linezolid 600 mg PO/IV twice daily or TMP-SMX 5 mg/kg/dose IV every 8–12 hours

Duration
- Meningitis: for 2 weeks
- Brain abscess, subdural empyema, spinal epidural abscess: for 4–6 weeks
- Septic thrombosis of cavernous or dural venous sinus: for 4–6 weeks

Interventions
- For CNS shunt infection—shunt removal, do not replace until CSF cultures are repeatedly negative
- For brain abscess, subdural empyema, spinal epidural abscess: incision and drainage by neurosurgery
- Septic thrombosis of cavernous or dural venous sinus: incision and drainage of contiguous sites of infection or abscess

TMP-SMX, Trimethoprim/sulfamethoxazole.

Osteomyelitis

Osteomyelitis is an infectious process with inflammation of the bone. Infection might spread from localized source (local wound/ulcer) or be secondary to hematogenic spread. It might be important in selecting empiric treatment since localized infections are frequently polymicrobial, while those caused by hematogenic spread are usually due to single organism.[25]

Diagnosis

- Laboratory tests: WBC, ESR, CRP, IL-6 (infection associated with joint prosthesis)
- Imaging
  - Plain X-ray not very sensitive especially early in the course
  - MRI is considered the main type of imaging, including early disease

  - o CT is of little utility in the diagnosis of acute infection
  - o Ultrasound reveals edema of soft tissue around the bones
  - o PET-CT has good specificity and sensitivity
  - o Nuclear bone scan (using indium is more specific than gallium or technetium)
- Pathology: bone biopsy with demonstration of pathogen in bone is a definitive test

---

ESR, Erythrocyte sedimentation rate; *IL-6*, interleukin-6; *MRI*, magnetic resonance imaging; *PET-CT*, positron emission tomography-computed tomography.

Classification Based on Chronicity

- Acute: initial episodes of osteomyelitis. Edema, formation of pus, vascular congestion, thrombosis of the small vessels

- Chronic: recurrence of acute cases. Large areas of ischemia, necrosis and bone sequestration

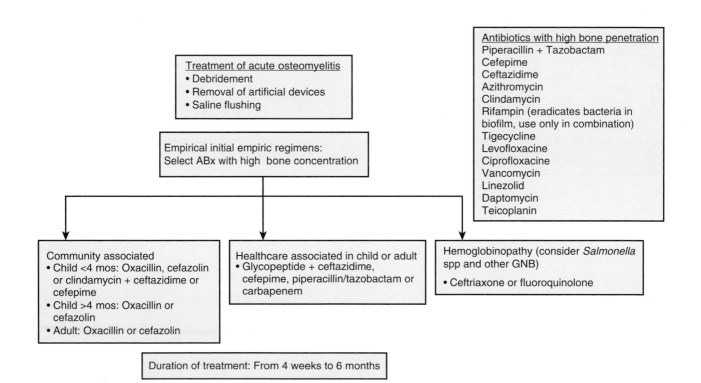

Treatment of Chronic Infections

- Extensive debridement, remove all devitalized tissue
- Wound closure by all means when vital structures are exposed
- Vacuum-assisted closure
- Remove synthetic materials
- Duration of antibiotics 3–6 months

MRSA Bone and Joint Infections

MRSA osteomyelitis and arthritis are relatively common and probably deserve special discussion. As in general case of osteomyelitis, the treatment is based on aggressive debridement and long course of antibiotics.[21]

MRSA Osteomyelitis

- MRI with gadolinium is the imaging modality of choice for osteomyelitis
- Debridement and drainage for osteomyelitis and septic arthritis
- IV or oral antibiotics can be used
  - IV:
    - Vancomycin
    - Daptomycin (6 mg/kg/dose daily)
- IV or oral:
  - TMP-SMX 4 mg/kg/dose (TMP component) BID in combination with rifampin 600 mg once daily
  - Linezolid 600 mg twice daily
  - Clindamycin 600 mg every 8 hours
  - Rifampin 600 mg daily or 300–450 mg PO twice daily might be added to any regimen above

Duration

- For septic arthritis 3–4 weeks of therapy
- Minimum 8 weeks for osteomyelitis
- For chronic infection or if debridement is not performed: 1–3 months (and possibly longer) of oral rifampin-based Rx

with TMP-SMX, doxycycline-minocycline, clindamycin, or a fluoroquinolone chosen on the basis of susceptibilities
- ESR and/or CRP levels can be used to guide response to therapy

Infective Endocarditis

Infective endocarditis diagnostic criteria[26]

Major criteria
- Isolation of *Streptococcus viridans*, *S. Bovis*, HACEK-group, or (in the absence of primary focus) community-acquired *S. aureus* or *Enterococcus* from two separate blood cultures or isolation of a microorganism consistent with endocarditis in
  - Blood cultures ≥12 h apart
  - All of three or most of four or more blood cultures, with first and last at least 1 h apart
- Evidence of endocarditis involvement on echo: Echocardiogram positive for IE (TEE recommended for patients with prosthetic valves, rated at least possible IE by clinical criteria, or complicated IE [paravalvular abscess]; TTE as first test in other patients)
- Single positive blood culture for *Coxiella burnetii* or anti–phase 1 IgG antibody titer ≥1:800

Minor criteria
- Risk factors: Predisposing lesion or IV drug use
- Fever ≥38.0°C
- Emboli: Major arterial emboli, septic pulmonary infarcts, mycotic aneurysm, intracranial hemorrhage, conjunctival hemorrhage, Janeway lesions
- Vasculitidis: Glomerulonephritis, Osler's node, Roth's spots, rheumatoid factor
- Culture: Positive blood cultures not meeting the major criterion or serologic evidence of active infection with organism that causes endocarditis

Definite IE
2 major + 0 minor
1 major + 3 minor
0 major + 5 minor

Possible IE
1 Major + 1 minor criterion, or 3 minor criteria

Definite IE	Possible IE
2 Major + 0 minor 1 Major + 3 minor 0 Major + 5 minor	1 Major + 1 minor criterion, or 3 minor criteria

Prevention of infective endocarditis (IE) is outside the scope of critical care; it is a primary care topic, but it is important for patient counseling, e.g., patients who recovered from a prior episode of IE should be advised to use prophylaxis prior to invasive procedures as discussed below.

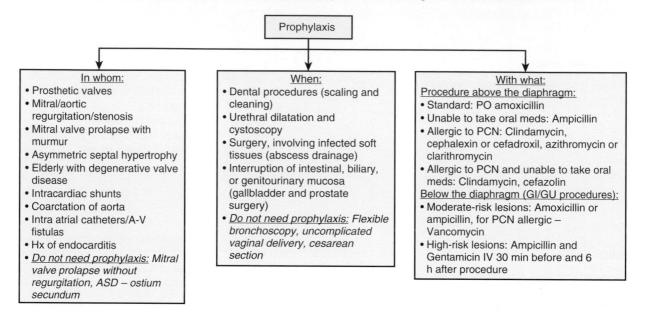

Prophylaxis

In whom:
- Prosthetic valves
- Mitral/aortic regurgitation/stenosis
- Mitral valve prolapse with murmur
- Asymmetric septal hypertrophy
- Elderly with degenerative valve disease
- Intracardiac shunts
- Coarctation of aorta
- Intra atrial catheters/A-V fistulas
- Hx of endocarditis
- *Do not need prophylaxis: Mitral valve prolapse without regurgitation, ASD – ostium secundum*

When:
- Dental procedures (scaling and cleaning)
- Urethral dilatation and cystoscopy
- Surgery, involving infected soft tissues (abscess drainage)
- Interruption of intestinal, biliary, or genitourinary mucosa (gallbladder and prostate surgery)
- *Do not need prophylaxis: Flexible bronchoscopy, uncomplicated vaginal delivery, cesarean section*

With what:
Procedure above the diaphragm:
- Standard: PO amoxicillin
- Unable to take oral meds: Ampicillin
- Allergic to PCN: Clindamycin, cephalexin or cefadroxil, azithromycin or clarithromycin
- Allergic to PCN and unable to take oral meds: Clindamycin, cefazolin
Below the diaphragm (GI/GU procedures):
- Moderate-risk lesions: Amoxicillin or ampicillin, for PCN allergic – Vancomycin
- High-risk lesions: Ampicillin and Gentamicin IV 30 min before and 6 h after procedure

Below is a simplified approach to empiric treatment of IE. It is important to note that *S. aureus* endocarditis incidence is growing, and it is now the leading cause of IE in developed countries.

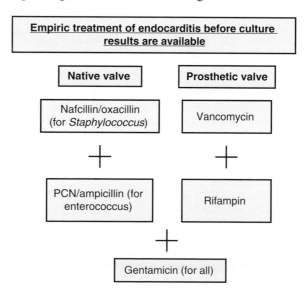

Empiric treatment of endocarditis before culture results are available

Native valve	Prosthetic valve
Nafcillin/oxacillin (for *Staphylococcus*)	Vancomycin
+	+
PCN/ampicillin (for enterococcus)	Rifampin

+

Gentamicin (for all)

Empiric Treatment of Infectious Endocarditis

Once blood culture is positive, antibiotic regimen is changed accordingly. Culture-negative endocarditis is treated based on epidemiological clues discussed below.[26]

Diagnostic clues for most likely causative organism based on clinical scenario/comorbidities/risk factors

Based on specific comorbidities

Genitourinary disorders, infection, and manipulation, including pregnancy, delivery, and abortion

- *Enterococcus* sp
- Group B streptococci (S agalactiae)
- *Listeria monocytogenes*
- Aerobic Gram-negative bacilli
- *Neisseria gonorrhoeae*

Chronic skin disorders, including recurrent infections

- *S. aureus*
- β-Hemolytic streptococci

Diabetes mellitus

- *S. aureus*
- β-Hemolytic streptococci
- *S. pneumoniae*

Pneumonia, meningitis

- *S. pneumoniae*

Burns

- *S. aureus*
- Aerobic Gram-negative bacilli, including *Pseudomonas aeruginosa*
- Fungi

Gastrointestinal lesions

- *S. gallolyticus (bovis)*
- *Enterococcus* sp.
- *Clostridium septicum*

Solid organ transplantation

- *S. aureus*
- *Aspergillus fumigatus*
- *Enterococcus* sp.
- *Candida* sp.

Valve replacement and cardiovascular indwelling devices

Indwelling cardiovascular medical devices

- *S. aureus*
- Coagulase-negative staphylococci
- Fungi
- Aerobic Gram-negative bacilli
- *Corynebacterium* sp.

Prosthetic valve placement

- Coagulase-negative staphylococci
- *S. aureus*
- Fungi
- *Corynebacterium* sp.
- *Legionella* sp. (within 1 year after placement)
- Aerobic Gram-negative bacilli (within 1 year after placement)
- *Viridans* group streptococci (>1 year after placement)
- *Enterococcus* species (>1 year after placement)

Based on social history and history of substance abuse

IVDU

- *S. aureus*, including community-acquired oxacillin-resistant strains
- Coagulase-negative staphylococci
- β-Hemolytic streptococci
- Fungi
- Aerobic Gram-negative bacilli, including *P. aeruginosa*
- Polymicrobial

Alcoholism, cirrhosis

- *Bartonella* sp.
- *Aeromonas* sp.
- *Listeria* sp.
- *S. pneumoniae*
- β-Hemolytic streptococci

Homeless, body lice

- *Bartonella* sp.
- AIDS *Salmonella* sp.
- *S. pneumoniae*
- *S. aureus*

Poor dental health, dental procedures

- *Viridans* group streptococci
- Nutritionally variant streptococci
- *Abiotrophia defectiva*
- *Granulicatella* sp.
- *Gemella* sp.
- HACEK organisms

History of exposure

Contact with contaminated milk or infected farm animals

- *Brucella* sp.
- *Coxiella burnetii*
- *Erysipelothrix* sp.

Dog or cat exposure

- *Bartonella* sp.
- *Pasteurella* sp.
- *Capnocytophaga* sp.

Surgical Treatment of Infectious Endocarditis

Antibiotics are the main component of therapy; in addition, surgery is indicated in many cases; it might need to be performed urgently or can be delayed in a selected patient population.[26]

Indications for surgery
- Refractory CHF
- Uncontrolled infection/relapse of infection following adequate course of ABx
- Severe valvular dysfunction/local suppurative complication by echo/evidence of intracardiac infection (block, abscess, heart failure, rupture of papillary muscle/chordae tendineae/valve)
- >1 serious systemic embolic event
- Mycotic aneurism
- Large vegetations
- Prosthetic valve endocarditis
- Endocarditis caused by fungi or Pseudomonas

Early surgery[27]
- High embolic risk
  - Vegetation >10 mm
  - Mobile vegetation
  - Mitral valve vegetation (anterior leaflet)
- Virulent species (e.g., *S. aureus*, fungal)
- Cerebral abscess
- Prosthetic valve endocarditis
- CHF

Delayed surgery[27]
- Decreased level of consciousness/coma
- Ongoing sepsis
- Low life expectancy/multi-organ failure
- Ruptured infectious aneurism

MRSA Bacteremia and Infective Endocarditis[21]

Above we discuss the management of endocarditis in general. Specific issues pertinent to management of MRSA-related bacteremia and endocarditis are also discussed here. Treatment of bacteremia (complicated and uncomplicated) and endocarditis is summarized in the following diagram. It is noted that there is no role for adding gentamycin or rifampin to vancomycin.

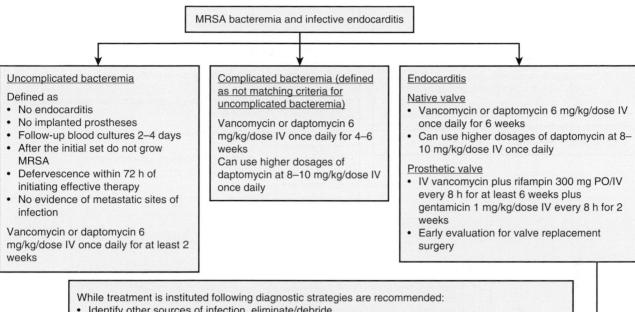

Selected UTI Scenarios

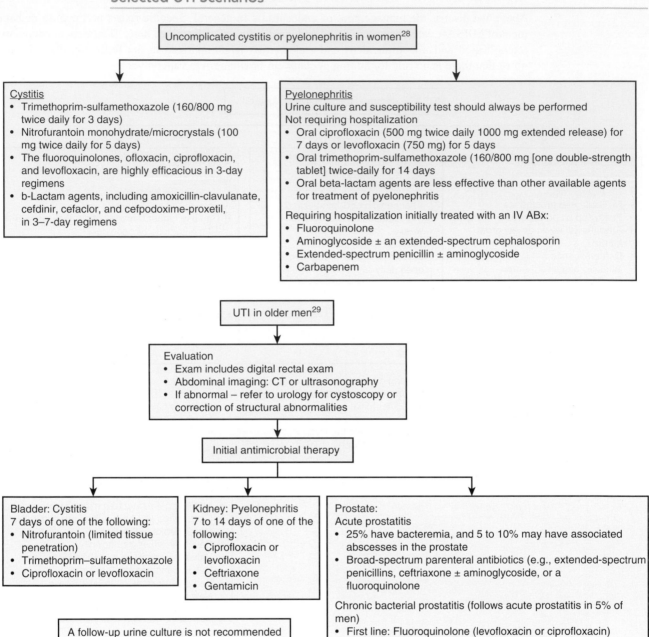

Catheter-Associated Bacteriuria and UTI

Please note the role of pyuria in the diagnosis of UTI; in the catheterized patient, pyuria must be present for the diagnosis but by itself is not sufficient to make a diagnosis.

- In the catheterized patient, pyuria (and odorous or cloudy urine) is not diagnostic of catheter associated (CA)-bacteriuria or CA-UTI; also it does not differentiate UTI from asymptomatic bacteriuria (ASB)
- Pyuria (and odorous or cloudy urine) without UTI should not be treated with ABx
- No UTI without pyuria

↓

CA-UTI vs CA-ASB

Diagnosis of catheter-associated UTI (CA-UTI)[30]
- Symptoms or signs compatible with UTI with no other identified source of infection
- ≥1000 colonyforming units (cfu)/mL of one bacterial species
- Urethral, suprapubic, or condom catheter has been removed within the previous 48 h

Diagnosis of catheter-associated ASB
- In a man with a condom catheter - presence of ≥100,000 cfu/mL of one bacterial species
- Freshly applied condom catheter
- No UTI symptoms
- Note: Screening for catheter-associated asymptomatic bacteriuria (CA-ASB) is not recommended

Symptoms of UTI
- In patients with catheter in place: New onset or worsening of fever, rigors, altered mental status, malaise, or lethargy with no other identified cause; flank pain; costovertebral angle tenderness; pelvic discomfort; acute hematuria;
- In those whose catheters have been removed: Dysuria, urgent or frequent urination, or suprapubic pain or tenderness
- In patients with spinal cord injury, increased spasticity, autonomic dysreflexia, or sense of unease are also compatible with CA-UTI

Treatment of CA-UTI
- Obtain urine culture prior to ABx start
- In CA-UTI remove or replace catheters that have been in place for >2 weeks
- Women ≤65 with CA-UTI, but without upper UTI symptoms – consider 3 days of Rx
- After start of ABx if prompt resolution of symptoms – treat for 7 days
- If delayed resolution of symptoms – treat for 10–14 days

Prevention of CA-UTI:
- Limit catheter use: e.g., incontinence is almost never an indication
- Remove catheter as soon as it is not required
- Insertion technique
- Consider condom catheter in men and intermittent catheterization as alternative to indwelling catheter
- Suprapubic rather than short-term indwelling catheter
- Unclear if suprapubic catheterization is better than long-term indwelling catheter and if intermittent catheterization is better than suprapubic
- Closed catheter system, preconnected system
- Antimicrobial coated catheters
- No role for systemic ABx prophylaxis

Skin and Soft Tissue Infections

Empiric treatment of skin and soft tissue infections targets *Staphylococci* in purulent infections and *Streptococci* in infections with nonpurulent presentation. In all cases of purulent infections (e.g., abscess), treatment involves incision and drainage.[31,33]

Treatment of skin and soft tissue infections

Purulent (abscess, furuncle, carbuncle) – target *Staphylococcus*

Empiric therapy
- I&D
- ABx
    - If severe: Vancomycin or daptomycin or linezolid or televancin or ceftaroline
    - If moderate: TMP/SMX or doxycycline
    - If mild: No ABx

Defined therapy
- MRSA
    - If severe – same as empiric Rx
    - If moderate – TMP/SMX
- MSSA
    - If severe – nafcillin or cefazolin or clindamycin
    - If moderate – dicloxacillin or cephalexin

Non-purulent (cellulitis, necrotizing infection, erysipelas) – target *Streptococcus*

Empiric therapy
- If severe: Surgical inspection/debridement, rule out necrotizing process, vancomycin + Zosyn
- If moderate: IV ABx penicillin or ceftriaxone or cefazoline or clindamycin
- If mild: Oral ABx penicillin or cephazolin or dicloxacillin or clindamycin

Defined therapy
- Monomicrobial
    - *Streptococcus pyogenes* or *Clostridia*: Penicillin plus clindamycin
    - *Vibrio vulnificus*: Doxycycline plus ceftazidime
    - *Aeromonas hydrophila*: Doxycycline plus ciprofloxacin
- Polymicrobial: Vancomycin + Zosyn

Some of the Newer Agents Used in Skin and Soft tissue Infections[32]	
Dalbavancin	Gram-positive organisms, including *S. aureus* (MSSA and MRSA), coagulase-negative staphylococci (CoNS), *Streptococcus* spp., and *Enterococcus* spp. In vitro activity against rarer Gram-positive pathogens (*L. monocytogenes*, *Micrococcus* spp., and *Corynebacterium* spp.). Eightfold and 16-fold greater in vitro activity against *S. aureus* than daptomycin and vancomycin, respectively
Oritavancin	Gram-positive organisms, including *S. aureus* (MSSA, MRSA, vancomycin-intermediate *S. aureus* [VISA], vancomycin-resistant *S. aureus* [VRSA]), CoNS, streptococci, and enterococci, including VRE. Also, *L. monocytogenes*, *Micrococcus* spp., and *Corynebacterium* spp.
Tedizolid	Staphylococci, streptococci, and enterococci
Retapamulin	Staph and Strep, including MRSA strains. Also *Propionibacterium*, *Fusobacterium*, and other Gram-positive cocci
Ozenoxacin	Gram-positive organisms including MRSA, CoNS, and streptococcal species
Delafloxacin	Gram-positive organisms, including MSSA and MRSA, Also, similar Gram-negative spectrum of activity to other fluoroquinolones and is also active against anaerobic organisms
Fosfomycin	MRSA, VRE, resistant Enterobacteriaceae, and *Pseudomonas aeruginosa*

MSSA, Methicillin-sensitive *S. aureus*; *VRE*, vancomycin-resistant enterococci.

MRSA Skin and Soft Tissue Infections[21]

Below we discuss skin and soft tissue infections caused specifically by MRSA, since it is common and requires aggressive treatment. As described above, drainage of the abscess is a necessary part of management; in addition, antibiotics are used in more severe cases.

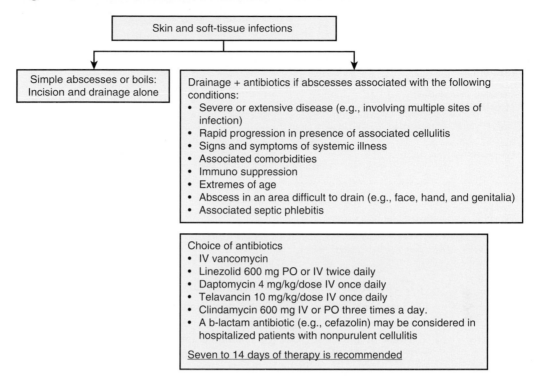

Necrotizing Fasciitis[33]

Necrotizing fasciitis is a special case of soft tissue infection; it is considered a medical as well as surgical emergency, needs to be quickly recognized, and requires prompt treatment with surgical debridement and antibiotics.

Necrotizing fasciitis	
Type 1 Polymicrobial infections usually caused by non–group A streptococcus, other aerobic and anaerobic micro organisms (e.g., *E. coli, A. hydrophila, V. vulnificus, Vibrio* spp. and *Aeromonas* spp)	**Type 2** Caused by *Streptococcus pyogenes* alone or with *Staphylococci* (predominant pathogens in the USA and Europe)

Predisposing Factors

- Immunosuppression
- DM
- Malignancy
- Drug abuse
- Chronic renal disease
- Liver cirrhosis and chronic hepatitis

Early Signs

- Pain, tenderness, swelling, erythema, and fever
- Pain out of proportion to physical presentation
- Cellulitis that does not respond to appropriate antibiotic therapy
- Bullae filled with serous fluid
- Crepitus

Diagnosis

- Plain X-rays of involved area may show evidence of soft tissue air
- CT and MRI are helpful in defining the presence and extent of infection
- Needle aspiration for gram stain and culture

Treatment

- Surgical debridement
- Hyperbaric oxygen therapy[34]
- Re-exploration
- Nutritional support
- Early soft tissue coverage as needed
- Antibiotics

Complications

- Disseminated intravascular coagulation
- Toxic shock syndrome

Clostridium difficile Infection (CDI)

Clostridium difficile is an anaerobic Gram-positive, spore-forming, toxin-producing bacillus that colonizes the large intestine when the protective effect of fecal microbiota is diminished (most often by use of antibiotics, old age, chemotherapy, and debilitated status). *C. difficile* produces two toxins TcdA and TcdB that cause symptoms, while the microorganism itself is not invasive and does not cause infection outside the colon.[35,36]

Clostridium difficile Colitis Risk Factor

- Antibiotic use (ampicillin, amoxicillin, cephalosporins, clindamycin, and fluoroquinolones)
- Older age
- Inpatient status
- Possibly gastric acid suppression
- Inflammatory bowel disease
- Immune deficiency or immunosuppression (organ transplantation, chemotherapy)
- Chronic kidney disease
- Exposure to an infant carrier or infected adult

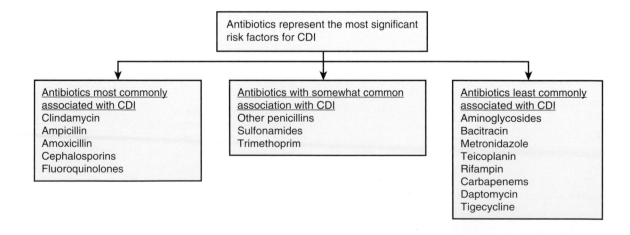

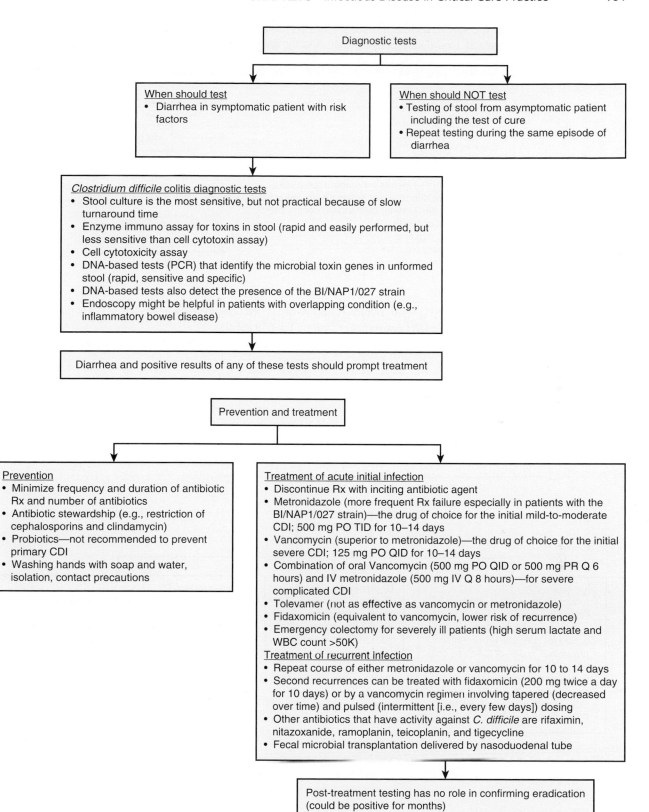

```
                          ┌─────────────────────────┐
                          │     Diagnostic tests     │
                          └─────────────────────────┘
```

When should test
- Diarrhea in symptomatic patient with risk factors

When should NOT test
- Testing of stool from asymptomatic patient including the test of cure
- Repeat testing during the same episode of diarrhea

***Clostridium difficile* colitis diagnostic tests**
- Stool culture is the most sensitive, but not practical because of slow turnaround time
- Enzyme immuno assay for toxins in stool (rapid and easily performed, but less sensitive than cell cytotoxin assay)
- Cell cytotoxicity assay
- DNA-based tests (PCR) that identify the microbial toxin genes in unformed stool (rapid, sensitive and specific)
- DNA-based tests also detect the presence of the BI/NAP1/027 strain
- Endoscopy might be helpful in patients with overlapping condition (e.g., inflammatory bowel disease)

Diarrhea and positive results of any of these tests should prompt treatment

Prevention and treatment

Prevention
- Minimize frequency and duration of antibiotic Rx and number of antibiotics
- Antibiotic stewardship (e.g., restriction of cephalosporins and clindamycin)
- Probiotics—not recommended to prevent primary CDI
- Washing hands with soap and water, isolation, contact precautions

Treatment of acute initial infection
- Discontinue Rx with inciting antibiotic agent
- Metronidazole (more frequent Rx failure especially in patients with the BI/NAP1/027 strain)—the drug of choice for the initial mild-to-moderate CDI; 500 mg PO TID for 10–14 days
- Vancomycin (superior to metronidazole)—the drug of choice for the initial severe CDI; 125 mg PO QID for 10–14 days
- Combination of oral Vancomycin (500 mg PO QID or 500 mg PR Q 6 hours) and IV metronidazole (500 mg IV Q 8 hours)—for severe complicated CDI
- Tolevamer (not as effective as vancomycin or metronidazole)
- Fidaxomicin (equivalent to vancomycin, lower risk of recurrence)
- Emergency colectomy for severely ill patients (high serum lactate and WBC count >50K)

Treatment of recurrent infection
- Repeat course of either metronidazole or vancomycin for 10 to 14 days
- Second recurrences can be treated with fidaxomicin (200 mg twice a day for 10 days) or by a vancomycin regimen involving tapered (decreased over time) and pulsed (intermittent [i.e., every few days]) dosing
- Other antibiotics that have activity against *C. difficile* are rifaximin, nitazoxanide, ramoplanin, teicoplanin, and tigecycline
- Fecal microbial transplantation delivered by nasoduodenal tube

Post-treatment testing has no role in confirming eradication (could be positive for months)

Management of Tuberculosis

Tuberculosis (TB) remains a significant healthcare issue and causes high morbidity and mortality. It reemerged in recent decades possibly due to HIV/AIDS epidemics (it is a leading cause of death among HIV-infected patients). TB is second only to HIV infection in terms of mortality; specifically, in the world, annual mortality from HIV/AIDS is 3 million people, from TB 2 million, and from malaria 1 million.[37] Below we discuss the diagnostic criteria, prophylaxis, and treatment of the TB.

Purified protein derivative (PPD) or tuberculin skin test considered (+) if:

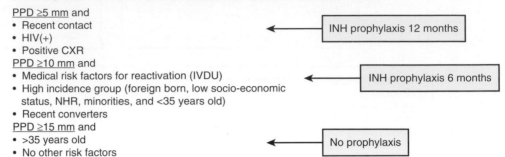

Purified protein derivative (PPD) or tuberculin skin test considered (+) if:

PPD ≥5 mm and
- Recent contact
- HIV(+)
- Positive CXR

PPD ≥10 mm and
- Medical risk factors for reactivation (IVDU)
- High incidence group (foreign born, low socio-economic status, NHR, minorities, and <35 years old)
- Recent converters

PPD ≥15 mm and
- >35 years old
- No other risk factors

← INH prophylaxis 12 months

← INH prophylaxis 6 months

← No prophylaxis

Prophylaxis

Isoniazid (INH) for 6 months (chest X-ray [CXR] negative) or 12 months (CXR positive)
    If possible INH resistance: rifampin for 6–9 months
    If possible multidrug resistance: pyrazinamide + ethambutol (EMB) or pyrazinamide + quinolone (6 months)

Diagnosis

Culture (both diagnosis and drug-susceptibility testing)
Molecular DNA–based diagnostics

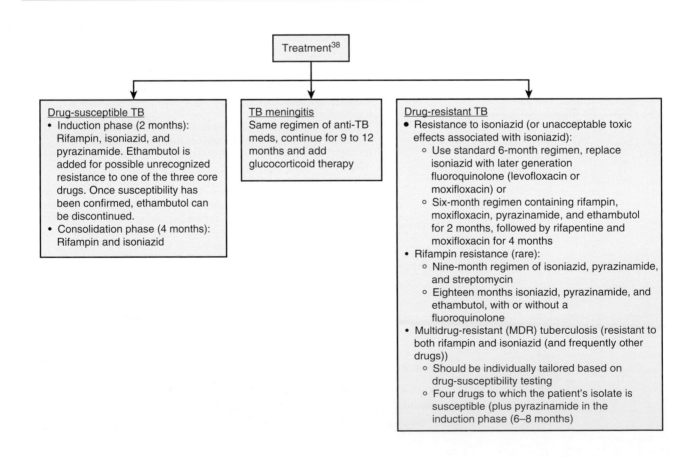

Treatment[38]

Drug-susceptible TB
- Induction phase (2 months): Rifampin, isoniazid, and pyrazinamide. Ethambutol is added for possible unrecognized resistance to one of the three core drugs. Once susceptibility has been confirmed, ethambutol can be discontinued.
- Consolidation phase (4 months): Rifampin and isoniazid

TB meningitis
Same regimen of anti-TB meds, continue for 9 to 12 months and add glucocorticoid therapy

Drug-resistant TB
- Resistance to isoniazid (or unacceptable toxic effects associated with isoniazid):
    ○ Use standard 6-month regimen, replace isoniazid with later generation fluoroquinolone (levofloxacin or moxifloxacin) or
    ○ Six-month regimen containing rifampin, moxifloxacin, pyrazinamide, and ethambutol for 2 months, followed by rifapentine and moxifloxacin for 4 months
- Rifampin resistance (rare):
    ○ Nine-month regimen of isoniazid, pyrazinamide, and streptomycin
    ○ Eighteen months isoniazid, pyrazinamide, and ethambutol, with or without a fluoroquinolone
- Multidrug-resistant (MDR) tuberculosis (resistant to both rifampin and isoniazid (and frequently other drugs))
    ○ Should be individually tailored based on drug-susceptibility testing
    ○ Four drugs to which the patient's isolate is susceptible (plus pyrazinamide in the induction phase (6–8 months)

MRSA Infection[21]

MRSA infection is common and sometimes difficult to treat. Both healthcare-acquired and community-acquired infections can be caused by MRSA. Earlier in this chapter we discussed MRSA infection in respective sections related to specific locations, e.g., skin and soft tissue infections, endocarditis, MRSA pneumonia, bone and joint infection, and CNS infection with MRSA.

Treatment discussion is mostly focused on vancomycin as it is probably the most commonly used antibiotic to treat MRSA infection at this time. Here we specifically discuss dosing of vancomycin and approach to persistent MRSA bacteremia or treatment failure.

Dosing of Vancomycin

- IV vancomycin 15–20 mg/kg/dose (actual body weight) every 8–12 hours, not to exceed 2 g per dose, in patients with normal renal function
- In seriously ill patients (e.g., sepsis, meningitis, pneumonia, or IE) with suspected MRSA infection, a loading dose of 25–30 mg/kg (actual body weight) may be considered (infusion time 2 hours; might use antihistamine prior to the loading dose)

- Serum trough concentrations should be prior to the fourth or fifth dose
- For serious infections (e.g., bacteremia, IE, osteomyelitis, meningitis, pneumonia, and severe SSTI) due to MRSA—vancomycin trough concentrations of 15–20 mcg/mL
- For most patients with SSTI with normal renal function, no obesity, doses of 1 g every 12 hours are adequate, and trough monitoring is not required

SSTI, Skin and soft tissue infection.

Persistent MRSA Bacteremia and Vancomycin Treatment Failure

If susceptible to daptomycin
- Search and removal of foci of infection
- High-dose daptomycin (10 mg/kg/day), if the isolate is susceptible, in combination with
  - Gentamicin 1 mg/kg IV every 8 hours or
  - Rifampicin 600 mg PO/IV daily or 300–450 mg PO/IV twice daily or

  - Linezolid 600 mg PO/IV BID or
  - TMP-SMX 5 mg/kg IV twice daily or
  - Beta-lactam antibiotic

If reduced susceptibility to vancomycin and daptomycin
- Quinupristin-dalfopristin 7.5 mg/kg/dose IV every 8 hours or
- TMP-SMX 5 mg/kg/ dose IV twice daily or
- Linezolid 600 mg PO/IV twice daily or
- Telavancin 10 mg/kg/dose IV once daily or
  These options may be administered as a single agent or in combination with other antibiotics.

Intravenous Catheter–Related Infections

IV devices are very common in hospital practice, especially in the ICU setting. They include peripheral arterial and venous catheters, central venous catheters, peripherally inserted central catheters (PICCs), pulmonary catheters, dialysis lines, and implantable devices. Catheter-related infection is common in ICU and may lead to persistent bacteremia and need to be quickly recognized or prevented.[39] Catheter-related bacteremia is always a suspect in a patient with IV device.

Catheter-Related Bloodstream Infection

Common Pathogens

Percutaneously inserted, noncuffed catheters (peripheral or central): CoNS, *S. aureus*, *Candida* species, enteric Gram-negative bacilli

Surgically implanted catheters and PICC lines: CoNS, enteric Gram-negative bacilli, *S. aureus*, and *P. aeruginosa*

Catheter-related bloodstream infection

Common pathogens
Percutaneously inserted, noncuffed catheters (peripheral or central): Coagulase-negative staphylococci, *S. aureus, Candida* species, enteric gram-negative bacilli
Surgically implanted catheters and PICC lines: Coagulase-negative staphylococci, enteric gram-negative bacilli, *S. aureus,* and *P. aeruginosa*

Treatment

Empiric systemic ABx therapy
- For suspected gram-positive: Vancomycin
- For suspected gram-negative: Fourth-generation cephalosporin, carbapenem, or b-lactam/b-lactamase combination, ± aminoglycoside
- Cover for *Pseudomonas* in neutropenic patients, severe sepsis, those with prior Hx of *Pseudomonas*
- For femoral catheter: Should include coverage for gram-negative bacilli and *Candida* species
- Suspect candidiasis if total parenteral nutrition, prolonged use of broad-spectrum antibiotics, hematologic malignancy, receipt of bone marrow or solid-organ transplant, femoral catheterization, or colonization due to *Candida* species at multiple sites. Use echinocandin or fluconazole

Should the catheter be removed?
- Antibiotic lock therapy is used as catheter salvage therapy (antibiotic solution into an intravascular catheter lumen) for – used in combination with systemic ABx therapy[40]
- Remove peripheral catheter for catheter-related bacteremia
- Remove long-term catheter if: Severe sepsis, tunnel infection or port abscess, suppurative thrombophlebitis; endocarditis; bacteremia despite >72 h of antimicrobial Rx, infections due to *S. aureus, P. aeruginosa,* fungi, or mycobacteria. Consider removal if exit site infection with *Pseudomonas,* also if bacteremia caused by: VRE, *Corynebacterium* JK, *Bacillus* spp, *Lactobacillus* spp
- Remove short-term catheter if: Any of the above or enterococci, gram-negative bacilli

Treatment for specific cases
- Suppurative thrombophlebitis, endocarditis: Catheter removal and 4–6 weeks of ABx
- Osteomyelitis: Catheter removal and 6–8 weeks of ABx
- Tunnel infection, port abscess in long-term catheters: Remove catheter and treat for 7–10 days
- Coagulase-negative *Staphylococcus*: 5–7 days if catheter removed, 10–14 days if catheter retained + ABx lock therapy for 10–14 days for long-term catheters
- *Staphylococcus aureus*: Remove catheter and treat for >14 days (4–6 weeks for long-term catheter)
- Enterococcus: Remove catheter and treat for 7–14 days if short-term catheter; may retain long-term catheter and treat for 7–14 days + ABx lock therapy for 7–14 days
- Gram-negative bacilli: Remove catheter and treat for 7–14 days. May attempt to salvage long-term catheter in some cases, then systemic ABx and lock therapy for 10–14 days
- *Candida*: Remove catheter and treat for 14 days after first negative blood culture. Four to 6 weeks of antibiotic therapy should be administered to patients with persistent fungemia or bacteremia after catheter removal (i.e., occurring >72 h after catheter removal)

Note: Duration of Rx starts from first negative blood culture

Catheter-related infection in hemodialysis patients with hemodialysis catheter

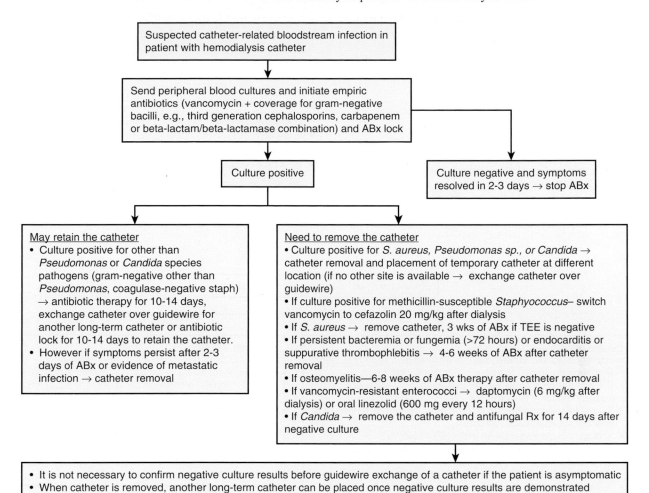

Antibiotic Dosing

Vancomycin 20 mg/kg loading dose during the last hour of dialysis and then 500 mg during last 30 minutes of each subsequent dialysis

Gentamicin or tobramycin 1 mg/kg not to exceed 100 mg after each dialysis session

Ceftazidime 1 g after each dialysis session
Cefazolin 20 mg/kg after each dialysis session
For *Candida*: echinocandin (caspofungin 70 mg IV loading dose followed by 50 mg IV daily; micafungin 100 mg IV daily; or anidulafungin 200 mg IV loading dose, followed by 100 mg IV daily); fluconazole (200 mg orally daily); or amphotericin B

Peritoneal Dialysis–Associated Infections

Peritoneal dialysis (PD) peritonitis is a frequent complication of PD which is potentially life-threatening and eventually leads to peritoneal membrane failure and need to switch to other dialysis modality.[41]

Prevention of PD Peritonitis

- Infection rates: continuous ambulatory PD (CAPD) > Continuous cycling PD (CCPD) > nocturnal
- Standard silicon Tenckhoff catheter is the best for prevention of peritonitis
- Prophylactic ABx (single dose IV) at the time of catheter insertion is beneficial

- Avoid trauma and hematoma during catheter placement
- Exit-site antibiotic protocols (e.g., mupirocin, gentamycin) against *S. aureus*
- ABx prophylaxis for invasive procedures (single oral dose of amoxicillin)
- Avoid constipation

Presentation and diagnosis of PD peritonitis

PD peritonitis presentation
- Presentation: Cloudy dialysate, abdominal pain (cloudy effluent should be presumed to be caused by peritonitis[42])
- Exit site infection presentation: Erythema (not very specific), purulent drainage from exit site
- Tunnel infection presentation: Erythema, edema, or tenderness over the subcutaneous pathway
- Abdominal pain might be an indicator of severity
- Dialysate WBC >100/mL, with at least 50% polymorphonuclear neutrophil cells
- If possible obtain cultures prior to starting ABx
- If very cloudy dialysate, add heparin to dialysis fluid, 500 units/L

Dialysate culture
- About 20% of peritonitis are culture negative
- Centrifugate 50 mL of peritoneal effluent at 3000g for 15 minutes, resuspend sediment in 3–5 L of NS and inoculate on solid culture media and into a standard blood culture medium (then only 5% are culture-negative)
- Solid media should be incubated in aerobic, microaerophilic, and anaerobic environments
- The majority of cultures will become positive after the first 24 hours

---

Causes of Cloudy Effluent (Other Than Bacterial Peritonitis)

- Chemical peritonitis
- Eosinophilia of the effluent

- Hemoperitoneum
- Malignancy (rare)
- Chylous effluent (rare)
- Specimen taken from "dry" abdomen

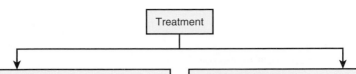

Empiric ABx selection
- Should provide both Gram(+) and Gram(−) coverage
- Start empiric ABx ASAP, before cell count or culture results are back
- Consider patient's and the program's history of micro-organisms and sensitivities.
- For gram-positive: Vancomycin or cephalosporin (cefazolin or cephalothin)
- For gram-negative: Third generation cephalosporin (ceftazidime, cefepime) or aminoglycoside or carbapenem. Quinolones only if supported by local sensitivities
- Monotherapy is possible: imipenem/cilastatin or cefepime or quinolone
- Delivery: Intraperitoneal route is preferable to IV

Catheter removal if
- Refractory peritonitis (failure to respond to appropriate antibiotics within 5 days)
- Relapsing peritonitis (within 4 weeks of completion of therapy with the same microorganism)
- Refractory exit-site and tunnel infection
- Fungal peritonitis
- Consider catheter removal if not responding to therapy
- Note that the priority is optimal treatment of the patient and protection of the peritoneum, and not saving the catheter
- Catheter replacement in a single procedure is safe, except should not be done in fungal and refractory peritonitis (2-3 weeks rest)

Subsequent management and specific pathogens
Minimum therapy for peritonitis is 2 weeks, or 3 weeks for more severe infections

- Coagulase-negative *Staphylococcus*: Can often be managed as an outpatient, first-generation cephalosporins. Relapsing course suggests formation of biofilm → catheter removal
- Streptococcal and enterococcal peritonitis: Tend to be severe, causes severe pain. Rx: IP ampicillin, aminoglycoside IP may be added for synergy for enterococcal. For VRE: ampicillin if sensitive, or linezolid or quinupristin-dalfopristin
- *S. Aureus*: Could be severe, often due to catheter infection (then Rx is catheter removal and rest period of 2 weeks). If MRSA – Vancomycin, might add rifampin for 1 week max. Alternatively - Teicoplanin, where available. If vancomycin-resistant → linezolid, daptomycin, or quinupristin-dalfopristin
- *Pseudomonas aeruginosa*: generally severe, catheter removal if catheter is infected, rest for min of 2 weeks on hemodialysis. Two anti-*Pseudomonas* ABx are necessary: oral quinolone + ceftazidime, cefepime, tobramycin, or piperacillin
- Other gram-negative (e.g., *E. coli, Klebsiella, Proteus*): Choice of ABx based on sensitivity and safety, e.g., cephalosporin, ceftazidime, or cefepime. High proportion of treatment failure and catheter loss
- Polymicrobial peritonitis: Higher risk of death, need surgical evaluation. If multiple gram-positive organisms – more benign course, generally respond to ABx; multiple gram-negative/enteric organisms – look for intraabdominal pathology (e.g., cholecystitis, ischemic bowel, appendicitis, diverticulitis). Rx: metronidazole + ampicillin and ceftazidime or an aminoglycoside. Good chance the catheter needs to be removed.
- Fungal: Immediate catheter removal, 25% mortality. ABx: combination of amphotericin B and flucytosine until the culture results are available. Other options: Caspofungin, fluconazole, or voriconazole. Continue treatment with oral agents for 10 days after catheter removal
- Mycobacteria (*Mycobacterium* tuberculosis or non-tuberculosis mycobacteria): Dx by culturing the sediment. Start Rx four drugs: rifampin (IP, 12 months), isoniazid for 12 months, pyrazinamide for 3 months, and ofloxacin for 3 months
- Culture negative peritonitis: Repeat cell count with differential, if not better, look for lipid dependent yeast, mycobacteria, *Legionella*, slow-growing bacteria, *Campylobacter*, fungi, *Ureaplasma, Mycoplasma*, and enteroviruses. If patient is improving – continue initial Rx for 2 weeks if good response. If no good response in 5 days – catheter removal.

Peritoneal Dialysis Catheter Exit-Site and Tunnel Infections[42,43]

Catheter tunnel and exit-site infections may lead to development of peritonitis, failure of dialysis catheter, and its removal (usually once peritonitis has developed). These infections need to be treated aggressively.

Catheter and Exit-Site Infection Presentation, Microbiology, and Diagnosis

- Exit-site infection presentation: erythema (not very specific), purulent drainage from exit site
- Positive culture in the absence of an abnormal appearance is indicative of colonization

- Tunnel infection presentation: erythema, edema, or tenderness over the subcutaneous pathway
- Microorganisms: *S. aureus* and *P. aeruginosa* are most common and most serious, but could also be diphtheroid, anaerobic organisms, nonfermenting bacteria, streptococci, *Legionella*, yeasts, and fungi
- Culture is important, ultrasound of the exit site and tunnel is helpful to determine the extent

Treatment

- Treatment: aiming at *S. aureus* and *P. aeruginosa*; oral antibiotic therapy is as effective as intraperitoneal (IP) therapy, except for MRSA; hypertonic saline dressings twice daily

- Minimum duration of ABx Rx is 2 weeks
- Catheter replacement in a single procedure under ABx coverage
- Exit-site infection + peritonitis -> catheter removal (except for coagulase-negative Staph)

Oral Antibiotics Used in Exit-Site and Tunnel Infection[42]

Amoxicillin 250–500 mg BID
Cephalexin 500 mg BID to TID
Ciprofloxacin 250 mg BID
Clarithromycin 500 mg loading dose, then 250 mg BID or QD
Dicloxacillin 500 mg QID
Erythromycin 500 mg QID
Flucloxacillin (or cloxacillin) 500 mg QID
Fluconazole 200 mg QD for 2 days, then 100 mg QD

Flucytosine 0.5–1 g/day titrated to response and serum trough levels (25–50 mg/mL)
INH 200–300 mg QD
Linezolid 400–600 mg BID
Metronidazole 400 mg TID
Moxifloxacin 400 mg daily
Ofloxacin 400 mg first day, then 200 mg QD
Pyrazinamide 25–35 mg/kg 3 times per week
Rifampicin 450 mg QD for <50 kg; 600 mg QD for >50 kg
TMP-SMX 80/400 mg QD

Infections in Immunocompromised Host

	Granulocytopenia (Absolute Neutrophil Count of <500/mm³)	Cellular Immune Dysfunction	Humoral Immune Dysfunction and Complement Deficiency
Clinical scenario	• Myelocytic leukemia • Cancer chemotherapy	• Lymphoma or lymphocytic leukemia • Steroids/cytotoxic drugs • Organ/bone marrow transplant • HIV • Anti-TNF treatment	• Multiple myeloma • Lymphoma, CLL • Splenectomy • Complement deficiencies (e.g., congenital, SLE) • HIV • Chemotherapy • Sickle cell disease
Most common pathogens	• G(−) rods (*Pseudomonas*) • G(+) cocci: alpha-Strep, coag(−) Staph, *S. aureus* • Fungi: *Candida* and *Aspergillus*	• Viruses: herpes, varicella, EBV • Bacteria: mycobacteria, *Legionella*, *Listeria*, *Salmonella*, *Nocardia* • Fungi: crypto, *Histoplasma*, *Coccidioides* • Protozoa: *Toxoplasma*, *Pneumocystis*, *Cryptosporidium*	• Encapsulated bacteria: • Pneumococci (*S. pneumoniae*) • Meningococci (*N. meningitidis*) • *H. influenzae* • Encapsulated Gram(−) rods (*Pseudomonas*, *Klebsiella*) • *Giardia* • *Capnocytophaga canimorsus*
Empiric treatment of febrile patient	High doses of IV broad-spectrum antibiotics: Ceftazidime Piperacillin/tazobactam Aztreonam Imipenem Antifungals: voriconazole, amphotericin B	Antiviral, Bactrim, antifungal (voriconazole or amphotericin)	Vancomycin plus third-or fourth-generation cephalosporin Levofloxacin if allergic

CLL, Chronic lymphatic leukemia; *SLE*, systemic lupus erythematosus.

Infections in Organ Transplant Recipients[44]

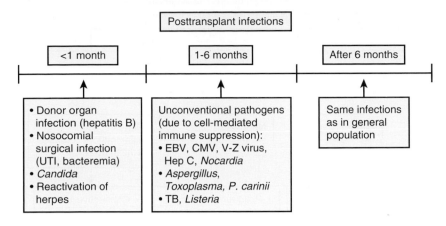

Fever of Unknown Origin (FUO)

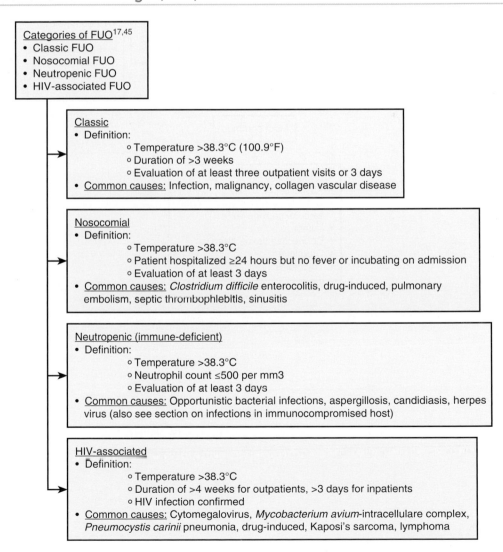

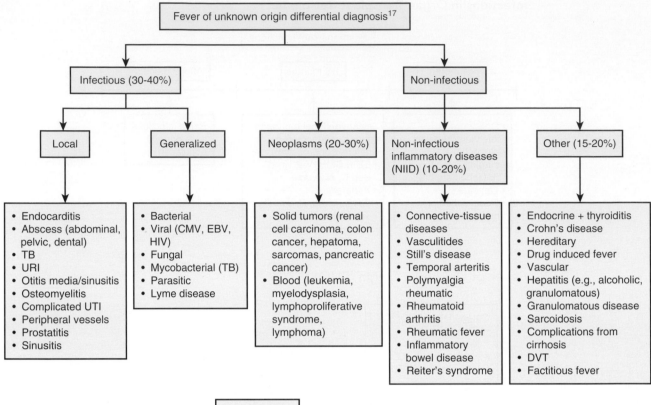

Fever of unknown origin differential diagnosis[17]

Infectious (30-40%)

Non-infectious

Local

Generalized

Neoplasms (20-30%)

Non-infectious inflammatory diseases (NIID) (10-20%)

Other (15-20%)

- Endocarditis
- Abscess (abdominal, pelvic, dental)
- TB
- URI
- Otitis media/sinusitis
- Osteomyelitis
- Complicated UTI
- Peripheral vessels
- Prostatitis
- Sinusitis

- Bacterial
- Viral (CMV, EBV, HIV)
- Fungal
- Mycobacterial (TB)
- Parasitic
- Lyme disease

- Solid tumors (renal cell carcinoma, colon cancer, hepatoma, sarcomas, pancreatic cancer)
- Blood (leukemia, myelodysplasia, lymphoproliferative syndrome, lymphoma)

- Connective-tissue diseases
- Vasculitides
- Still's disease
- Temporal arteritis
- Polymyalgia rheumatic
- Rheumatoid arthritis
- Rheumatic fever
- Inflammatory bowel disease
- Reiter's syndrome

- Endocrine + thyroiditis
- Crohn's disease
- Hereditary
- Drug induced fever
- Vascular
- Hepatitis (e.g., alcoholic, granulomatous)
- Granulomatous disease
- Sarcoidosis
- Complications from cirrhosis
- DVT
- Factitious fever

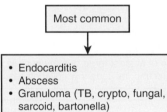

Most common

- Endocarditis
- Abscess
- Granuloma (TB, crypto, fungal, sarcoid, bartonella)
- Tumor
- Connective tissue disease
- Drug fever
- Thyroiditis

Workup of FUO

Workup depends on the individual patient and clinical suspicion that comes from history and exam. In general, diagnostic workup can be represented as below.

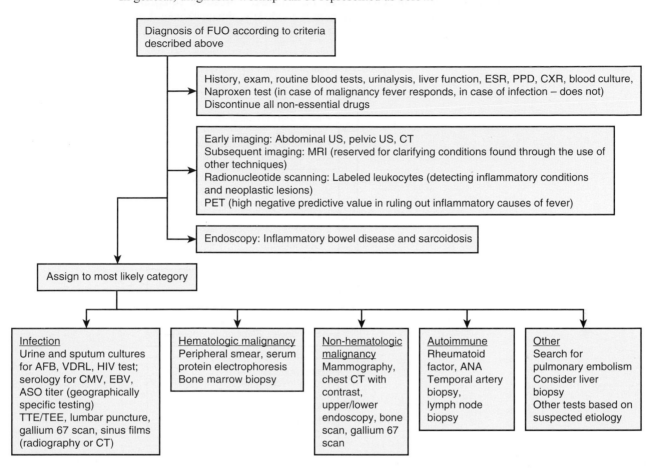

Empiric treatment is not recommended except in the following cases[45]:

- Antibiotics for suspected culture-negative endocarditis
- TB treatment in suspected active TB

- Glucocorticoids for suspected temporal arteritis with the risk of vision loss
- Antipyretic therapy is OK most of the time

Most Common Causes in Returning Travelers[46]

- Malaria
- Dengue
- Enteric fever caused by *Salmonella typhi* or *Salmonella paratyphi*

- Rickettsial disease
- Mononucleosis syndromes (EBV, CMV)
- Acute HIV infection
- Toxoplasmosis

CMV, Cytomegalovirus; *EBV*, Epstein-Barr virus.

Opportunistic Infections in HIV/AIDS

Special attention needs to be paid to patients infected with HIV in the diagnosis and treatment of potential opportunistic infections. Most opportunistic infections (OIs) are diagnosed in those with CD4 cell counts <200/mm^3, though there is a risk of esophageal candidiasis, Kaposi's sarcoma, and pulmonary TB even in those with CD4 counts >200/mm^3.[47,48]

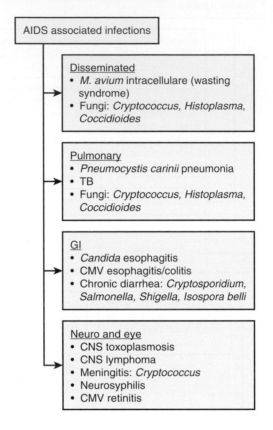

Stage	CD4 Count	Opportunistic Infection
Early	CD4 >500	Uncommon
Intermediate	CD4 200–500	Mycobacteria TB Herpes (recurrent herpes zoster, mucocutaneous herpes simplex) Oral and esophageal candidiasis Bacteremia (*S. pneumoniae, Salmonella*) Kaposi's sarcoma
Late	CD4 50–200	*Pneumocystis carinii* pneumonia Esophageal candidiasis
Advanced	CD4 <50	Cerebral toxoplasmosis Cryptococcal meningitis *Mycobacterium avium* Disseminated CMV, invasive aspergillosis, disseminated histoplasmosis, coccidioidomycosis, bartonellosis, progressive multifocal leukoencephalopathy
Terminal	CD4 <5	

CNS Lesions in HIV-Positive Patients

	Toxoplasmosis	CNS Lymphoma	Progressive Multifocal Leukoencephalopathy
Presentation	Hemiparesis, aphasia, visual defects, cranial nerve palsies, tremor, seizures	Seizures, focal findings	Focal neurologic examination
Neuroimaging	Multiple bilateral hypodense lesions enhanced with contrast, typically involving basal ganglia or corticomedullary junction	Single or several hypodense lesions	White matter disease without mass lesion

Management of Opportunistic Infections in Patients With HIV/AIDS[47,48]

Opportunistic Infection	Risk Factors	Diagnosis	Prophylaxis	Rx	When to Start ART
Latent TB: LTBI in HIV-infected individuals is defined as a tuberculin skin test (TST) with >5 mm of induration without clinical or radiographic evidence of active disease	CD4 <500	• If TST is negative in patients with CD4 cell count <200/mm³—repeat after ART and immune reconstitution • Interferon-gamma release assays (IGRAs)		• INH daily for 9 months • Alternatively: once-weekly INH and rifapentine by directly observed therapy for 3 months	
Active TB	CD4 <500	• Detecting *Mycobacterium tuberculosis* in smear or culture (sputum or other samples) • Acid-fast bacilli (AFB) • GeneXpert MTB/RIF (real-time PCR) • Lipopolysaccharide antigen lipoarabinomannan (LAM) in urine		Same treatment as HIV-negative individuals consisting of intensive phase and continuation phase	• Start ART in all people with HIV and active TB regardless of CD4 cell count • TB treatment should be started first, followed by ART • CD4 cell count < 50/mm³—within 2 weeks after starting TB Rx • CD4 cell count > 50/mm³—within 8–12 weeks after starting TB Rx

Opportunistic Infection	Risk Factors	Diagnosis	Prophylaxis	Rx	When to Start ART
CMV disease, disseminated CMV	CD4 <50	Viremia by PCR or antigen assays		• CMV retinitis: oral valganciclovir, IV ganciclovir, IV ganciclovir followed by oral valganciclovir, IV foscarnet, IV cidofovir, and the ganciclovir intraocular implant coupled with valganciclovir • Colitis or esophagitis: IV ganciclovir or foscarnet • Pneumonitis: IV ganciclovir, foscarnet, or cidofovir	Start along with anti-CMV treatment
Varicella-zoster	CD4 <500	• Swabs from a fresh lesion for viral culture • Direct fluorescent antigen testing • PCR	Varicella vaccination, post-exposure varicella-zoster immune globulin, acyclovir	• Oral acyclovir (20 mg/kg body weight up to a maximum dose of 800 mg 5 times daily) • Valacyclovir (1 g PO TID) • Famciclovir (500 mg PO TID) for 5–7 days • IV acyclovir for 7–10 days for severe disease	
Herpes simplex	CD4 <500	Viral culture, HSV DNA PCR, and HSV antigen		• Orolabial lesions: oral valacyclovir, famciclovir, or acyclovir for 5–10 days • Severe mucocutaneous HSV lesions: initial treatment with IV acyclovir • Genital HSV: oral valacyclovir, famciclovir, or acyclovir for 5–14 days	
Oral and esophageal candidiasis	CD4 <200, but sometimes <500	• Clinical diagnosis • Potassium hydroxide (KOH) preparation • Esophageal candidiasis requires endoscopic visualization of lesions	Fluconazole can reduce the risk for mucosal candidiasis	• Oral fluconazole • Initial episodes of oropharyngeal candidiasis topical therapy (clotrimazole troches, nystatin suspension, or pastilles) • Itraconazole oral solution for 7–14 days (as effective as oral fluconazole) • Systemic antifungals for esophageal candidiasis: 14–21-day course of either fluconazole (oral or IV) or oral itraconazole; micafungin and anidulafungin	

continued

Opportunistic Infection	Risk Factors	Diagnosis	Prophylaxis	Rx	When to Start ART
Bacteremia (**S. pneumoniae**, **Salmonella**)	CD4 <500		Vaccination against **S. pneumoniae**	Same treatment as in non–HIV-infected patients	
HHV-8 (associated with KS and Castleman disease)	CD4 <500	• Serologic assays (immunofluorescence, ELISA, Western blot) • In situ DNA hybridization and PCR) • Diagnosis of KS requires biopsy/pathology	• Early initiation of ART, suppression of HIV replication • Antiviral use for prevention of KS is not currently recommended	• Cytotoxic chemotherapy for KS, liposomal doxorubicin or paclitaxel • Suppression of HIV replication with ART • In Castleman disease: anti–herpesvirus drugs (IV ganciclovir or oral valganciclovir)	ART recommended for all HIV patients with active KS and other HHV-8–associated malignant lymphoproliferative disorders
P. carinii pneumonia	CD4 <200	• Microscopic examination of induced sputum, BAL, or tissue • Elevated LDH (nonspecific marker) • Beta-glucan	Start prophylaxis if: • CD4 cell count <200/mm^3 • Oropharyngeal candidiasis • CD4 cell percentage <14% • History of AIDS-defining illness • CD4 cell count >200 but <250/mm^3 if CD4 cell count monitoring not feasible • In Pts on HAART primary and secondary prophylaxis can be discontinued after the CD4 increased to 200 for more than 3 monthsAgents: Bactrim, dapsone, atovaquone	Bactrim 5mg/kg IV Q6	Within ~2 weeks of initiating OI treatment
Cerebral toxoplasmosis (toxoplasmic encephalitis)	CD4 <50	Anti–toxoplasma immunoglobulin G (IgG) antibodies	• Start in seropositive patients with CD4 <100 • Bactrim • Dapsone-pyrimethamine plus leucovorin • Atovaquone with or without pyrimethamine/leucovorin • Stop if ART → increase in CD4+ counts to >200 cells/µL for >3 months	• Pyrimethamine plus sulfadiazine plus leucovorin: • Clarithromycin plus pyrimethamine • 5-Fluorouracil plus clindamycin • Dapsone plus pyrimethamine plus leucovorin • Acute therapy for TE should be continued for at least 6 weeks, if there is clinical and radiologic improvement	

Opportunistic Infection	Risk Factors	Diagnosis	Prophylaxis	Rx	When to Start ART
Cryptococcal meningitis	CD4 <50	• Serum or CSF cryptococcal antigen (CrAg) or culture • India ink staining of CSF		• Induction phase (at least 2 weeks): liposomal amphotericin B at 3–4 mg/kg/day in combination with flucytosine 100 mg/kg • Consolidation therapy with fluconazole 400 mg daily for at least 8 weeks divided into four equal doses daily for at least 2 weeks • May stop if received at least 12 months of fluconazole maintenance therapy, have CD4 cell counts ≥100/mm^3, and undetectable HIV RNA for ≥3 months on ART	Approximately 5 weeks after starting antifungal therapy
MAC	CD4 <50	Isolation of MAC from cultures of blood, lymph node, bone marrow, or other normally sterile tissue or body fluids	• Azithromycin or clarithromycin is the preferred prophylactic agent or rifabutin • Discontinue if responded to ART with an increase in CD4+ counts to >100 cells/μL for >3 months	Two or more antimycobacterial drugs: clarithromycin + EMB ± rifabutin	
Disseminated histoplasmosis	CD4 <50	• Histoplasma antigen in blood or urine • Histoplasma capsulatum cultured from blood, bone marrow, respiratory secretions, or other involved sites	Itraconazole can reduce the risk of histoplasmosis	IV lipid formulation of amphotericin B for >2 weeks (or till clinical improvement) followed by oral itraconazole (200 mg 3 times daily for 3 days and then 200 mg twice daily for a total of >12 months)	
Coccidioidomycosis	CD4 <50	• Culture of the organism from clinical specimens or by demonstration of the typical spherule on histopathologic examination of involved tissue • Coccidioidal IgM and IgG serology • Complement fixation IgG antibody is frequently detected in the CSF in coccidioidal meningitis	Questionable benefit in patients living in endemic areas: oral fluconazole 400 mg daily or itraconazole 200 mg BID if IgM or IgG serology and CD4 <250 cells/μL	• Fluconazole or itraconazole 400 mg daily • Posaconazole and voriconazole if failed to respond	

continued

Opportunistic Infection	Risk Factors	Diagnosis	Prophylaxis	Rx	When to Start ART
Invasive aspergillosis	CD4 <50	• Repeated isolation of Aspergillus spp. from cultures or respiratory secretions • Finding of dichotomously branching septate hyphae consistent with *Aspergillus* spp. in respiratory or other samples • Histological evidence of tissue invasion by hyphae with a positive culture for *Aspergillus* spp.	Posaconazole has been effective in patients with hematologic malignancy and neutropenia	• Voriconazole or • Amphotericin B	
Progressive multifocal leukoencephalopathy (PML)	CD4 <50, though possible with CD4 >100/mm^3			No effective antiviral agent against JC virus	As part of initial therapy for the OI
Bartonellosis	CD4 <100	• Histopathologic examination of biopsied tissue • Serologic test	Primary chemoprophylaxis for *Bartonella*-associated disease is not recommended	• Erythromycin and doxycycline • Doxycycline ± rifamycin for bartonellosis involving the CNS • For severe infection—all three	

ART, Antiretroviral therapy; *ELISA*, enzyme-linked immunosorbent assay; *HAART*, highly active antiretroviral therapy; *HHV-8*, human herpesvirus 8; *HSV*, herpes simplex virus; *JC*, John Cunningham; *KS*, Kaposi's sarcoma; *LTBI*, latent TB infection; *MAC*, *M. avium* complex; *TE*, toxoplasmic encephalitis.

Infections Endemic to Certain Geographic Regions in America

Geographic Region	Infection
Northeast	Lyme disease (*Borrelia burgdorferi*)
Desert Southwest	Plaque (*Yersinia pestis*)
Southwest US and Northern Mexico	*C. immitis*
Mississippi and Ohio valleys	Histoplasmosis
Arkansas, Missouri	Tularemia (*Francisella tularensis*) Ehrlichiosis
South East US, Oklahoma, mid-Atlantic	Rocky Mountain spotted fever
Andes mountains (Peru)	Bartonellosis (*Bartonella bacilliformis*)—"Oroya fever"
South America	Chagas disease

REFERENCES

1. Marik PE. Early management of severe sepsis: concepts and controversies. *Chest*. 2014;145(6):1407–1418.
2. Angus DC, van der Poll T. Severe sepsis and septic shock. *N Engl J Med*. 2013;369(9):840–851.
3. Hilton AK, Bellomo R. A critique of fluid bolus resuscitation in severe sepsis. *Crit Care*. 2012;16(1):302.
4. Bark BP, Persson J, Grande PO. Importance of the infusion rate for the plasma expanding effect of 5% albumin, 6% HES 130/0.4, 4% gelatin, and 0.9% NaCl in the septic rat. *Crit Care Med*. 2013;41(3):857–866.
5. Yunos NM, Bellomo R, Hegarty C, Story D, Ho L, Bailey M. Association between a chloride-liberal vs chloride-restrictive intravenous fluid administration strategy and kidney injury in critically ill adults. *J Am Med Assoc*. 2012;308(15):1566–1572.
6. Boniatti MM, Cardoso PR, Castilho RK, Vieira SR. Is hyperchloremia associated with mortality in critically ill patients? A prospective cohort study. *J Crit Care*. 2011;26(2):175–179.
7. Perner A, Haase N, Guttormsen AB, et al. Hydroxyethyl starch 130/0.42 versus Ringer's acetate in severe sepsis. *N Engl J Med*. 2012;367(2):124–134.
8. Marik PE, Corwin HL. Efficacy of red blood cell transfusion in the critically ill: a systematic review of the literature. *Crit Care Med*. 2008;36(9):2667–2674.
9. Varpula M, Tallgren M, Saukkonen K, Voipio-Pulkki LM, Pettila V. Hemodynamic variables related to outcome in septic shock. *Intensive Care Med*. 2005;31(8):1066–1071.
10. Jellema WT, Groeneveld AB, Wesseling KH, Thijs LG, Westerhof N, van Lieshout JJ. Heterogeneity and prediction of hemodynamic responses to dobutamine in patients with septic shock. *Crit Care Med*. 2006;34(9):2392–2398.
11. Sandifer JP, Jones AE. Is the addition of vasopressin to norepinephrine beneficial for the treatment of septic shock? *Ann Emerg Med*. 2013;62(5):534–535.
12. Dellinger RP, Levy MM, Rhodes A, et al. Surviving sepsis campaign: international guidelines for management of severe sepsis and septic shock: 2012. *Crit Care Med*. 2013;41(2):580–637.
13. Kopcinovic LM, Culej J. Pleural, peritoneal and pericardial effusions—a biochemical approach. *Biochem Med*. 2014;24(1):123–137.
14. Seidman AJ, Limaiem F. Synovial Fluid Analysis; 2019 In *StatPearls*. StatPearls Publishing: Treasure Island, FL, USA; 2019.
15. Deisenhammer F, Bartos A, Egg R, et al. Routine cerebrospinal fluid (CSF) analysis. In Gilhus NE, Barnes MP, Brainin M, eds. *European Handbook of Neurological Management,* 2nd ed. Blackwell Publishing Ltd, USA; 2011:5–17.
16. Mandell LA, Wunderink RG, Anzueto A, et al. Infectious Diseases Society of America/American Thoracic Society consensus guidelines on the management of community-acquired pneumonia in adults. *Clin Infect Dis*. 2007;44(suppl 2):S27–S72.
17. Roth AR, Basello GM. Approach to the adult patient with fever of unknown origin. *Am Fam Physician*. 2003;68(11):2223–2228.
18. Mandell LA, Wunderink RG, Anzueto A, et al. Infectious Diseases Society of America/American Thoracic Society consensus guidelines on the management of community-acquired pneumonia in adults. *Clin Infect Dis*. 2007;44(suppl 2):S27–S72.
19. Kalil AC, Metersky ML, Klompas M, et al. Management of adults with hospital-acquired and ventilator-associated pneumonia: 2016 clinical practice guidelines by the Infectious Diseases Society of America and the American Thoracic Society. *Clin Infect Dis*. 2016;63(5):e61–e111.
20. Walaszek M, Kosiarska A, Gniadek A, et al. The risk factors for hospital-acquired pneumonia in the Intensive Care Unit. *Przegl Epidemiol*. 2016;70(1):15–20, 107-110.
21. Liu C, Bayer A, Cosgrove SE, et al. Clinical practice guidelines by the infectious diseases society of America for the treatment of methicillin-resistant Staphylococcus aureus infections in adults and children. *Clin Infect Dis*. 2011;52(3):e18–e55.
22. Hersi K, Kondamudi NP. Meningitis. In: *StatPearls*. Treasure Island, FL: StatPearls; 2017.
23. Viallon A, Botelho-Nevers E, Zeni F. Clinical decision rules for acute bacterial meningitis: current insights. *Open Access Emerg Med*. 2016;8:7–16.
24. Vaziri S, Mansouri F, Sayad B, et al. Meta-analysis of studies comparing adjuvant dexamethasone to glycerol to improve clinical outcome of bacterial meningitis. *J Res Med Sci*. 2016;21:22.
25. Lima AL, Oliveira PR, Carvalho VC, et al. Recommendations for the treatment of osteomyelitis. *Braz J Infect Dis*. 2014;18(5):526–534.
26. Baddour LM, Wilson WR, Bayer AS, et al. Infective endocarditis in adults: diagnosis, antimicrobial therapy, and management of complications: a scientific statement for healthcare professionals from the American Heart Association. *Circulation*. 2015;132(15):1435–1486.
27. Yanagawa B, Pettersson GB, Habib G, et al. Surgical management of infective endocarditis complicated by embolic stroke: practical recommendations for clinicians. *Circulation*. 2016;134(17):1280–1292.
28. Gupta K, Hooton TM, Naber KG, et al. International clinical practice guidelines for the treatment of acute uncomplicated cystitis and pyelonephritis in women: a 2010 update by the Infectious Diseases Society of America and the European Society for Microbiology and Infectious Diseases. *Clin Infect Dis*. 2011;52(5):e103–e120.
29. Schaeffer AJ, Nicolle LE. Clinical practice. Urinary tract infections in older men. *N Engl J Med*. 2016;374(6):562–571.
30. Hooton TM, Bradley SF, Cardenas DD, et al. Diagnosis, prevention, and treatment of catheter-associated urinary tract infection in adults: 2009 international clinical practice guidelines from the Infectious Diseases Society of America. *Clin Infect Dis*. 2010;50(5):625–663.

31. Stevens DL, Bisno AL, Chambers HF, et al. Practice guidelines for the diagnosis and management of skin and soft tissue infections: 2014 update by the Infectious Diseases Society of America. *Clin Infect Dis*. 2014;59(2):e10–e52.

32. McClain SL, Bohan JG, Stevens DL. Advances in the medical management of skin and soft tissue infections. *BMJ*. 2016;355:i6004.

33. Wang JM, Lim HK. Necrotizing fasciitis: eight-year experience and literature review. *Braz J Infect Dis*. 2014;18(2):137–143.

34. Riseman JA, Zamboni WA, Curtis A, Graham DR, Konrad HR, Ross DS. Hyperbaric oxygen therapy for necrotizing fasciitis reduces mortality and the need for debridements. *Surgery*. 1990;108(5):847–850.

35. Leffler DA, Lamont JT. Clostridium difficile infection. *N Engl J Med*. 2015;372(16):1539–1548.

36. Cohen SH, Gerding DN, Johnson S, et al. Clinical practice guidelines for Clostridium difficile infection in adults: 2010 update by the society for healthcare epidemiology of America (SHEA) and the Infectious Diseases Society of America (IDSA). *Infect Control Hosp Epidemiol*. 2010;31(5):431–455.

37. Sandhu GK. Tuberculosis: current situation, challenges and overview of its control programs in India. *J Glob Infect Dis*. 2011;3(2):143–150.

38. Horsburgh Jr CR, Barry 3rd CE, Lange C. Treatment of tuberculosis. *N Engl J Med*. 2015;373(22):2149–2160.

39. Mermel LA, Allon M, Bouza E, et al. Clinical practice guidelines for the diagnosis and management of intravascular catheter-related infection: 2009 Update by the Infectious Diseases Society of America. *Clin Infect Dis*. 2009;49(1):1–45.

40. Fortun J, Grill F, Martín-Dávila P, et al. Treatment of long-term intravascular catheter-related bacteraemia with antibiotic-lock therapy. *J Antimicrob Chemother*. 2006;58(4):816–821.

41. Piraino B, Bailie GR, Bernardini J, et al. Peritoneal dialysis-related infections recommendations: 2005 update. *Perit Dial Int*. 2005;25(2):107–131.

42. Li PK, Szeto CC, Piraino B, et al. Peritoneal dialysis-related infections recommendations: 2010 update. *Perit Dial Int*. 2010;30(4):393–423.

43. Piraino B. Peritoneal catheter exit-site and tunnel infections. *Adv Ren Replace Ther*. 1996;3(3):222–227.

44. Fishman JA. Infections in immunocompromised hosts and organ transplant recipients: essentials. *Liver Transpl*. 2011;17(suppl 3):S34–S37.

45. Unger M, Karanikas G, Kerschbaumer A, Winkler S, Aletaha D. Fever of unknown origin (FUO) revised. *Wien Klin Wochenschr*. 2016;128(21–22):796–801.

46. Korzeniewski K, Gawel B, Krankowska D, Wasilczuk K. Fever of unknown origin in returning travellers. *Int Marit Heal*. 2015;66(2):77–83.

47. Zanoni BC, Gandhi RT. Update on opportunistic infections in the era of effective antiretroviral therapy. *Infect Dis Clin North Am*. 2014;28(3):501–518.

48. Kaplan JE, Benson C, Holmes KK, Brooks JT, Pau A, Masur H. Guidelines for prevention and treatment of opportunistic infections in HIV-infected adults and adolescents. *Morb Mortal Wkly Rep*. 2009;58(RR-4):1–207.

CHAPTER 7

Critical Care Gastroenterology

Alexander Goldfarb-Rumyantzev

Abdominal Signs Pertinent to ICU

A number of symptoms related to gastrointestinal (GI) problems need to be recognized and addressed in Intensive Care Unit (ICU) patients, most of them quite obvious based on history and physical examination. Important points regarding GI signs are discussed below.[1]

Abdominal Pain

- Visceral pain is often poorly localized (distension or spasm of a hollow organ)

- Parietal pain is very well localized and sharp (peritoneal irritation, e.g. acute appendicitis)
- Referred pain is perceived to be near the surface of the body and aching (e.g., basal pneumonia)

Abdominal Distention

Increase in intraabdominal volume due to
- ascites

- bowel edema
- hematoma
- bowel distension, or ileus

Diarrhea (See Diarrhea Section for Details)

- Defined as ≥3 loose/liquid stools per day with a stool weight >200–250 g per day (or >250 mL/day)

- Risk factors: enteral nutrition itself, hypoalbuminemia, intestinal ischemia, medications (antibiotics, laxatives)
- Consequences: fluid and electrolyte loss, hemodynamic instability

Abnormal Bowel Sounds

- Diminished or absent bowel peristalsis is common in mechanically ventilated patients receiving sedatives, opiates, and/or catecholamines

- Excessive and tinkling bowel sounds in bowel obstruction

Vomiting

- Multiple causes including increased intraabdominal pressure

- Complications: aspiration pneumonia, dehydration, malnutrition, disruption of the surgical site

Gastric Residual Volume

- Gastric residual volume (GRV) is high if a single volume is >200 mL or a total gastric aspirate volume is >1000 mL per 24 hours

- Increasing the cut-off for normal GRV to 500 mL is not associated with increased adverse effects of enteral nutrition (EN), GI complications, or in outcome variables
- Although high GRV requires specific attention, tube enteral feeding should not be automatically discontinued

Paralytic Ileus

- Due to impaired peristalsis
- Inevitable after abdominal surgery and lasts usually 3–5 days
- Other contributing factors:
  - mechanical ventilation
  - increased intracranial or intraabdominal pressure
  - volume overload

- sedation
- sepsis
- hypotension
- use of drugs with known inhibitory effects on GI motility (catecholamines, opioids)
- Importantly, in patients receiving analgesics and sedation, who are mechanically ventilated, GI paralysis may be the only sign of ongoing peritonitis

Bowel Dilatation

- Colonic diameter is >6 cm (>9 cm for caecum) or small bowel diameter is >3 cm
- It could be a sign of obstruction at any level of the GI tract

- It may also appear without an obstruction (as in toxic megacolon or acute colonic pseudo-obstruction = Ogilvie's syndrome)
- Predisposing factors for Ogilvie's syndrome: nonoperative abdominal trauma, infections, and cardiac diseases

Jaundice

- Prehepatic jaundice—hemolysis (e.g., malaria, sickle cell anemia)

- Intrahepatic jaundice—parenchymal disease of the liver (e.g., acute hepatitis, liver cirrhosis, liver cancer)
- Posthepatic jaundice—biliary obstruction (e.g., bile duct cancer, gallstones)

Dysphagia

- Neurological disorders (multiple sclerosis, myasthenia gravis, cerebral palsy, stroke)

- Motility disorders (achalasia, esophageal spasm, esophagitis)
- Structural problems and obstruction (rings, webs, strictures, malignancy, external compression)

Abdominal Pain

Abdominal pain is a frequent symptom and can be caused by a number of conditions, not necessarily limited to abdominal organs. Due to innervation of abdominal and thoracic organs, while the location of the pain is very helpful, it is not always specific to location of the cause of symptoms. Below we discuss the approach to diagnostic steps in patients presenting with abdominal pain. While history and physical examination are very important in evaluation of any medical condition, they are crucial in diagnostic approach to patients with abdominal pain.[2]

Causes of Abdominal Pain

- History (characteristics of pain, other elements of the history)
- Physical examination
- Labs and imaging studies

History: Characteristics of the Pain (PQRST Mnemonic)[2]

- P3—Positional, palliating, and provoking factors
  - Jarring motions such as coughing or walking exacerbate the pain, suggesting peritoneal irritation; in peritonitis often increased pain with jolts or bumps in the road
  - Pleuritic pain may signify chest disease
  - Peptic ulcer disease may be exacerbated (gastric) or relieved (duodenal) by eating
  - Mesenteric ischemia may be precipitated by eating
  - Pain of intermittently symptomatic gallstones is often associated with fatty meals
- Q—Quality
  - Viscerally innervated organs: dull, poorly localized, aching, or gnawing pain
  - Parietal peritoneum or other somatically innervated structures sharp, more defined, and localized somatic pain
- R3—Region, radiation, referral
  - Location
    - Perceived as epigastric: stomach, pancreas, liver, biliary system, and the proximal duodenum
    - Perceived as periumbilical: small bowel and the proximal third of the colon including the appendix
    - Perceived as suprapubic: bladder, and distal two-thirds of the colon, pelvic genitourinary organs
  - Radiation
    - Diaphragmatic irritation → shoulder pain (Kehr's sign); biliary disease → ipsilateral scapula pain
    - In general: remember that deep musculoskeletal structures (especially of the back) are innervated by visceral sensory fibers with similar qualities to those arising from intra-abdominal organs (these fibers converge in the spinal cord, giving rise to "sclerotomes")
- S—Severity
  - Severe pain: concern for a serious underlying cause
  - Descriptions of milder pain cannot be relied on to exclude serious illness, especially in older patients
- T3—Temporal factors (time and mode of onset, progression, previous episodes)
  - Onset:
    - Severe acute-onset pain: concern for potential intraabdominal catastrophe (e.g., vascular emergency such as a ruptured abdominal aortic aneurysm, aortic dissection; perforated ulcer, volvulus, mesenteric ischemia, and torsion)
    - Gradual onset: infectious or inflammatory process
    - Pain that awakens the patient from sleep: serious until proven otherwise
  - Duration
    - Persistent worsening pain is worrisome
    - Pain that is improving is typically favorable
    - Migration of pain (e.g., appendicitis)
    - Paroxysmal or steady (e.g., gallbladder pain is not paroxysmal, almost never lasts <1 hour, with an average of 5–16 hours' duration, and up to 24 hours)
    - Small bowel obstruction: typically progresses from an intermittent ("colicky") pain to more constant pain when distention occurs

Cause of Abdominal Pain Based on Location

Along with other elements of the history, pain location is crucial in determining the cause and next diagnostic and therapeutic step.[3]

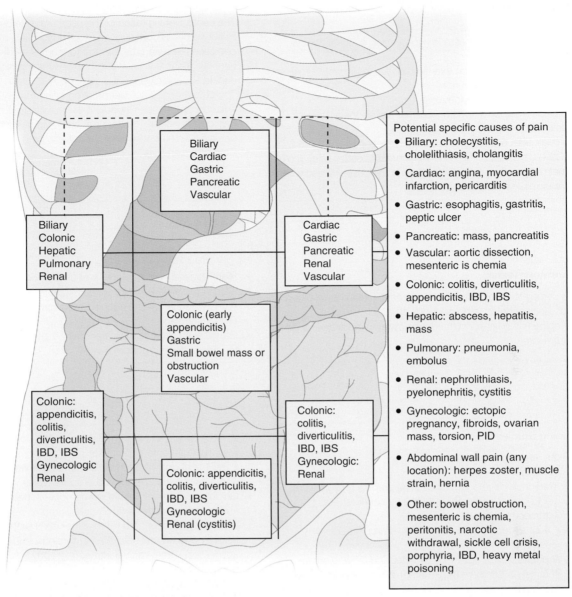

Potential specific causes of pain
- Biliary: cholecystitis, cholelithiasis, cholangitis
- Cardiac: angina, myocardial infarction, pericarditis
- Gastric: esophagitis, gastritis, peptic ulcer
- Pancreatic: mass, pancreatitis
- Vascular: aortic dissection, mesenteric ischemia
- Colonic: colitis, diverticulitis, appendicitis, IBD, IBS
- Hepatic: abscess, hepatitis, mass
- Pulmonary: pneumonia, embolus
- Renal: nephrolithiasis, pyelonephritis, cystitis
- Gynecologic: ectopic pregnancy, fibroids, ovarian mass, torsion, PID
- Abdominal wall pain (any location): herpes zoster, muscle strain, hernia
- Other: bowel obstruction, mesenteric ischemia, peritonitis, narcotic withdrawal, sickle cell crisis, porphyria, IBD, heavy metal poisoning

(IBD) Irritable Bowel Disease, *(IBS)* Irritable Bowel Syndrome, *(PID)* Pelvic inflammatory disease

Other Elements of the History[2]
- Associated symptoms
  - Vomiting
    - Vomiting: almost any abdominal disease (e.g., small bowel obstruction)
    - Presence of bile or blood (e.g., massive hematemesis in a patient with a prior AAA repair ?aorto-enteric fistula)
    - Vomiting from more benign causes (e.g., viral or food-borne illness) is self-limited
  - Anorexia in appendicitis
  - Diarrhea
    - Infectious
    - Noninfectious: mesenteric ischemia, appendicitis, colonic obstruction, early small bowel obstruction
  - The urge to defecate + acute abdominal pain—?serious disease (e.g., ruptured aneurysm in the older patient or ruptured ectopic pregnancy in younger female patients)
  - Pyuria and dysuria: UTI, but also appendicitis, cholecystitis, pancreatitis, or any inflammatory process involving bowel
  - Cardiopulmonary symptoms (cough and dyspnea): ?non-abdominal cause of abdominal pain
  - Syncope: ?disease originating in the chest (pulmonary embolism, dissection) or abdomen (acute aortic aneurysm, ectopic pregnancy)
- Medical/surgical history
  - Hx of surgery → adhesions
  - Diabetic ketoacidosis, hypercalcemia, Addison's disease, and sickle cell crisis, uremia, lead poisoning, methanol intoxication, hereditary angioedema, porphyria -> acute abdominal pain
- Medications: steroids, Non-steroidal anti-inflammatory drugs (NSAIDs), immunosuppressive medications
- Social history: drugs, alcohol (e.g., cocaine → bowel/cardiac ischemia); domestic violence → trauma

AAA, abdominal aortic aneurysm; *NSAIDs*, Nonsteroidal antiinflammatory drugs; *UTI*, urinary tract infection.

Physical Examination Clues[2,3]

- Fever suggests infection
- Tachycardia and orthostatic hypotension suggest hypovolemia
- Pulmonary and cardiac examination are important to rule out nonabdominal source
- Specific signs and maneuvers
- Carnett's sign: confirms abdominal wall as the source of pain
- Cough test: evidence of peritoneal irritation
- Closed eyes sign: indicator of nonorganic cause of abdominal pain (positive if the patient keeps their eyes closed when abdominal tenderness is elicited)
- Murphy's sign: cholecystitis
- The psoas sign: irritation of the psoas muscle by an inflammatory process contiguous to the muscle (inflammatory conditions involving the retroperitoneum, including pyelonephritis, pancreatitis, and psoas abscess; positive on the right in appendicitis)
- The obturator sign: presence of an inflammatory process adjacent to the muscle deep in lateral walls of the pelvis (pelvic appendicitis [on the right only], sigmoid diverticulitis, pelvic inflammatory disease, or ectopic pregnancy)
- Rovsing's sign (appendicitis)

Laboratory Tests[3]

- A complete blood count is appropriate if infection or blood loss is suspected (e.g., appendicitis)
- If epigastric pain—simultaneous amylase and lipase measurements
- Right upper quadrant pain—liver chemistries
- Hematuria, dysuria, or flank pain—urinalysis
- A urine pregnancy test should be performed in females of childbearing age
- Females at risk of sexually transmitted infections—testing for chlamydia and gonorrhea

Imaging Studies[4]

- Right upper quadrant pain
  - Ultrasonography
  - Radionuclide imaging (cholescintigraphy) is slightly better to detect acute cholecystitis (generally should follow ultrasonography)
  - CT of abdomen with contrast is appropriate in some cases
  - If pulmonary symptoms—d-dimer and CT angiogram
  - If urinary symptoms (e.g., hematuria)—consider CT for nephrolithiasis
- Left upper quadrant
  - CT (imaging of the pancreas, spleen, kidneys, intestines, and vasculature)
  - If stomach is suspected—upper endoscopy or upper GI series
- Right lower quadrant
  - CT with IV contrast media (if fever, leukocytosis consider appendicitis or peritonitis)
  - Ultrasonography of abdomen sometimes is appropriate with graded compression
  - Ultrasonography of pelvis is appropriate in females with pelvic pain
- Left lower quadrant
  - CT with oral and IV contrast media (sigmoid diverticulitis is the most common cause)
  - MRI of abdomen and pelvis with and/or without contrast media may be appropriate in some cases
- Left lower quadrant pain in women of childbearing age—abdominal or transvaginal ultrasonography. If ectopic pregnancy is suspected (or for other GYN pathology: as fibroids, ovarian masses, ovarian torsions, and tubo-ovarian abscesses)—transvaginal ultrasonography
- Suprapubic
  - Ultrasonography
- Acute nonlocalized abdominal pain and fever (suspected abdominal abscess)
  - CT of abdomen and pelvis with contrast media
  - In some cases ultrasonography of abdomen or MRI (e.g., in pregnant patients).
  - In some cases radiography of abdomen to evaluate for bowel perforation (free air under the diaphragm)
- Role for plain radiography
  - An upright radiograph of the chest or abdomen can detect free air under the diaphragm
  - Abnormal calcifications also can be seen on a plain radiograph (10% of gallstones, 90% percent of kidney stones, and appendicoliths in 5% of patients with appendicitis)

CT, Computed tomography; *IV*, intravenous; *MRI*, magnetic resonance imaging; *GYN*, gynecology.

Dysphagia

Dysphagia or swallowing dysfunction is a frequent symptom in critically ill patients. It is associated with aspiration into airway (potentially leading to aspiration pneumonia). Some patients present with dysphagia, but dysphagia may present a new problem in the ICU patients who survived critical illness.[5] Patients might not be aware of dysphagia and aspiration, therefore it should be suspected and screened for.

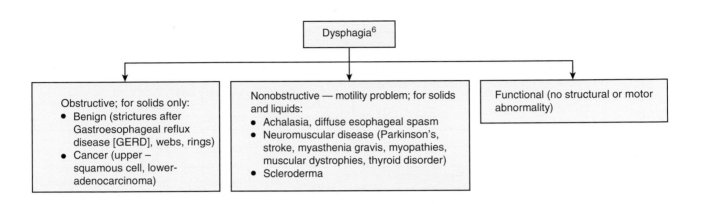

Dysphagia[6]

Obstructive; for solids only:	Nonobstructive — motility problem; for solids and liquids:	Functional (no structural or motor abnormality)
• Benign (strictures after Gastroesophageal reflux disease [GERD], webs, rings) • Cancer (upper – squamous cell, lower-adenocarcinoma)	• Achalasia, diffuse esophageal spasm • Neuromuscular disease (Parkinson's, stroke, myasthenia gravis, myopathies, muscular dystrophies, thyroid disorder) • Scleroderma	

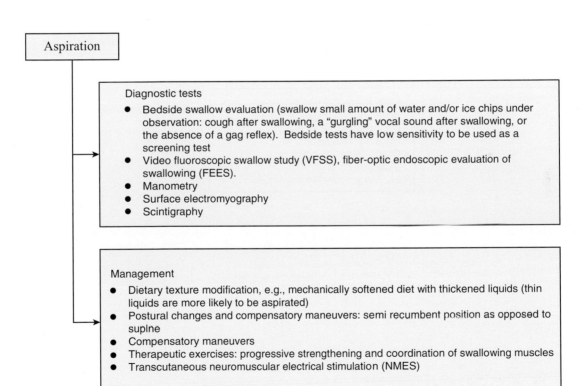

Aspiration

Diagnostic tests

- Bedside swallow evaluation (swallow small amount of water and/or ice chips under observation: cough after swallowing, a "gurgling" vocal sound after swallowing, or the absence of a gag reflex). Bedside tests have low sensitivity to be used as a screening test
- Video fluoroscopic swallow study (VFSS), fiber-optic endoscopic evaluation of swallowing (FEES).
- Manometry
- Surface electromyography
- Scintigraphy

Management

- Dietary texture modification, e.g., mechanically softened diet with thickened liquids (thin liquids are more likely to be aspirated)
- Postural changes and compensatory maneuvers: semi recumbent position as opposed to supine
- Compensatory maneuvers
- Therapeutic exercises: progressive strengthening and coordination of swallowing muscles
- Transcutaneous neuromuscular electrical stimulation (NMES)

Diarrhea

Diarrhea is defined by increased frequency of bowel movements (usually more than three per day) and/or a change in consistency of stool, the latter potentially being watery or just loose stools. Similar to some other abdominal symptoms, diarrhea has many potential causes which are discussed below.

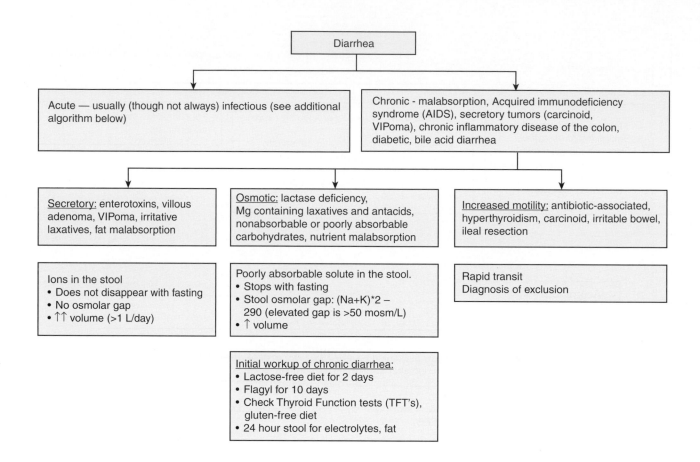

Management of Acute Diarrhea[7,8]

Non inflammatory (enterotoxigenic), secretory diarrhea
Stool most of the time grows normal flora, tends to involve upper GI tract, more voluminous, watery, non-bloody stool, that do not contain Polymorphonuclear (PMN) leukocytes. It is generally milder, though severe fluid loss can still occur, especially in malnourished patients

Inflammatory (invasive), exudative
Abnormal flora on stool culture and sensitivity (C&S), tends to involve lower GI tract, relatively small volume, purulent or bloody stool, accompanied by fever, presence of fecal leukocytes. It is generally more severe

Likely noninfectious
(clinically suggestive of noninfectious process)
Workup: stool culture, ova and parasites, sometimes endoscopy and colonic biopsy in difficult case

Likely infectious: bacterial or parasitic
additional workup and treatment as below

Likely food poisoning with preformed toxins
(several persons with a common food exposure experience symptoms within 16 hours of exposure)
Self-limited; supportive therapy (treat symptoms, provide hydration)

- Community-acquired or traveler's diarrhea: test for *Salmonella, Shigella, Campylobacter,* Shiga toxin–producing *E. coli* (enterohemorrhagic *E. coli;* if history of hemolytic uremic syndrome), *C. difficile* toxins A and B (if treated with antibiotics or chemotherapy in recent weeks)
- Nosocomial (after >3 days in the hospital or other facility) or if Abx were used within 3 months: test for *C. difficile* toxins A and B, *Salmonella, Shigella, Campylobacter,* and Shiga toxin–producing *E. coli*
- Persistent diarrhea of more than 7 days (especially if patient is immunocompromised): consider testing for *Giardia, Cryptosporidium, Cyclospora,* and *Isospora belli,* and inflammatory screening (fecal lactoferrin)
- In immunocompromised add testing for *Microsporida, Mycobacterium avium* intracellulare complex, *Cytomegalovirus, C. difficile* if chemotherapy

Potential infectious etiologies:
- Enterotoxigenic *Escherichia coli* (24–72 h after ingestion): Cipro, azithromycin, Bactrim
- *Clostridium perfringes* (8–14 h after ingestion)
- *Staphylococcus aureus* (2–6 h after exposure)
- *Bacillus cereus* (emetic form — Staphylococcus type of enterotoxin, diarrheal form — *E. coli* type of enterotoxin)
- *Vibrio cholerae* (12–48 h after ingestion): doxycycline, azithromycin, tetracycline, Bactrim
- *Cryptosporidium:* nitazoxanide
- *Giardia:* metronidazole
- *Cyclospora* or *Isospora:* Bactrim
- Viral (nonbloody, watery stool; mild disease; afebrile): Rotavirus (children under 3: vomiting <24 hours, diarrhea, low grade fever), Norwalk-like viruses, Adenovirus, Astrovirus, Coronavirus. Treat with fluid replacement, loperamid

More details on specific infections and therapy
- *Campylobacter jejuni* (Raw milk. 2–6 days after ingestion): azithromycin, erythromycin, cipro
- Shigellosis (Incub - 1–7 days): cipro, Bactrim, azithromycin, ceftriaxone
- Shiga toxin producing *E.Coli* (0157:H7 or Non-0157): cipro, Bactrim
- *C. difficile* (see Infectious Disease section for details): metronidazole, vancomycin
- *Vibrio parahaemolyticus* (raw or undercooked seafood Incubation 4 hours to 4 days)
- *Entamoeba histolitica:* metronidazole
- Salmonellosis (Incubation 24–48 hours, typhoid fever: 10 days). Typhoid fever: cipro, Bactrim, azithromycin
- *Yersinia:* doxycycline, Bactrim, cipro

Consider non infectious causes
- Ischemia
- Ulcerative colitio
- Crohn's disease

Jaundice Workup

Yellow skin color is caused by elevated plasma bilirubin (>3 mg/dL), which can be caused either by increased production of bilirubin (e.g., hemolytic anemia) or decreased excretion due to diminished conjugation or obstruction. The cause of jaundice/elevated bilirubin and its workup are discussed below.[9]

Initial Workup

- Fractionated bilirubin (differentiate between conjugated and unconjugated hyperbilirubinemia)
- Complete blood count (hemolysis, anemia of chronic disease, thrombocytopenia in liver cirrhosis)

- Alanine transaminase, aspartate transaminase (hepatocellular damage)
- Gamma-glutamyltransferase, alkaline phosphatase (biliary obstruction and parenchymal liver disease, though nonspecific)
- Prothrombin time, INR, albumin, and protein (liver synthetic function)

INR, International normalized ratio.

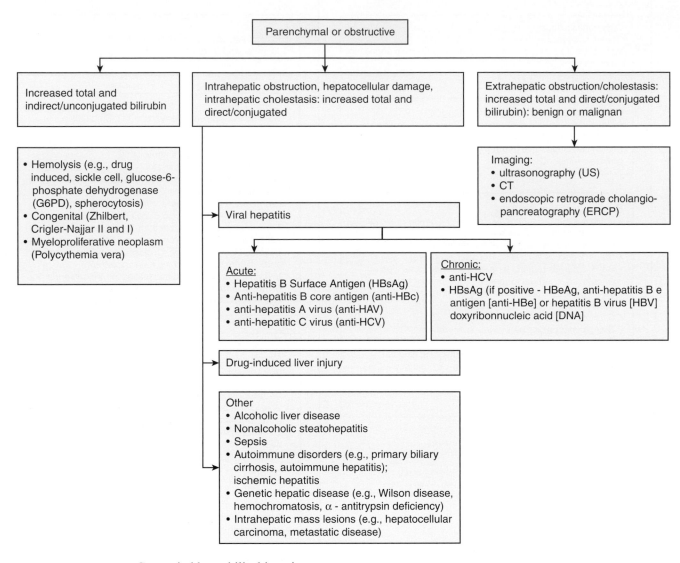

Congenital hyperbilirubinemias

↑ Unconjugated	↑ Conjugated
• Zhilbert—defect in uptake and conjugation • Crigler-Najjar II and I	• Dubin-Johnson—↓transport in hepatocyte and across membrane • Rotor—storage problem

Upper GI Bleeding

Upper GI bleeding defined as intraluminal bleeding proximal to the Treitz ligament and is divided into variceal and nonvariceal.[10] Upper GI bleeding might vary significantly in their severity; in certain cases, patients will need ICU level of care, and occasionally require intubation mostly for airway protection as discussed below.

Treatment of Upper GI Bleeding[10–12]

- Fluid resuscitation: obtain two peripheral venous access for crystalloid infusion, infuse intravenous fluid (IVF), the goal is SBP 90–100, HR <100
- Blood transfusion: decision based on comorbidities, hemodynamic conditions, markers of tissue hypoxia; maintain Hb >7–8 g/dL[12]
- Coagulation: platelet transfusion, correction of coagulation disorders (fresh frozen plasma [FFP], vitamin K, or protamine sulfate) when severe bleeding, in patients on antiplatelet drugs and/or blood thinners. In liver cirrhosis: if active bleeding and severe thrombocytopenia (<50,000/μL) or coagulopathy (INR > 1.5) consider platelet and/or plasma transfusion
- Gastric lavage is controversial
- Prokinetic agents (erythromycin 250 mg IV 30–60 minutes before endoscopy) to empty the stomach before endoscopy
- High dose of proton pump inhibitors IV infusion (bolus of 80 mg, followed by 8 mg/h for 72 hours). No role for H2-receptor antagonists.
- Test for Helicobacter pylori

- Antibiotic prophylaxis for a short period in patients with cirrhosis (e.g., Cipro 500 mg PO Q12 hours or norfloxacin 400 mg PO Q12 hours or ceftriaxone 1 g/day for 7 days)
- Vasoactive drugs if suspected variceal bleeding (e.g., somatostatin, octreotide, vasopressin)—decreasing variceal blood flow by mesenteric and splenic vein constriction; no role for somatostatin or octreotide in nonvariceal bleeding except may be considered in those with massive unresponsive bleeding
- Endoscopy (in the first 24 hours after admission in patients with suspected nonvariceal upper gastrointestinal bleeding [UGB]) and within 12 hours in those with variceal bleeding ± endoscopic treatment. Endoscopy may be delayed in rare patients (e.g., suspected perforation or active acute coronary syndrome)
  - nonvariceal bleed: cautery, thermocoagulation, clips, or injection; epinephrine injection alone provides suboptimal efficacy, combine with another modality such as clips, thermal, or sclerosant injection
  - variceal bleed: endoscopic sclerotherapy and variceal ligation
- Routine second-look endoscopy is not recommended

HR, Heart rate; *SBP*, systolic blood pressure.

Who Should Be Admitted to the ICU

- Elderly
- High comorbidity level

- Suspicion of variceal hemorrhage
- Initial presentation with active bleeding
- Hemodynamic instability

Consider Intubation in the Following Cases

- Massive bleeding
- Hematemesis

- Respiratory failure
- Altered level of consciousness

Risk Stratification: Predictors of Rebleeding and Mortality[11]

- High comorbidities
- Low initial hemoglobin levels
- Transfusion requirements

- Finding of fresh red blood upon rectal examination or nasogastric aspirate or in the emesis
- Age over 65 years
- Poor overall health status
- Endoscopic predictors: active bleeding, ulcer size larger than 2 cm, ulcer location, and the presence of high-risk stigmata

Persistent Bleeding or Rebleeding

- Second endoscopic attempt: consider a different endoscopic method for hemostasis
- Rescue therapy:
  - Sengstaken-Blakemore tube for up to 24 hours; intubation is recommended for airway protection prior to balloon tamponade

  - Transarterial embolization
  - Transjugular intrahepatic portosystemic shunt (TIPS) for variceal bleed refractory to endoscopic treatment
  - Surgery (shunt surgery reserved only for patients with variceal bleeding refractory to clinical and endoscopic therapy)
  - Self-expanding metal stents (SEMS) for variceal bleeding

Lower GI Bleeding

Lower GI bleeding occurs from the colon, rectum, or anus, and it presents with bright red blood (hematochezia) or melena.[13]

Causes (in the Order of Frequency)

- Diverticulosis
- Hemorrhoids
- Ischemic
- IBD
- Post-polypectomy
- Colon cancer/polyps
- Rectal ulcer
- Vascular ectasia
- Radiation colitis/proctitis

IBD, Inflammatory bowel disease.

Initial Management (Prior to Endoscopy)

- Resuscitation with isotonic crystalloid solutions to maintain SBP >100 mm Hg
- Blood transfusion to maintain Hb above 9–10 g/dL (some data for lower threshold of 7 g/dL[4])
- Keep platelets >50,000/mm^3
- Keep INR at 1.5 or less

Diagnostic Options

- Endoscopy
- Radionuclide scintigraphy (detect bleeding at a rate as low as 0.04 mL/min)
- CT angiography (the bleeding rate must be at least 0.3–0.5 mL/min)
- Capsule endoscopy
- Enteroscopy: double-balloon enteroscopy/push enteroscopy

Therapeutic options to stop lower GI bleeding[9]

Endoscopy
- Colonoscopy if diverticular bleed is suspected
- Sigmoidoscopy if suspect
  o Solitary rectal ulcer
  o Ulcerative colitis
  o Radiation proctitis
  o Infectious colitis
  o Ischemic colitis
  o Post polypectomy bleeding in cases of polyp(s) removed only from the rectum and/or left colon
  o Internal hemorrhoids

Endoscopic treatment options
- Injecting epinephrine
- Thermal probe to cauterize the diverticular edge
- Endoscopic clips
- Endoscopic band ligation

Angiography
- Endovascular embolization of arterial branches (with gelatin sponges, particles, coils, microcoils, glue)[14]
- Indications for embolization:
  o Hemodynamic instability or patientswho are stabilized with fluid resuscitation
  o Failed medical Rx or endoscopy
- Potential complications:
  o Bowel ischemia
  o Hematoma
  o Femoral artery thrombosis
  o Contrast reaction
  o Acute kidney injury (AKI)
  o TIA

Surgery
- Rarely necessary
- Indications:
  o Malignancy
  o Diffuse bleeding that fails to cease with medical therapy (as in ischemic or ulcerative colitis) or embolization
  o Recurrent bleeding from a diverticulum

Acute Pancreatitis

Acute inflammation of pancreatic tissue might be caused by several factors including common bile duct obstruction (distal to the pancreatic duct joining), alcohol, and other factors. Acute pancreatitis may be a single event; it may be recurrent, or it may progress to chronic pancreatitis. Workup and treatment of acute pancreatitis are discussed below. Since the outcome of acute pancreatitis might range from quick recovery to severe course and be extremely unfavorable, the prognostic algorithms are described separately to help identify patients at higher risk of poor outcome.

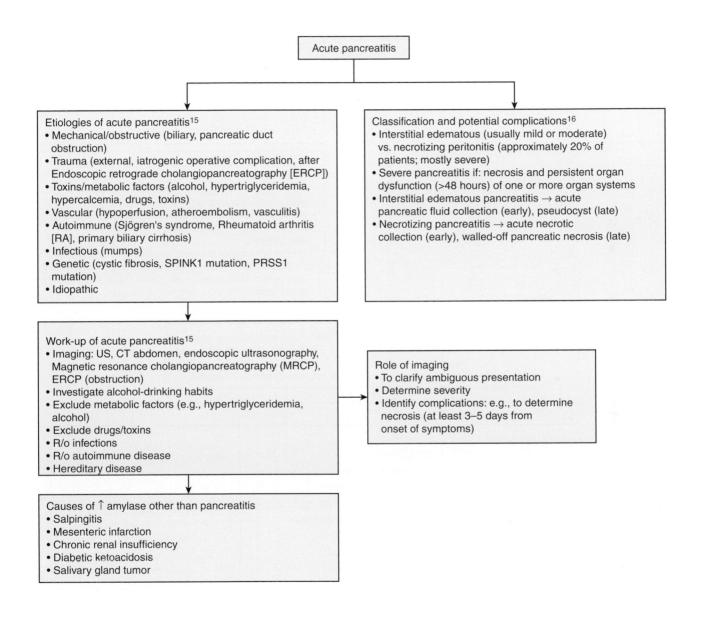

Acute pancreatitis

Etiologies of acute pancreatitis[15]
- Mechanical/obstructive (biliary, pancreatic duct obstruction)
- Trauma (external, iatrogenic operative complication, after Endoscopic retrograde cholangiopancreatography [ERCP])
- Toxins/metabolic factors (alcohol, hypertriglyceridemia, hypercalcemia, drugs, toxins)
- Vascular (hypoperfusion, atheroembolism, vasculitis)
- Autoimmune (Sjögren's syndrome, Rheumatoid arthritis [RA], primary biliary cirrhosis)
- Infectious (mumps)
- Genetic (cystic fibrosis, SPINK1 mutation, PRSS1 mutation)
- Idiopathic

Classification and potential complications[16]
- Interstitial edematous (usually mild or moderate) vs. necrotizing peritonitis (approximately 20% of patients; mostly severe)
- Severe pancreatitis if: necrosis and persistent organ dysfunction (>48 hours) of one or more organ systems
- Interstitial edematous pancreatitis → acute pancreatic fluid collection (early), pseudocyst (late)
- Necrotizing pancreatitis → acute necrotic collection (early), walled-off pancreatic necrosis (late)

Work-up of acute pancreatitis[15]
- Imaging: US, CT abdomen, endoscopic ultrasonography, Magnetic resonance cholangiopancreatography (MRCP), ERCP (obstruction)
- Investigate alcohol-drinking habits
- Exclude metabolic factors (e.g., hypertriglyceridemia, alcohol)
- Exclude drugs/toxins
- R/o infections
- R/o autoimmune disease
- Hereditary disease

Role of imaging
- To clarify ambiguous presentation
- Determine severity
- Identify complications: e.g., to determine necrosis (at least 3–5 days from onset of symptoms)

Causes of ↑ amylase other than pancreatitis
- Salpingitis
- Mesenteric infarction
- Chronic renal insufficiency
- Diabetic ketoacidosis
- Salivary gland tumor

Treatment of acute pancreatitis

Supportive care of acute pancreatitis[17]
• Aggressive fluid resuscitation in the first 48–72 hours
• Pain control
• Bowel rest
• ERCP in biliary pancreatitis or concomitant cholangitis
• No role currently for prophylactic antibiotics
  (unless cholangitis or extrahepatic infection)
• Early enteral nutrition within 48 hours (vial postpyloric
  feeding tube, e.g., naso-jejunal). Using Total parenteral
  nutrition (TPN) has worse outcome than enteral nutrition

Management of complications

Infected pancreatic necrosis (2–4 weeks after symptom
onset)
• Antibiotics with Gram-negative coverage
  (carbapenems, metronidazole, fluoroquinolones,
  selected cephalosporines)
• CT-guided aspiration
• Debridement or drainage (open surgery, videoassisted
  retroperitoneal debridement, endoscopic
  transmural debridement)

Hemorrhage into pancreatic necrosis (into retroperitoneum
or peritoneal cavity)
• Life-threatening complication
• Diagnosed by noting a drop in Hb
• Treatment: IR embolization or surgery

Inflammation and abdominal compartment syndrome
• Inflammation causing blocking nearby structures
  (e.g., biliary compression, hydronephrosis, bowel or
  gastric outlet obstruction)
• Abdominal compartment syndrome (caused by fluid
  collection, ascites, ileus, overly aggressive fluid
  resuscitation)
• Monitor abdominal pressure (bladder pressure sensor),
  if >20 mm Hg → decompression by nasogastric or rectal
  tube, sedation/paralysis, minimize IV fluids, drain ascites,
  laparotomy

Prognosis of acute pancreatitis[18]
• Signs of organ failure within 24 hours of admission significantly increase
  the risk of death
• In addition several severity scores have association with the outcome

Ranson's criteria of acute pancreatitis
severity

At presentation
• Age >55 years
• WBC count >16,000/mm^3
• Blood glucose >200 mg/dL
• Lactate dehydrogenase (LDH) >350 U/L
• ALT/AST >250 U/L

At 48 hours
• Hematocrit decrease by 10%
• Blood urea nitrogen increase by 5
  mg/dL
• Calcium below 8 mg/dL
• PaO2 below 60 mm Hg
• Base deficit >4 meq/L
• Fluid sequestration >6000 mL

Scoring:1 point for each positive
criterion
Score >3 at 48 hours is associated with
higher mortality major complications,
pancreatic necrosis

Imrie scoring system
At 48 hours
• Age >55 years
• WBC >15,000/mm^3
• Blood glucose >180 mg/ dL in
  patients wit hout diabetes
• Serum LDH >600 U/L
• AST/ALT >100 U/L
• Calcium <8 mg/dL
• PaO2 <60 mm Hg
• Serum albumin <3.2 g/dL
• Serum urea >45 mg/dL

Scoring: 1 point for each positive
criterion 48 hours after admission
Score ≥3 is associated with higher
mortality, major complications,
pancreatic necrosis

CT severity index (72 hours after
admission)
• CT grade:
  ○ grade A, i.e., normal = 0 points;
  ○ grade B (edematous) = 1 point;
  ○ grade C (= B plus mild
    extrapancreatic changes) = 2
    points;
  ○ grade D (severe extrapancreatic
    changes plus one fluid
    collection) = 3 points;
  ○ grade E (multiple or extensive
    fluid collections) = 4 points
• Necrosis score:
  ○ None = 0 points
  ○ <⅓ = 2 points
  ○ >⅓ but <½ = 4 points
  ○ >½ = 6 points

Scoring: CT grade + necrosis score:
score of 5 or greater correlated with
prolonged hospitalization and higher
rates of mortality (15 times higher) and
morbidity

Ischemic Colitis

Ischemic Colitis vs. Mesenteric Ischemia (Ischemic Bowel). Two similar terms used to describe two separate entities: (1) ischemic colitis (a result of ischemia) and (2) mesenteric ischemia or ischemic bowel, which is a result of embolic event. The latter has sudden onset and blood supply to affected segment is totally blocked. It presents with abdominal pain out of proportion to clinical findings and requires urgent surgery. Ischemic colitis on the other hand presents with more gradual onset (over hours), its cause is multifactorial (including embolic), and blood supply loss is transient. It presents with moderate abdominal pain and tenderness and bloody diarrhea and requires conservative treatment.[19]

Ischemic colitis
(acute, transient compromise in blood flow, below that required for the metabolic needs of the colon)

Causes
- Systemic (Congestive heart failure [CHF], systemic inflammatory response syndrome, atherosclerosis)
- Embolic (atrial fibrillation)
- Thrombotic (malignancy, hematological disorders)
- Pharmacological (chemotherapy, sex hormones, interferon therapy, pseudoephedrine, cardiac glycosides, diuretics, statins, non-steroidal, NSAIDs, immunosuppressive drugs, vasopressors)
- Surgical (AAA repair)
- Endoscopy (colonoscopy and bowel preparation media for colonoscopy)

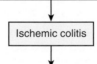

Ischemic colitis

Symptoms

- Diarrhea, rectal bleeding, and colicky abdominal pain, tenderness and voluntary guarding
- Systemic inflammatory response syndrome (SIRS): tachycardia, hypotension, tachypnea, fever
- Shock, leading on to multiorgan failure

Diagnosis

- DDx: infective colitis, inflammatory colitis
- Labs: elevated C-Reactive protein (CRP), lactate and neutrophil count (non-specific)
- CT with contrast (wall thickening, abnormal or absent wall enhancement, dilatation, mesenteric stranding, venous engorgement, ascites, pneumatosis, portal venous gas)
- Colonoscopy to visualize mucosa (petechial hemorrhages, edematous and fragile mucosa, segmental erythema, scattered erosions, longitudinal ulcerations, sharply defined segment of involvement)
- NO role for abdominal X ray and ultrasound

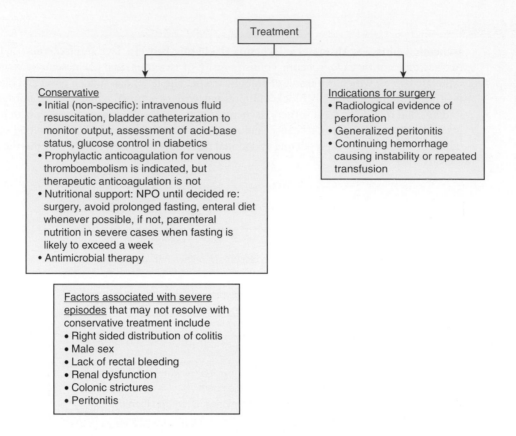

Intraabdominal Hypertension and Abdominal Compartment Syndrome

Intraabdominal pressure (IAP) is a steady-state pressure concealed within the abdominal cavity. Since abdominal cavity is a closed space and relatively nonexpandable compartment, elevated pressure might eventually lead to abdominal compartment syndrome (ACS) and severe organ dysfunction.[20]

IAP Definitions

- Normal—5–7 mm Hg
- IAH—IAP ≥12 mm Hg without organ dysfunction

- ACS—sustained IAP >20 mm Hg that is associated with single or multiple organ failure that was not previously present
- Abdominal perfusion pressure (APP)—difference between mean arterial pressure (MAP) and IAP (APP = MAP – IAP)

IAH, Intraabdominal hypertension.

Risk Factors for IAH[20,21]

- Abdominal wall factors: diminished abdominal wall compliance, abdominal surgery, prone positioning major trauma, major burns
- Intra-abdominal factors: gastroparesis, ileus, hemoperitoneum, acute pancreatitis, intra-abdominal tumor or infection, ascites, peritoneal dialysis

- Increased intravascular volume: massive fluid resuscitation, polytransfusion (>10 units of blood per 24 hours), oliguria
- Capillary leak: sepsis, acidosis, hypothermia, damage control laparotomy
- Other risk factors: anemia, coagulopathy, increased head of bed angle, mechanical ventilation, obesity, PEEP >10, pneumonia, shock, or hypotension

---

PEEP, Positive end-expiratory pressure.

Pathophysiology[20]

- Immediate effects: elevation of diaphragm, vascular compression (IVC, aorta, systemic vasculature)
- Consequences
  - Pulmonary: increased intrathoracic and pulmonary pressure, ARDS
  - Vascular: increased intrathoracic pressure → increased CVP, PCWP, pulmonary vascular resistance
  - Cardiac: decreased stroke volume, cardiac output, and hypotension
  - Intra-abdominal organs: vascular compression → bowel ischemia, AKI
  - Renal: IAP of ≥15 mm Hg is associated with renal impairment
  - Infection: bowel ischemia → bacterial translocation and sepsis. Note that intestinal mucosa lacks effective autoregulatory control (unlike kidneys or brain) and is particularly susceptible to hypotension coupled with elevated IAP
  - Inflammation: activation of inflammatory mediators, increased extravascular fluid loss via capillary leak, and subsequently increased intraabdominal volume and pressure

AKI, Acute kidney injury; *ARDS,* acute respiratory distress syndrome; *CVP,* central venous pressure; *IVC,* inferior vena cava; *PCWP,* pulmonary capillary wedge pressure.

Measuring IAP

- Intravesical pressure
- Iliac/IVC CVP
- Continuous IAP measurement with three-way bladder catheter, continuous saline infusions, and a transducer

Management[20,21]

- Evacuate intraluminal contents
  - nasogastric and/or rectal drainage
  - prokinetic motility agents
  - correction of electrolyte abnormalities
  - enteral nutrition in the critically ill (e.g., early enteral nutrition in acute pancreatitis) to stimulate motility
  - minimize enteral nutrition
- Evacuate intraabdominal space–occupying lesion (i.e., hemoperitoneum, ascites, intra-abdominal abscess, retroperitoneal hematoma, and free air)
- Improve abdominal wall compliance
  - address abdominal wall or third-space edema
  - constrictive bandages and/or tight abdominal closures
  - treat pain, agitation, ventilator dyssynchrony
  - neuromuscular blockers to reduce abdominal muscle tone
  - supine patient position
- Optimize fluid administration (see below)
- Optimize systemic and regional tissue perfusion (see below)

Steps to Optimize Fluid Administration

- Goals
  - Balance between achieving adequate tissue perfusion and oxygenation, avoiding organ dysfunction associated with volume overload
  - Avoid hypotension as bowel lacks effective autoregulatory control and is susceptible to hypotension coupled with elevated IAP
  - On the other hand, hypervolemia should be avoided. It has frequently been identified as an independent predictor for the development of ACS
- Volume resuscitation/management strategies
  - Avoid excessive fluid resuscitation
  - Use diuretics
  - Use colloids and hypertonic saline in patients with elevated IAP
  - Use biologically active colloids (e.g., fresh-frozen plasma) address both posttrauma coagulopathy and intravascular volume
  - Damage control resuscitation: permissive hypotension, limiting crystalloid intravenous fluids and delivering higher ratios of plasma, platelets, and red blood cells
  - Administer vasopressors if hemodynamically unstable to limit reducing the absolute volume of resuscitation fluid required during shock management
  - Combine colloids and diuretics to mobilize third-space edema and achieve negative fluid balance
  - Intermittent hemodialysis or Continuous renal replacement therapy (CRRT)

Steps to Optimize Systemic/Regional Tissue Perfusion

- Early goal-directed therapy: correction of hypovolemia with defined resuscitation endpoints
- Hemodynamic monitoring to guide resuscitation

- Note: traditional barometric measurements (e.g., CVP, pulmonary artery occlusion pressure) are less accurate in IAH/ACS patients (they reflect the sum of both intravascular pressure and intrapleural pressure)

Inflammatory Bowel Disease

Patients with ulcerative colitis and Crohn's disease have a higher risk for being critically ill and admitted to ICU than the general population. Furthermore, they have increased mortality 1 year after admission.[22] We briefly discuss management of inflammatory bowel disease (IBD).

Ulcerative colitis Rx			
Topical mesalamine or corticosteroids	Oral 5-aminosalicylic acid (5-ASA)	Oral corticosteroids at tapering dose	IV corticosteroids, IV cyclosporine
Mild to moderate	*Mild more extensive*	*Unresponsive / moderate to severe*	*Severe / toxic symptoms*

Toxic megacolon Rx:
- NPO
- Suction
- Rotation
- Broad spectrum antibiotics
- IVF

Indications for total colectomy
- Unresponsive severe colitis
- Intractable symptoms
- Corticosteroid side effects
- Colonic perforation
- Severe hemorrhage
- Mucosal dysplasia colon carcinoma

Crohn's disease Rx	
Oral 5-ASA ± metronidazole 10–20 mg/kg/day	Oral corticosteroids, if abscess: drainage + antibiotics
Mild to moderate	*Moderate to severe*

Indications for surgery
- Irreversible obstruction Severe disease unresponsive to medical Rx
- Drainage of abscess
- Resection of fistulas

Management of acute diarrhea [3]
- Hydration (oral or IV)
- Nutrition (dietary restrictions are usually not beneficial and may be harmful)
- Symptomatic treatment
- Antibiotics in some cases

REFERENCES

1. Reintam Blaser A, Starkopf J, Malbrain MLNG. Abdominal signs and symptoms in intensive care patients. *Anaesthesiol Intensive Ther*. 2015;47(4):379–387.
2. Macaluso CR, McNamara RM. Evaluation and management of acute abdominal pain in the emergency department. *Int J Gen Med*. 2012;5:789–797.
3. Cartwright SL, Knudson MP. Evaluation of acute abdominal pain in adults. *Am Fam Physician*. 2008;77(7):971–978.
4. Cartwright SL, Knudson MP. Diagnostic imaging of acute abdominal pain in adults. *Am Fam Physician*. 2015;91(7):452–459.
5. Macht M, White SD, Moss M. Swallowing dysfunction after critical illness. *Chest*. 2014;146(6):1681–1689.
6. O'Horo JC, Rogus-Pulia N, Garcia-Arguello L, Robbins J, Safdar N. Bedside diagnosis of dysphagia: a systematic review. *J Hosp Med*. 2015;10(4):256–265.
7. Barr W, Smith A. Acute diarrhea. *Am Fam Physician*. 2014;89(3):180–189.
8. Brandt KG, de Castro Antunes MM, da Silva GAP. Acute diarrhea: evidence-based management. *J Pediatr*. 2015;91(6 suppl 1):S36–S43.

9. Fargo MV, Grogan SP, Saguil A. Evaluation of jaundice in adults. *Am Fam Physician.* 2017;95(3):164–168.
10. Franco C, Nakao FS, Rodrigues R, Maluf-Filho F, de Paulo GA, Della Libera E. Proposal of a clinical care pathway for the management of acute upper gastrointestinal bleeding. *Arq Gastroenterol.* 2015;52(4):283–292.
11. Greenspoon J, Barkun A. A summary of recent recommendations on the management of patients with nonvariceal upper gastrointestinal bleeding. *Pol Arch Med Wewn.* 2010;120(9):341–346.
12. Villanueva C, Colomo A, Bosch A, et al. Transfusion strategies for acute upper gastrointestinal bleeding. *N Engl J Med.* 2013; 368:11-21.
13. Ghassemi KA, Jensen DM. Lower GI bleeding: epidemiology and management. *Curr Gastroenterol Rep.* 2013;15(7):333.
14. Ierardi AM, Urbano J, De Marchi G, et al. New advances in lower gastrointestinal bleeding management with embolotherapy. *Br J Radiol.* 2016;89(1061):20150934.
15. da Silva S, Rocha M, Pinto-de-Sousa J. Acute pancreatitis etiology investigation: a workup algorithm proposal. *GE Port J Gastroenterol.* 2017;24(3):129–136.
16. Chua TY, Walsh RM, Baker ME, Stevens T. Necrotizing pancreatitis: diagnose, treat, consult. *Cleve Clin J Med.* 2017;84(8):639–648.
17. Bruno MJ, Dutch Pancreatitis Study Group. Improving the outcome of acute pancreatitis. *Dig Dis.* 2016;34(5):540–545.
18. Carroll JK, Herrick B, Gipson T, Lee SP. Acute pancreatitis: diagnosis, prognosis, and treatment. *Am Fam Physician.* 2007;75(10):1513–1520.
19. Trotter JM, Hunt L, Peter MB. Ischaemic colitis. *BMJ.* 2016;355:i6600.
20. Rastogi P, Iyer D, Aneman A, D'Amours S. Intra-abdominal hypertension and abdominal compartment syndrome: pathophysiological and non-operative management. *Minerva Anestesiol.* 2014;80(8):922–932.
21. Kirkpatrick AW, Roberts DJ, De Waele J, et al. Intra-abdominal hypertension and the abdominal compartment syndrome: updated consensus definitions and clinical practice guidelines from the World Society of the Abdominal Compartment Syndrome. *Intensive Care Med.* 2013;39(7):1190–1206.
22. Marrie RA, Garland A, Peschken CA, et al. Increased incidence of critical illness among patients with inflammatory bowel disease: a population-based study. *Clin Gastroenterol Hepatol.* 2014;12(12):2063–2070.e1–e4.

CHAPTER 8

Hematology and Oncology Aspects of Critical Care

Alexander Goldfarb-Rumyantzev

Red Cell Disorders. Anemias, Hemoglobin Disorders

Identifying the exact etiology of anemia is crucial to treatment. In addition to careful history (specifically the duration of anemia, e.g., long-standing anemia might indicate congenital factors; medications, blood loss, comorbidities, alcohol use, recent surgery), three diagnostic steps indicated below should be helpful in establishing the diagnosis.[1] Initial anemia workup and some considerations for specific types of anemia are presented below. In general, considering that red blood cells (RBCs) stay in circulation for approximately 120 days, the degree of anemia development may help to differentiate between anemias caused by RBC underproduction (relatively slow progression) and those caused by RBC loss, e.g., bleeding or hemolysis (relatively fast progression).[2]

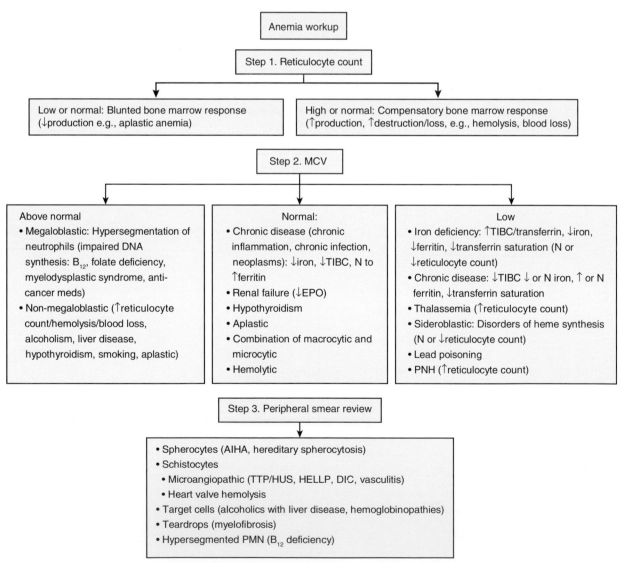

N, Normal; *HELLP,* Hemolysis, Elevated Liver enzymes and Low Platelets

Important Definitions

- TIBC—total iron binding capacity
- Measured serum iron = iron bound to transferrin

- Transferrin saturation (%) = (Iron/TIBC) × 100%
- Corrected reticulocytes—what reticulocyte % would it be if patient was not anemic; Corrected reticulocytes = (Ht/45) × patient's reticulocytes

Abnormal Red Cell Morphology and Corresponding Conditions

- Target cell—thalassemia
- Basophilic stippling—thalassemia, P5'N deficiency
- Hb H inclusion body—Hb H disease
- Heinz body—unstable hemoglobin, G6PD deficiency

- Schistocyte—microangiopathy (TP, HUS, DIC, prosthetic cardiac valve, vasculitis, malignant HTN, eclampsia)
- Spherocyte—hereditary spherocytosis
- Elliptocyte—hereditary elliptocytosis
- Piculated cell—uremia, spur cell anemia

DIC, Disseminated intravascular coagulation; *HTN*, hypertension; *HUS*, hemolytic uremic syndrome; *P5'N*, pyrimidine 5'-nucleotidase; *GP6D*, glucose 6-phosphate dehydrogenase; *TTP*, thrombotic thrombocytopenic purpura.

Iron Deficiency Anemia vs. Anemia of Inflammation (Anemia of Chronic Disease)

Three main components of red cell production regulation are erythropoietin, hepcidin, and iron. Below we demonstrate the interaction between those factors.[3] Iron is a necessary component for erythropoiesis and its level is regulated by hepcidin that blocks iron absorption and release from storage. Hepcidin is under feedback regulation by iron, but can also be stimulated by inflammation.[4] On the other hand, erythropoietin, the most powerful stimulus for erythropoiesis, is being produced by kidneys under conditions of ischemia or hypoxia triggering stabilization of hypoxia-inducible factor (HIF).

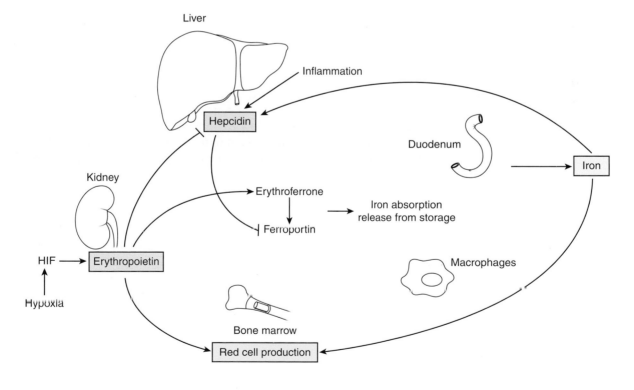

Anemia can be caused by a dysfunction of any of the above factors, or their combination, as in anemia of chronic kidney disease (CKD), which is caused by decreased erythropoietin production, inhibitory effect of uremia on the erythropoietin effect on bone marrow, increased level of hepcidin caused by decreased clearance and inflammation, leading to functional iron deficiency. Furthermore, uremia and inflammatory state might have direct effects on differentiation of progenitors, suppression of HIF, and potentially other components of erythropoiesis. In addition, blood loss in CKD patients leads to iron deficiency as well.[3]

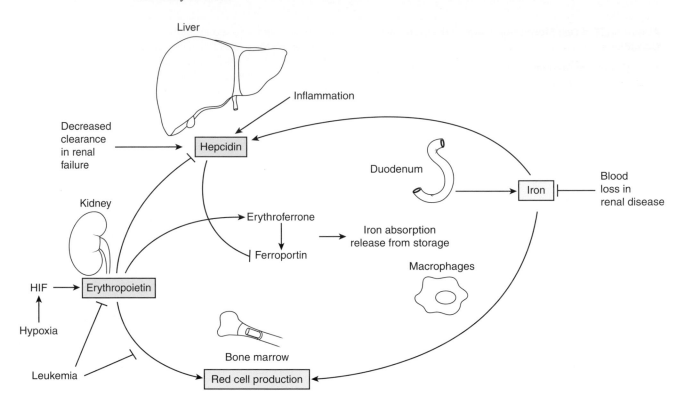

The differential diagnosis of two very common etiologies of anemia—iron deficiency and anemia of inflammation (chronic disease)[5]—is based on several factors: anemia of inflammation is typically normocytic and normochromic, while iron deficiency anemia is usually microcytic and hypochromic. Iron deficiency is associated with low ferritin, which is normal or high in anemia of inflammation. The latter however depends on the definition of low ferritin, which is not consistent across sources. When iron deficiency is suspected the therapeutic trial of iron supplementation is reasonable.[6]

	Iron	TIBC	Transferrin Saturation	Ferritin	Bone Marrow Iron Storages	Hepcidin	Treatment
Iron deficiency	↓	↑	↓	↓	↓	↓	Iron supplement
Anemia of inflammation	N or ↓	↓ or N	↓ or N	N or ↑	N or ↑	↑	Treat the cause, might use erythropoiesis-stimulating agents

Hemolytic Anemia

The diagnosis of hemolytic anemia is suggested by increased reticulocyte count, increased bilirubin, lactate dehydrogenase (LDH), and low haptoglobin. There are several types of hemolysis that can be separated by site (i.e., intravascular and extravascular, the latter by red cells being taken out of circulation and destructed by macrophages in the spleen and liver),[7] morphology of red cells (spherocytic and non-spherocytic), and mechanism (immune mediated and nonimmune mediated, intrinsic and extrinsic to the RBC).[2]

Potential causes of hemolytic anemia

Membrane problems (membranopathies)
- Intrinsic (inherited) abnormalities of erythrocyte membrane[7]: Spherocytosis, elliptocytosis, paroxysmal nocturnal hemoglobinuria, drug-associated reactions of abnormal erythrocyte membrane
- Extrinsic (acquired): Further differential is based on the results of direct antiglobulin test (Coombs test)
  - Coombs (−): Splenomegaly, mechanical trauma/fragmentation (DIC, TTP, HUS, mechanical heart valve, malignant hypertension), infection (malaria, babesiosis, Bartonella, clostridium toxin, Hemophilus influenzae), toxins (e.g., drugs, snake bites, ingestion of strong acid)
  - Coombs (+) (autoimmune):
    - Warm-mediated autoimmune hemolytic anemia: IgG – specific for Rh group (Rx: steroids with or without rituximab, immunosuppression and or splenectomy);
    - Cold-medicated autoimmune hemolytic anemia: IgM – specific for ABO group (Rx: plasma exchange, steroids with or without rituximab, immunosuppression)[8]
  - Transfusion reaction (could be Coombs negative)

Coombs test:
- Direct: Patient RBC's + anti-IgG/anti-C3 – to detect IgG or C3 on the surface of patient's red cells
- Indirect: Normal RBC + patient's serum + anti-IgG – to detect serum antibodies

Congenital abnormal hemoglobin (hemoglobinopathies)
- Sickling Hb
- Thalassemia
- Other hemoglobinopathies: Unstable hemoglobin, methemoglobins

Cytosolic enzymes
- Decreased reduction of normally produced methemoglobin: G6PD, methemoglobin reductase deficiency, pyruvate kinase deficiency
- Decreased ATP production: Pyruvate kinase deficiency, deficiency of other enzymes in anaerobic glycolysis

Hemolytic anemia is suggested by presence of anemia, ↑reticulocyte count, ↑bilirubin

Confirm Hemolysis
- ↑Bilirubin
- ↑LDH
- ↑Urobilinogen
- ↓Haptoglobin
- ↑Reticulocytosis
- Erythroid hyperplasia of bone marrow

Cause of hemolysis by type[9]
• Consider the cause by type (spherocytic versus non-spherocytic)
• Site (intramedullary versus extramedullary; intravascular versus extravascular),
• Mechanism (immune-mediated versus nonimmune-mediated; intrinsic versus extrinsic to the RBC).

Peripheral smear (red cell morphology)
• Spherocytes: Implies loss of membrane, either by inherited (e.g., hereditary spherocytosis) or acquired (e.g., antibody-mediated) mechanisms
• Schistocytes (suggest fragmentation hemolysis, as in micro- or macroangiopathic hemolytic anemias): TTP, HUS, DIC, eclampsia, preeclampsia, malignant hypertension, prosthetic valve
• Sickle cells

History
• Immune hemolysis suggested by
  • Drug intake (suspect G6PD deficiency, antibiotic exposure, etc)
  • Blood transfusion
  • Underlying disease (cancer, lymphoproliferative disease, autoimmune disease)
• Family history
• Infections, fever, recent travel: Thick and thin blood smears, Babesia serologies, bacterial cultures
• History suggestive of mechanical destruction: TTP, HUS, DIC, eclampsia, malignant hypertension, prosthetic valve

Additional laboratory tests
• Red cell indices (e.g., macrocytic vs microcytic, normochromic vs hypochromic)
• Osmotic fragility (hereditary spherocytosis)
• Autoantibody: Antiglobulin test/Coombs test (autoimmune hemolytic anemia); cold agglutinin (cold agglutinin disease)
• Ham test and sugar water test (paroxysmal nocturnal hemoglobinuria)
• Membrane protein analysis (membrane protein defect)
• Hb analysis: Electrophoresis (unstable hemoglobin hemolysis anemia, thalassemia)
• Red cell enzyme analysis (enzymopathy, e.g., G6PD deficiency)

Aplastic Anemia

Aplastic anemia is caused by bone marrow failure to generate blood cells. It is frequently related to immune-mediated destruction of hematopoietic cells,[10] hence treatment sometimes is based on immunosuppression. Hematopoietic growth factors do not seem to have a role.[11] Noticeably, aplastic anemia is frequently associated with pancytopenia.

Diagnosis of Aplastic Anemia (suspect in patients with pancytopenia)

• Bone marrow studies
  ○ Biopsy (e.g., MDS, leukemia, metastatic cancer)
  ○ Aspirate (e.g., cytogenetics: chromosomal abnormalities, cytology to confirm absence of blasts)
  ○ Examine peripheral blood
  ○ Human leukocyte antigen (HLA) typing for the purpose of future bone marrow transplant

MDS, Myelodysplastic syndrome.

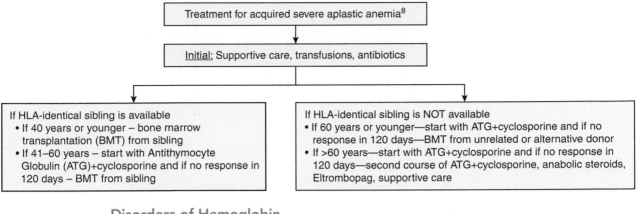

Treatment for acquired severe aplastic anemia[8]

↓

Initial: Supportive care, transfusions, antibiotics

If HLA-identical sibling is available
- If 40 years or younger – bone marrow transplantation (BMT) from sibling
- If 41–60 years – start with Antithymocyte Globulin (ATG)+cyclosporine and if no response in 120 days – BMT from sibling

If HLA-identical sibling is NOT available
- If 60 years or younger—start with ATG+cyclosporine and if no response in 120 days—BMT from unrelated or alternative donor
- If >60 years—start with ATG+cyclosporine and if no response in 120 days—second course of ATG+cyclosporine, anabolic steroids, Eltrombopag, supportive care

Disorders of Hemoglobin

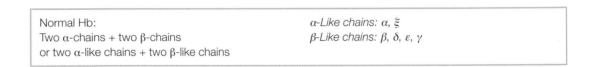

Normal Hb: Two α-chains + two β-chains or two α-like chains + two β-like chains	α-Like chains: α, ξ β-Like chains: β, δ, ε, γ

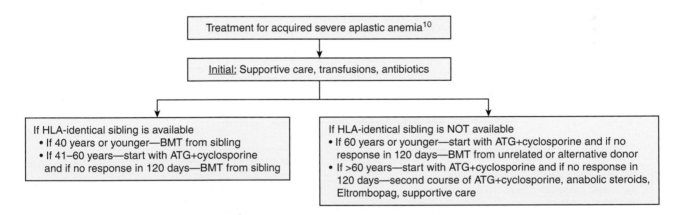

Treatment for acquired severe aplastic anemia[10]

↓

Initial: Supportive care, transfusions, antibiotics

If HLA-identical sibling is available
- If 40 years or younger—BMT from sibling
- If 41–60 years—start with ATG+cyclosporine and if no response in 120 days—BMT from sibling

If HLA-identical sibling is NOT available
- If 60 years or younger—start with ATG+cyclosporine and if no response in 120 days—BMT from unrelated or alternative donor
- If >60 years—start with ATG+cyclosporine and if no response in 120 days—second course of ATG+cyclosporine, anabolic steroids, Eltrombopag, supportive care

Sickle Cell Disease

Sickle cell disease is caused by structural defect in hemoglobin (sickle Hb—Hb S). It is a result of single amino acid substitution. Hb S forms insoluble polymers when deoxygenated.[12,13]

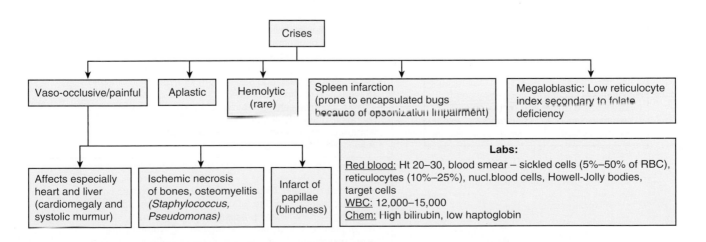

Crises

- Vaso-occlusive/painful
- Aplastic
- Hemolytic (rare)
- Spleen infarction (prone to encapsulated bugs because of opsonization impairment)
- Megaloblastic: Low reticulocyte index secondary to folate deficiency

Vaso-occlusive/painful:
- Affects especially heart and liver (cardiomegaly and systolic murmur)
- Ischemic necrosis of bones, osteomyelitis (*Staphylococcus, Pseudomonas*)
- Infarct of papillae (blindness)

Labs:
Red blood: Ht 20–30, blood smear – sickled cells (5%–50% of RBC), reticulocytes (10%–25%), nucl.blood cells, Howell-Jolly bodies, target cells
WBC: 12,000–15,000
Chem: High bilirubin, low haptoglobin

Consequences of the Sickle Cell Disease[13]

- Cardiothoracic: dysrhythmias and sudden death, CHF, pulmonary HTN, restrictive lung disease, acute chest syndrome
- Nervous: ischemic or hemorrhagic stroke, venous sinus thrombosis, retinopathy, orbital infarction, cognitive impairment, chronic pain

- Reticuloendothelial: anemia, hemolysis, splenic sequestration
- Musculoskeletal: avascular necrosis, leg skin ulceration
- Urogenital: renal failure, proteinuria, hematuria, papillary necrosis, priapism
- GI: mesenteric vaso-occlusion, cholelithiasis, hepatopathy
- Infections: due to splenic dysfunction

CHF, Congestive heart failure.

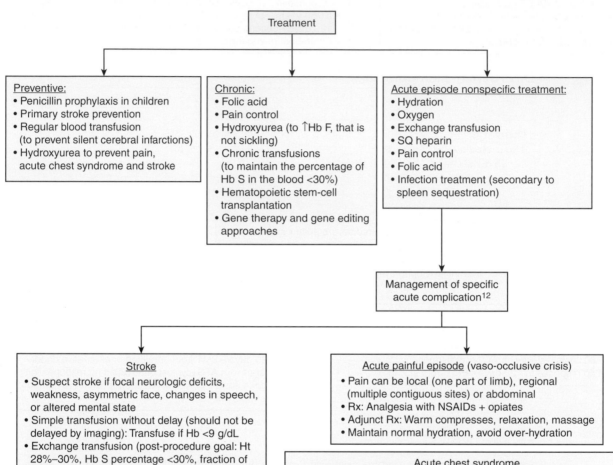

Treatment

Preventive:
- Penicillin prophylaxis in children
- Primary stroke prevention
- Regular blood transfusion (to prevent silent cerebral infarctions)
- Hydroxyurea to prevent pain, acute chest syndrome and stroke

Chronic:
- Folic acid
- Pain control
- Hydroxyurea (to ↑Hb F, that is not sickling)
- Chronic transfusions (to maintain the percentage of Hb S in the blood <30%)
- Hematopoietic stem-cell transplantation
- Gene therapy and gene editing approaches

Acute episode nonspecific treatment:
- Hydration
- Oxygen
- Exchange transfusion
- SQ heparin
- Pain control
- Folic acid
- Infection treatment (secondary to spleen sequestration)

Management of specific acute complication[12]

Stroke
- Suspect stroke if focal neurologic deficits, weakness, asymmetric face, changes in speech, or altered mental state
- Simple transfusion without delay (should not be delayed by imaging): Transfuse if Hb <9 g/dL
- Exchange transfusion (post-procedure goal: Ht 28%–30%, Hb S percentage <30%, fraction of cells remaining <0.3)
- Erythrocytapheresis (better long-term outcomes than simple transfusion)

Acute painful episode (vaso-occlusive crisis)
- Pain can be local (one part of limb), regional (multiple contiguous sites) or abdominal
- Rx: Analgesia with NSAIDs + opiates
- Adjunct Rx: Warm compresses, relaxation, massage
- Maintain normal hydration, avoid over-hydration

Acute anemic events
- Acute anemic event is an exacerbation of chronic, partially compensated hemolytic anemia
- Commonly occur as a consequence of parvovirus B19 infection, acute splenic sequestration, or a "hyperhemolytic" event
- Rx: transfusion

Acute chest syndrome
- New chest x ray (CXR) infiltrate + fever and respiratory signs and symptoms
- Triggers of ACS: Infection (viruses, *Mycoplasma, Chlamydia, Streptococcus pneumoniae*), pulmonary vascular occlusion, hypoventilation/atelectasis, pulmonary edema, bronchospasm, and surgery or general anesthesia
- Infection treatment/prophylaxis: Empiric antibiotic therapy with a cephalosporin (e.g., ceftriaxone) and a macrolide (e.g., azithromycin)
- Transfusion (or exchange transfusion) for hypoxemia or acute exacerbation of chronic anemia
- Other supportive care: Correction of hypoxemia, maintenance of normal hydration, adequate analgesia, bronchodilators for wheezing, and support of ventilation for severe disease
- Adjunct Rx: Incentive spirometry

Priapism
- Home management: Oral hydration, warm compresses or showers, exercise, voiding, oral analgesics and pseudoephedrine
- Seek urgent care for any priapism lasting >4 hours
- Rx for prolonged priapism: IV analgesia, IV hydration, oral pseudoephedrine, local injection of pseudoephedrine, urologic consultation for aspiration and irrigation
- Acute transfusion not shown to be helpful
- Prevention of recurrent priapism: Optimize disease-modifying therapies (hydroxyurea, chronic transfusions)

Stem Cell Disorders

Stem cell disorders cover a wide spectrum of the hematological problems from hypoproliferation (e.g., aplastic anemia, pancytopenia) to hyperproliferation (e.g., polycythemia, leukemia). We will discuss issues most pertinent to critical care, which mostly have to do with aplastic anemia (discussed above).

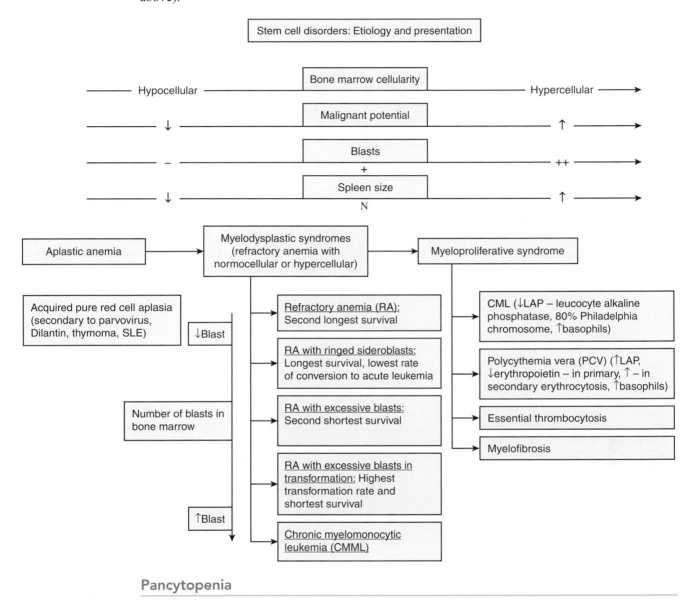

Pancytopenia

Pancytopenia

1. Aplastic anemias
   a. Cytotoxic therapy (azathioprine, mycophenolate mofetil, OKT3), viral (hepatitis, parvovirus) and other medications (ganciclovir, gold, Dilantin)
   b. Chemicals (benzene, chloramphenicol)
   c. Alcohol
2. Hematologic neoplasias (leukemia, lympho- and myeloproliferative disorders)
3. Marrow infiltration/replacement
   a. Infection (TB, fungal)
   b. Solid tumor
   c. Osteoporosis
   d. Gaucher disease, etc.
4. Nutritional deficiencies (vitamin B_{12}, folate)
5. Other (graft-versus-host disease, bacterial sepsis, SLE, thymoma, sarcoidosis, viral infection, hypersplenism, HIV, babesiosis)

SLE, Systemic lupus erythematosus; *TB*, tuberculosis; *HIV*, human immunodeficiency virus.

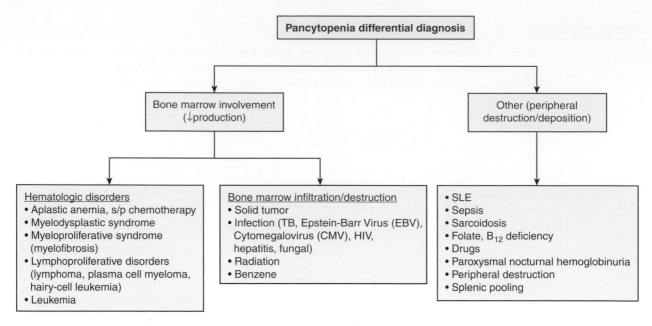

Myelodysplastic Syndromes

A group of diseases that have to do with impaired maturation of blood cells is called myelodysplastic syndrome (MDS). There are a number of risk factors, most of them directly affecting bone marrow (e.g., autoimmune reaction, chemotherapy, radiation, benzene, heavy metals).

Cause	Mechanism
Genetic aberrations, immunologic aberrations (e.g., aberrant immune attack on myeloid progenitors), secondary MDS (e.g., after exposure to chemotherapy, radiation therapy, heavy metals)	Ineffective hematopoiesis due to excessive apoptosis of hematopoietic precursors leading to hypercellular bone marrow and peripheral blood cytopenias[14]

Diagnosis	
• Presents with anemia and cytopenias: evaluate further if symptomatic or progressive anemia, especially if associated with other cytopenias	• Rule out other causes of anemia • Bone marrow evaluation: cellularity, cell maturation, dysplasia, percentage of blasts, iron stores and sideroblasts, cytogenetics, MDS-specific fluorescence in situ hybridization (FISH) panels, flow cytometry, and other special testing[14]

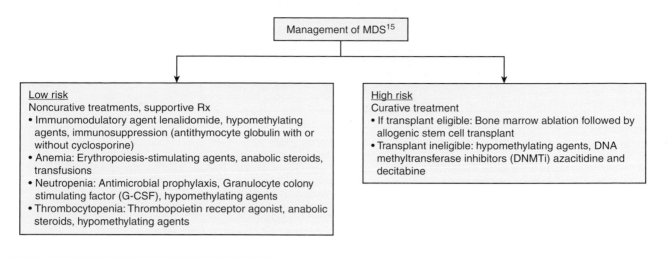

Management of MDS[15]

Low risk
Noncurative treatments, supportive Rx
- Immunomodulatory agent lenalidomide, hypomethylating agents, immunosuppression (antithymocyte globulin with or without cyclosporine)
- Anemia: Erythropoiesis-stimulating agents, anabolic steroids, transfusions
- Neutropenia: Antimicrobial prophylaxis, Granulocyte colony stimulating factor (G-CSF), hypomethylating agents
- Thrombocytopenia: Thrombopoietin receptor agonist, anabolic steroids, hypomethylating agents

High risk
Curative treatment
- If transplant eligible: Bone marrow ablation followed by allogenic stem cell transplant
- Transplant ineligible: hypomethylating agents, DNA methyltransferase inhibitors (DNMTi) azacitidine and decitabine

Platelet Disorders

A group of platelet disorders consist of quantitative (thrombocytopenia and thrombocytosis) and qualitative (disorders of aggregation, adhesion, secretion, etc.) platelet issues.

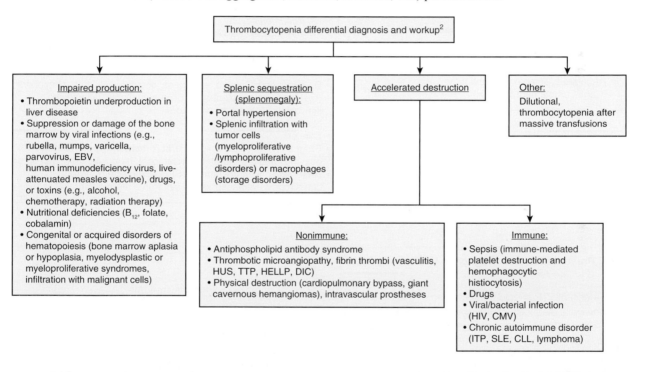

Thrombocytopenia differential diagnosis and workup[2]

Impaired production:
- Thrombopoietin underproduction in liver disease
- Suppression or damage of the bone marrow by viral infections (e.g., rubella, mumps, varicella, parvovirus, EBV, human immunodeficiency virus, live-attenuated measles vaccine), drugs, or toxins (e.g., alcohol, chemotherapy, radiation therapy)
- Nutritional deficiencies (B_{12}, folate, cobalamin)
- Congenital or acquired disorders of hematopoiesis (bone marrow aplasia or hypoplasia, myelodysplastic or myeloproliferative syndromes, infiltration with malignant cells)

Splenic sequestration (splenomegaly):
- Portal hypertension
- Splenic infiltration with tumor cells (myeloproliferative /lymphoproliferative disorders) or macrophages (storage disorders)

Accelerated destruction

Other:
Dilutional, thrombocytopenia after massive transfusions

Nonimmune:
- Antiphospholipid antibody syndrome
- Thrombotic microangiopathy, fibrin thrombi (vasculitis, HUS, TTP, HELLP, DIC)
- Physical destruction (cardiopulmonary bypass, giant cavernous hemangiomas), intravascular prostheses

Immune:
- Sepsis (immune-mediated platelet destruction and hemophagocytic histiocytosis)
- Drugs
- Viral/bacterial infection (HIV, CMV)
- Chronic autoimmune disorder (ITP, SLE, CLL, lymphoma)

Differences Between ITP and TTP	
Idiopathic Thrombocytopenic Purpura	**Thrombotic Thrombocytopenic Purpura/HUS**
May be associated with HIV, lupus, sarcoidosis, CLL, solid tumors	Primary
Immuno: antibodies to one's platelets	Nonimmune (small vessels occluded by hyaline material)
Relatively benign	Complicated by nephritis, arthritis, abdominal pain, GI bleeding, CNS complications
Management: • Steroids • Splenectomy • Cytotoxic drugs • Immunoglobulin	Management: • Plasmapheresis with FFP or cryo-supernatant • Corticosteroids • Splenectomy • Vincristine in combination with plasmapheresis[16]

CLL, chronic lymphocytic leukemia; *FFP*, fresh frozen plasma; *GI*, Gastrointestinal; *ITP*, idiopathic thrombocytopenic purpura; *TTP*, thrombotic thrombocytopenic purpura.

Thrombotic Microangiopathy (TMA)[17–20]

> Pathogenesis of TMA can be viewed as
> - Primary or secondary
> - Complement dysregulation or non–complement initiated

Primary
- TTP caused by
  a severe deficiency of the enzyme *ADAMTS13* (10%)
  - Congenital/hereditary (mutations of *ADAMTS13* gene)
  - Aquired (impaired *ADAMTS13* activity and inhibitor/antibodies)
- Hemolytic uremic syndrome
  - Typical HUS: Related to Shiga toxin–producing *Escherichia coli* (STEC), follows a diarrheal illness caused by STEC (positive stool cultures or polymerase chain reaction testing for Shiga toxin)
  - Atypical HUS. Complement dysregulation (genetic mutations in complement regulatory proteins, anti–complement-factor-H autoantibodies) or coagulation gene mutation
    - Hereditary: Complement gene mutations/deletions (C3, SD46, others)
    - Coagulation protein gene mutations (plasminogen, thrombomodulin)
    - Acquired: Complement antibody (anti-complement factor H)

Secondary TMA
- Malignant hypertension
- Pregnancy-associated TMA, preeclampsia/eclampsia, HELLP
- Drugs and toxins (e.g., calcineurin inhibitors, quinine, ticlopidine)
- Infections (e.g., influenza, HIV, EBV, parvovirus)
- Autoimmune disease (e.g., systemic lupus erythematosus)
- Organ transplantation
- Disseminated intravascular coagulation
- Cancer
- Metabolic (e.g., cobalamin C deficiency)

Other (usually apparent clinically)
- Renal or stem cell transplant
- Disseminated intravascular coagulation associated with infection (*S. Pneumoniae*, HIV)
- TMA associated with infections, typically viral (cytomegalovirus, adenovirus, herpes simplex virus), or severe bacterial (meningococcus, pneumococcus), fungal
- DIC in cancer, trauma, pancreatitis
- Drug-induced: Quinine, estrogens, cocaine, calcineurin inhibitors (cyclosporine, tacrolimus), sirolimus, penicillin, ticlopidine, simvastatin, interferon, and more
- Malignant HTN
- Cancer
- Pregnancy-associated, e.g., HELLP (hemolysis, elevated liver enzymes and low platelets), eclampsia, hemolytic uremic syndrome
- Rheumatologic/autoimmune (SLE, acute scleroderma, catastrophic antiphospholipid syndrome, vasculitis)

Clinical Presentation and Diagnostic Features in Acute TTP

The diagnosis of TTP should be treated as a medical emergency; the initial diagnosis of TTP should be made on clinical history, examination, and routine laboratory parameters.[18]
- Thrombocytopenia
- Schistocytic anemia (typically schistocytes >1% of red cells in the smear)
- Hemolysis (jaundice, pallor, anemia, elevated LDH, indirect bilirubin, decreased haptoglobin, reticulocytosis)
- Organ damage
  - AKI
  - Central neurological symptoms
  - Heart failure
  - Hypotension
  - Fever
  - Sometimes other clinical features: unexplained bloody diarrhea, nausea, vomiting
- Abdominal pain

AKI, Acute kidney injury.

Differential Diagnosis[1,2]

- Serological tests for HIV, hepatitis B virus and hepatitis C virus, autoantibody screen, and when appropriate, a pregnancy test should be performed at presentation
- Pretreatment samples should be obtained to measure ADAMTS13 activity levels and to detect anti-ADAMTS13 antibodies. Measurement of ADAMTS13 antigen levels is also useful in congenital TTP case
- Other initial diagnostic tests: liver function, hemolysis labs, coagulopathy labs (PT, PTT, direct antiglobulin test, homocysteine), blood smear, complement panel
- Rule out HUS: stool cultures or polymerase chain reaction testing for Shiga toxin
- Once HUS is ruled out, focus on TTP, TMA associated with compliment dysregulation or coagulopathy, other causes
- Suspect hereditary if <2 years age of onset

PT, Prothrombin time; *PTT*, partial thromboplastin time; *TMA*, thrombotic microangiopathy.

Histologic Findings

- Microangiopathy

- Red cell fragmentation (i.e., schistocytes)
- Microthrombi leading to ischemic tissue injury

Treatment of TMA[14]

Treatment for TTP

In view of the high risk of preventable, early deaths in TTP, treatment with TPE should be initiated as soon as possible, preferably within 4–8 hours, regardless of the time of day at presentation, if a patient presents with a microangiopathic hemolytic anemia (MAHA) and thrombocytopenia in the absence of any other identifiable clinical cause[13]

- Therapeutic plasma exchange ASAP
- If any delay in starting TPE then give FFP infusion (watch for fluid overload)
- Transfuse packed red cells when necessary to correct anemia
- Platelet transfusions are contraindicated; transfuse ONLY in those with serious bleeding due to thrombocytopenia
- If HIV-positive, start HAART immediately
- Prednisone if congenital TTP is unlikely (1 mg/kg with quick taper)
- Indicator of response: Platelets ≥150 for 2 days with normalizing LDH and stable or improving organ function – stop TPE and taper steroids
- If neurological or cardiac involvement, start rituximab
- If no response in 7 days, other options: Add rituximab, TPE twice a day, TPE with cryoprecipitate-reduced plasma
- Folic acid supplementation
- Consider antiplatelet agents to prevent ongoing platelet aggregation and minimize microthrombus formation
- For atypical HUS – eculizumab

Refractory TTP
- Continue, resume or intensify plasma exchange
- Start or increase dose of corticosteroids
- Rituximab 375 mg/m^2 × 4 weekly doses
- Consider additional therapies (e.g., cyclosporine, cyclophosphamide, vincristine, bortezomib or splenectomy)

Treatment for TMA with complement dysregulation
TPE
Depending on the type there is a potential role for plasma infusion, prednisone, rituximab or eculizumab

---

Treatment for TMA in renal transplant recipients
- TPE
- Rule out acute rejection (biopsy, donor-specific antibodies)
- Check for complement dysregulation, if positive treat for it

---

Treatment for TMA with hyper-homocysteinemia
- If homocysteine <3 × ULN – look for other causes
- If homocysteine ≥3 × ULN: Might still be other causes, if B$_{12}$, folate deficient – replace, if plasma methionine low (cobalamin C deficiency) – folate, hydroxocobalamin, betaine

---

Treatment for TMA secondary to other factors
- If drug induced – discontinue
- If infection/DIC – supportive care

TPE regimen for treatment of the TMA
- Start TPE with 1.5 plasma volume exchanges, using plasma in all age groups and reassessed daily
- Reduce volume to 1.0 PV when the clinical condition and laboratory test results are stabilizing
- Intensification in frequency and or volume of TPE procedures should be considered in life-threatening
- Continue daily TPE for a minimum of 2 days after platelet count has been >150 and then stop

Heparin-Induced Thrombocytopenia

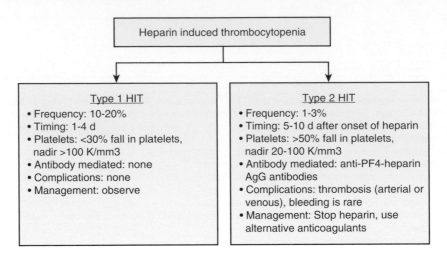

Clinical Presentation and Diagnostic Features

- Much more common with unfractionated heparin compared to LMW heparin
- More common after major surgery, e.g., cardiac surgery
- Diagnosis:
  - o decrease in platelet count by 50% or thrombosis 5–10 days after starting the heparin
  - o presence of platelet-activating HIT antibodies
  - o anti–PF4-heparin enzyme immunoassays (excellent negative predictive value, but not positive predictive value)
  - o duplex ultrasonography to rule out subclinical deep-vein thrombosis

HIT, Heparin-induced thrombocytopenia; *LMW*, low molecular weight.

Treatment[21]

- Stop heparin and initiate an alternative anticoagulant at a therapeutic dose
- Vitamin K antagonists (e.g., warfarin and phenprocoumon) should not be given until HIT has abated (e.g., the platelet count has increased to >150K/mm³), as they can decrease the level of protein C and increase the risk of venous limb gangrene and limb loss
- When vitamin K antagonists are initiated, overlap with an alternative anticoagulant is needed
- Approved medications: argatroban (direct thrombin inhibitor), danaparoid (antithrombin-dependent factor Xa inhibitor)
- Not approved, but used successfully: fondaparinux and bivalirudin (can be reliably monitored by anti–factor Xa assays)
- Uncertainty regarding use of dabigatran, rivaroxaban, and apixaban
- Patients who have HIT with thrombosis require ≥3 months therapeutic-dose anticoagulation, those without thrombosis at least until the platelet count has reached a stable plateau (ideally >150K/mm³)

If patient needs cardiac surgery

- Postponing surgery until platelet-activating anti–PF4-heparin antibodies disappear, then using heparin intraoperatively is safe
- Another option in urgent situations: plasmapheresis to remove platelet-activating anti–PF4-heparin antibodies
- Otherwise, bivalirudin is a compatible anticoagulant for cardiac surgery if platelet-activating anti–PF4-heparin antibodies are present

Thrombocytosis

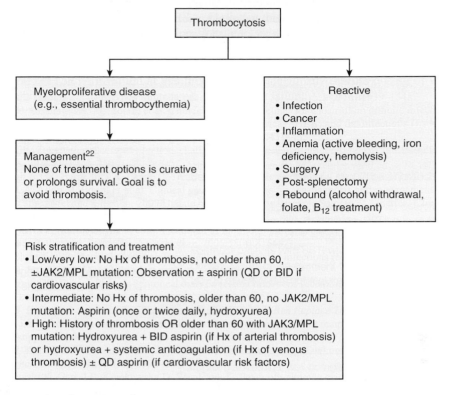

Thrombocytosis

Myeloproliferative disease
(e.g., essential thrombocythemia)

Management[22]
None of treatment options is curative
or prolongs survival. Goal is to
avoid thrombosis.

Risk stratification and treatment
• Low/very low: No Hx of thrombosis, not older than 60,
  ±JAK2/MPL mutation: Observation ± aspirin (QD or BID if
  cardiovascular risks)
• Intermediate: No Hx of thrombosis, older than 60, no JAK2/MPL
  mutation: Aspirin (once or twice daily, hydroxyurea)
• High: History of thrombosis OR older than 60 with JAK3/MPL
  mutation: Hydroxyurea + BID aspirin (if Hx of arterial thrombosis)
  or hydroxyurea + systemic anticoagulation (if Hx of venous
  thrombosis) ± QD aspirin (if cardiovascular risk factors)

Reactive
• Infection
• Cancer
• Inflammation
• Anemia (active bleeding, iron
  deficiency, hemolysis)
• Surgery
• Post-splenectomy
• Rebound (alcohol withdrawal,
  folate, B_{12} treatment)

Qualitative Platelet Disorders

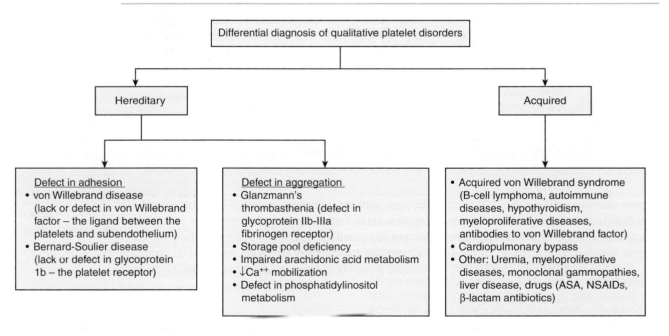

Differential diagnosis of qualitative platelet disorders

Hereditary

Acquired

Defect in adhesion
• von Willebrand disease
  (lack or defect in von Willebrand
  factor – the ligand between the
  platelets and subendothelium)
• Bernard-Soulier disease
  (lack or defect in glycoprotein
  1b – the platelet receptor)

Defect in aggregation
• Glanzmann's
  thrombasthenia (defect in
  glycoprotein IIb-IIIa
  fibrinogen receptor)
• Storage pool deficiency
• Impaired arachidonic acid metabolism
• ↓Ca++ mobilization
• Defect in phosphatidylinositol
  metabolism

• Acquired von Willebrand syndrome
  (B-cell lymphoma, autoimmune
  diseases, hypothyroidism,
  myeloproliferative diseases,
  antibodies to von Willebrand factor)
• Cardiopulmonary bypass
• Other: Uremia, myeloproliferative
  diseases, monoclonal gammopathies,
  liver disease, drugs (ASA, NSAIDs,
  β-lactam antibiotics)

Treatment[23]

• Transfusion of platelet concentrates

• Patients with abnormalities of their platelet
  surface receptors (might develop an immune
  response to platelet transfusion)—recombinant
  factor VIIa (rFVIIa)

Coagulopathies

Coagulation is a process involving multiplicity of factors, both humoral and cellular, and involves activation, adhesion and aggregation of platelets, and deposition and maturation of fibrin resulting in hemostasis. The diagram below represents the cascade of factor activation leading to formation of clot. Intrinsic, extrinsic, and common pathways are recognized. Intrinsic pathway abnormalities are reflected in abnormal activated partial thromboplastin time (aPTT), while prothrombin time (PT) reflects extrinsic pathway abnormalities and thrombin time (TT) is affected by extrinsic and common pathways.

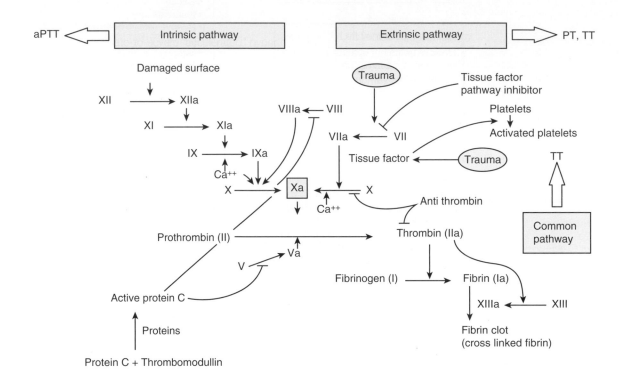

Hemostatic Disorder	Clinical Presentation
Hemostatic plug disorder (problems with forming a stable fibrin clot)	• Cutaneous bleeding (petechiae, purpura, ecchymoses) • Mucous membrane bleeding (epistaxis, menorrhagia, oropharyngeal bleeding)
Coagulation factor defect	• Deep hematomas, hemarthroses • Delayed bleeding after surgery/trauma
Thrombocytopenia/endothelial cell injury	• Petechiae, purpura alone

Bleeding time—platelet aggregation	TT—conversion from fibrinogen to fibrin

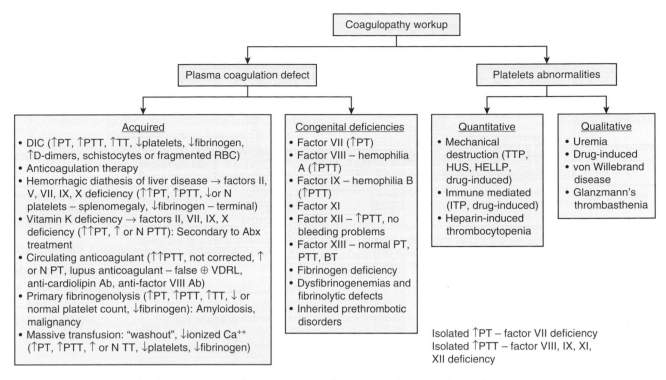

Isolated ↑PT – factor VII deficiency
Isolated ↑PTT – factor VIII, IX, XI, XII deficiency

Brief Summary of Treatment of Acquired Coagulopathies

DIC	• Treat underlying cause • FFP, cryoprecipitate • Low-dose IV heparin (bolus 25 U/kg, then 5–10 U/kg/h) • Antifibrinolytic agents (e-aminocaproic acid [EACA]) • Plasma protein concentrates of antithrombin III, activated protein C • No platelets or give platelets + heparin
TTP and HUS	• Plasma infusion, plasmapheresis with FFP or cryo-supernatant • Antiplatelet agents • Corticosteroids, vincristine, high-dose IV IgG • Splenectomy for refractory patients
Primary fibrinogenolysis	• Antifibrinolytic agents (EACA, tranexamic acid) • Cryoprecipitate for severe hypofibrinogenemia (≤75–100)
Liver disease/vitamin K deficiency	• Vitamin K • FFP
Massive transfusion syndrome ("washout")	• Transfusion of 1 U FFP and platelets (or 1 U of fresh whole blood) for every 5–10 U of stored PRBCs
Warfarin overdose	• Withhold further warfarin • FFP or vitamin K
Heparin overdose	• Withhold further heparin administration • Protamine sulfate (1 mg for 100 U of heparin)
Quantitative platelet disorders	• Transfuse platelets if <10,000–20,000 dose 1 unit/10 kg of body mass
Qualitative platelet disorder	• von Willebrand factor deficiency—desmopressin (↑synthesis and secretion of von Willebrand factor), von Willebrand factor–rich factor VIII concentrate • Uremia—desmopressin, estrogen, ↑dialysis time, RBC transfusion

IgG, Immunoglobulin G; *PRBCs*, packed red blood cells.

Thrombophilia (Predisposition to Developing Thrombosis)

Thrombosis can occur in arterial or venous system. Arterial thrombosis usually results from atherosclerotic plaque rupture or other cause of endothelial damage with subsequent formation of the clot. Venous thrombosis on the other hand has multiple causes and risk factors. Venous thrombosis/thromboembolism usually presents with deep venous thrombosis or pulmonary embolism (PE).[24]

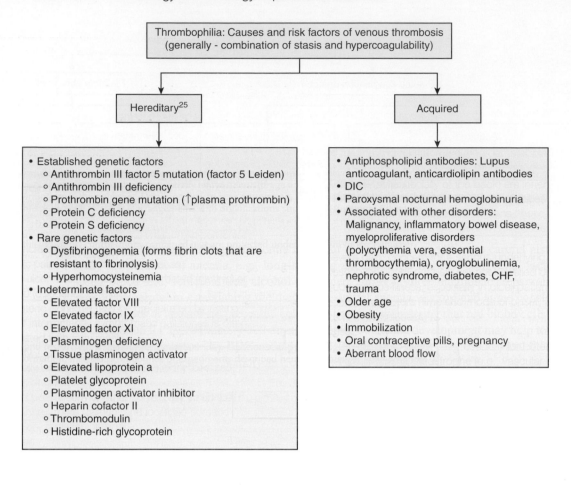

Thrombophilia: Causes and risk factors of venous thrombosis
(generally - combination of stasis and hypercoagulability)

Hereditary[25]

- Established genetic factors
  - Antithrombin III factor 5 mutation (factor 5 Leiden)
  - Antithrombin III deficiency
  - Prothrombin gene mutation ($\uparrow$plasma prothrombin)
  - Protein C deficiency
  - Protein S deficiency
- Rare genetic factors
  - Dysfibrinogenemia (forms fibrin clots that are resistant to fibrinolysis)
  - Hyperhomocysteinemia
- Indeterminate factors
  - Elevated factor VIII
  - Elevated factor IX
  - Elevated factor XI
  - Plasminogen deficiency
  - Tissue plasminogen activator
  - Elevated lipoprotein a
  - Platelet glycoprotein
  - Plasminogen activator inhibitor
  - Heparin cofactor II
  - Thrombomodulin
  - Histidine-rich glycoprotein

Acquired

- Antiphospholipid antibodies: Lupus anticoagulant, anticardiolipin antibodies
- DIC
- Paroxysmal nocturnal hemoglobinuria
- Associated with other disorders: Malignancy, inflammatory bowel disease, myeloproliferative disorders (polycythemia vera, essential thrombocythemia), cryoglobulinemia, nephrotic syndrome, diabetes, CHF, trauma
- Older age
- Obesity
- Immobilization
- Oral contraceptive pills, pregnancy
- Aberrant blood flow

Hypercoagulable state has to be worked up if:

- <40 years old with thrombotic events
- Strong family history of thrombosis

- Recurrent thrombosis at different sites
- Skin necrosis
- Recurrent fetal loss
- Thrombosis at unusual sites

Initial Workup of Hypercoagulable State

- Antithrombin III
- Protein C and S activity levels

- Fibrinogen concentration
- Dilute TT
- Activated protein C resistance time
- Homocysteine level

CHA$_2$DS$_2$-VASc prediction score of stroke[26]

For atrial fibrillation (AF), anticoagulation is indicated if score = 1 for males and 2 for females.

CHA$_2$DS$_2$-VASC SCORE		CHA$_2$DS$_2$-VASC SCORE AND RISK OF STROKE PER YEAR WITHOUT ANTICOAGULATION	
Risk factor	Points	Score	Percent
Heart failure	1	0	0%
Hypertension	1	1	1.30%
Resting blood pressure >140/90 mm Hg (at least two measurements) or current antihypertensive treatment			
Age 75 years or older	2	2	2.20%
Diabetes mellitus	1	3	3.20%
Fasting blood glucose >125 mg/dL (7 mmol/L) or treatment with oral antidiabetic drugs and/or insulin			
Prior stroke, transient ischemic attack, or thromboembolic event	2	4	4.00%
Vascular disease	1	5	6.70%
Prior myocardial infarction, peripheral vascular disease, or aortic plaque			
Age 65–74 years	1	6	9.80%
Sex category	1	7	9.60%
Female		8	6.70%
Maximum score	9	9	15.20%

Anticoagulation

Drug	Therapeutic Effect	Adverse Effects
Aspirin	Antiplatelet (inhibition of platelet cyclooxygenase with blockade of platelet thromboxane A$_2$ synthesis)	GI bleeding
Clopidogrel, ticlopidine (rarely used)	Antiplatelet	Neutropenia, TTP, rash, diarrhea, ↑cholesterol
Warfarin	↓Prothrombin and factor X	Major bleeding (especially GI bleeding), Rx of bleedings—vitamin K, FFP
Standard heparin	Binds to antithrombin III so that it avidly binds and neutralizes thrombin and other clotting factors	Bleeding, HIT
Target-specific oral anticoagulants (TSOACs)/ non–vitamin K oral anticoagulants (NOACs)	Discussed below	

Newer Drugs (Target-Specific Oral Anticoagulation)

- Available agents:
  - Factor IIa/thrombin inhibitors dabigatran (Pradaxa), argatroban
  - Factor Xa inhibitors: rivaroxaban (Xarelto), apixaban (Eliquis), edoxaban (Savaysa), and betrixaban (Bevyxxa)
- Benefits:
  - Compared to warfarin, newer drugs have wider therapeutic windows, faster onset and offset of action, and fewer drug and food interactions
  - Favorable risk-benefit profile with reductions in stroke, intracranial hemorrhage, and mortality with similar overall major bleeding rates, except for a possible increase in GI bleeding
- Challenges:
  - May be associated with a higher incidence of GI bleeding than warfarin
  - Lack reversal agents that can be used to manage an acute bleeding event (dabigatran is dialyzable)
- Additional considerations:
  - In patients with significant renal impairment, the choice of agent will be limited to a vitamin K antagonist
  - In the elderly (age 75 years and older) TSOACs did not cause excess bleeding and were associated with at least equal efficacy compared with vitamin K antagonists
  - TSOACs may be beneficial in patients who have challenges in achieving INR targets
  - Potential concern that a patient may occasionally miss a dose; given the rapid onset and offset of action might, this might bring levels to the subtherapeutic range

INR, International normalized ratio.

FDA-Approved Indications for Oral Anticoagulants[27]

Warfarin	Prophylaxis and treatment of venous thrombosis and its extension, PE Prophylaxis and treatment of thromboembolic complications associated with AF or cardiac valve replacement Reduction in the risk of death, recurrent myocardial infarction, and thromboembolic events
Dabigatran	Stroke prevention in patients with nonvalvular AF Treatment of DVT and PE after 5–10 days of parenteral anticoagulation Reduction in the risk of recurrence of DVT and PE in previously treated patients
Rivaroxaban	Stroke prevention in patients with nonvalvular AF Prevention of venous thromboembolism in patients undergoing hip or knee replacement Acute treatment of DVT/PE Secondary prevention of DVT/PE
Apixaban	Stroke prevention in patients with nonvalvular AF Acute treatment of DVT/PE Secondary prevention of DVT/PE

DVT, Deep-vein thrombosis.

AF (vitamin K antagonist [VKA] or non–vitamin K oral anticoagulant [NOAC]), venous thromboembolism (VKA or NOAC), and mechanical valves (VKA) are the main indications for oral anticoagulation.[26]

Goals and Duration of Anticoagulation[28]

Indication	Target INR range	Duration of Therapy
Most cases of venous thromboembolism	2–3	3–6 months
First unprovoked episode of venous thromboembolism or recurrent venous thromboembolism, as well as active malignancy	2–3	Lifelong
Antiphospholipid antibody syndrome with history of arterial or venous thromboembolic event	2–3	Lifelong
Bioprosthetic mitral valve	2–3	3 months
Mechanical aortic valve	2–3	Lifelong
Aortic mechanical prostheses who are also at higher risk for thromboembolic events (e.g., with AF, previous thromboembolism, and a hypercoagulable state)	2.5–3.5	Lifelong
Mechanical mitral valve	2.5–3.5	Lifelong
Mechanical combined mitral and aortic valve	2.5–3.5	Lifelong

HAS-BLED score: bleeding risk with anticoagulation[26]

HAS-BLED SCORE		HAS-BLED SCORE AND BLEEDING RATE PER YEAR WITH ANTICOAGULATION	
Risk factor	Points	Score	Percent
Hypertension	1	0	0.90%
Abnormal renal and liver function	1 or 2	1	3.40%
Stroke	1	2	4.10%
Bleeding	1	3	5.80%
Labile INRs	1	4	8.90%
Age > 65 years	1	5	9.10%
Drugs that predispose bleeding/alcohol	1 or 2	6–9	Insufficient data
Maximum score	9		

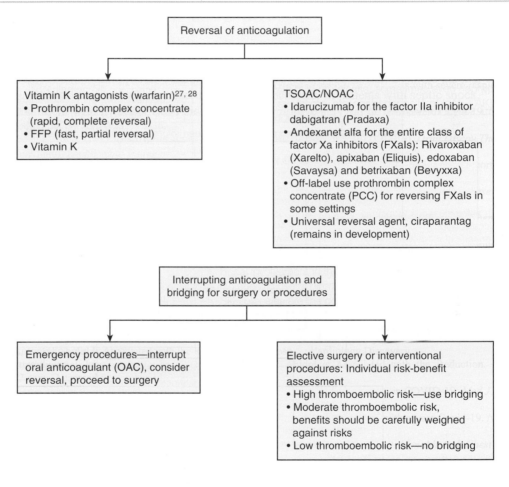

Reversal of anticoagulation

Vitamin K antagonists (warfarin)[27, 28]
- Prothrombin complex concentrate (rapid, complete reversal)
- FFP (fast, partial reversal)
- Vitamin K

TSOAC/NOAC
- Idarucizumab for the factor IIa inhibitor dabigatran (Pradaxa)
- Andexanet alfa for the entire class of factor Xa inhibitors (FXaIs): Rivaroxaban (Xarelto), apixaban (Eliquis), edoxaban (Savaysa) and betrixaban (Bevyxxa)
- Off-label use prothrombin complex concentrate (PCC) for reversing FXaIs in some settings
- Universal reversal agent, ciraparantag (remains in development)

Interrupting anticoagulation and bridging for surgery or procedures

Emergency procedures—interrupt oral anticoagulant (OAC), consider reversal, proceed to surgery

Elective surgery or interventional procedures: Individual risk-benefit assessment
- High thromboembolic risk—use bridging
- Moderate thromboembolic risk, benefits should be carefully weighed against risks
- Low thromboembolic risk—no bridging

Resuming Anticoagulation After Hemorrhagic Event[29]

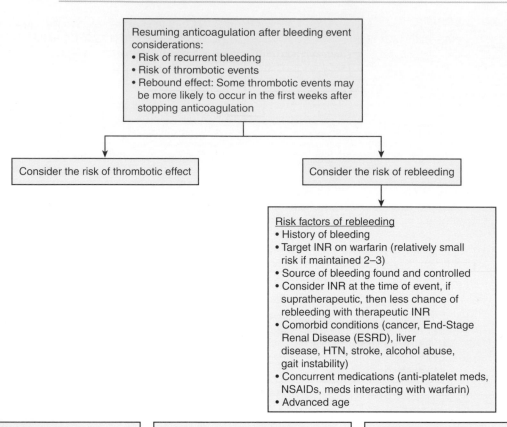

Resuming anticoagulation after bleeding event considerations:
- Risk of recurrent bleeding
- Risk of thrombotic events
- Rebound effect: Some thrombotic events may be more likely to occur in the first weeks after stopping anticoagulation

Consider the risk of thrombotic effect

Consider the risk of rebleeding

Risk factors of rebleeding
- History of bleeding
- Target INR on warfarin (relatively small risk if maintained 2–3)
- Source of bleeding found and controlled
- Consider INR at the time of event, if supratherapeutic, then less chance of rebleeding with therapeutic INR
- Comorbid conditions (cancer, End-Stage Renal Disease (ESRD), liver disease, HTN, stroke, alcohol abuse, gait instability)
- Concurrent medications (anti-platelet meds, NSAIDs, meds interacting with warfarin)
- Advanced age

High risk indications to resume anticoagulation
- Mechanical mitral valve
- Hypercoagulable state (e.g., antiphospholipid antibody syndrome with recurrent thromboembolic events.)
- High risk of embolic event (e.g., CHADS2 score >5, CHA2DS2-VASc score >6)

Moderate-risk indications
- After a partial course of anticoagulation for provoked venous thromboembolism
- Lack of strong evidence supporting the use of anticoagulation (e.g., heart failure, pulmonary hypertension, or splanchnic and hepatic vein thrombosis)

Low risk indications - delay anticoagulation
- No absolute indication for ongoing anticoagulation
- Atrial fibrillation with low CHA2DS2-VASc score
- Near completion of planned anticoagulation course (e.g., after 6 months of anticoagulation for unprovoked deep vein thrombosis.)
- High risk of rebleeding or presence of additional risk factors for bleeding
- Anticipated high risk of morbidity or death if rebleeding occurs

Timing of Anticoagulation Restart

- Why restart earlier
  - Rebound effect—increased risk of PE and AF-related stroke during the first 90 days of interruption of therapy
  - In patients with intracranial hemorrhage—increased risk of arterial and venous thromboembolic events
  - In anticoagulation-associated retroperitoneal bleeding— increased risk of DVT from compression
- Why restart later
  - In small studies first 2 months after warfarin-associated

GI bleeding, there is substantial risk of rebleeding when anticoagulation is resumed, but has not shown in larger series
- Recommendations:
  - After GI bleeding resume anticoagulation after 4–7 days of interruption, re-initiation with warfarin or apixaban therapy may present the lowest risk of recurrent GI rebleeding[28]
  - After soft tissue hemorrhage—resume after 4 days
  - After intracranial hemorrhage—see separate discussion below

Anticoagulation After Intracranial Hemorrhage

- Prophylactic anticoagulation to prevent venous thrombosis
  - Guidelines suggest starting prophylactic-dosed anticoagulation early in all intracranial hemorrhage patients, including those not previously on warfarin[30,31]
  - Low-dose subcutaneous heparin the day after an intracranial hemorrhage decreased the risk of thromboembolism without increasing the risk of rebleeding

Resuming long-term anticoagulation[30,31]

- In nonvalvular AF, long-term anticoagulation should be avoided after spontaneous lobar hemorrhage; antiplatelet agents can be considered instead[30]

- In nonlobar hemorrhage, consider anticoagulation depending on strength of indication 7–10 days after the onset[30]
- Patients with strong indications for anticoagulation/high risk of thromboembolism—restart on warfarin 10–14 days after the event, depending on the risk of thromboembolism and recurrent intracranial hemorrhage[31] or in 7 days by other recommendations[29]
- In patients at lower risk of thromboembolism, restart after at least 14 days[29]
- Agent to use: the risk of rebleeding may be lower if a TSOAC (factor Xa or direct thrombin inhibitors) is used

Coagulopathy in Sepsis[32]

In sepsis, the hemostatic balance is shifted toward a pro-coagulation state

Mechanism of coagulopathy in sepsis has to do with inflammation and hemostasis being closely tied

- Monocytes-macrophages aberrant expression of tissue factor

- The impairment of anticoagulant pathways caused by dysfunctional endothelial cells
- Overproduction of plasminogen activator inhibitor-1 (PAI-1) by endothelial cells and thrombin-mediated suppression of fibrinolysis

Clinical Presentation

Ranges from subclinical activation of blood coagulation to acute DIC:

- Widespread microvascular thrombosis
- Consumption of platelets and coagulation proteins
- Bleeding

Therapeutic Options

- Heparin (unfractionated or LMW heparin)
- Recombinant human thrombomodulin
- Antithrombin

Approach to Cancer Patients Requiring ICU or Mechanical Ventilation

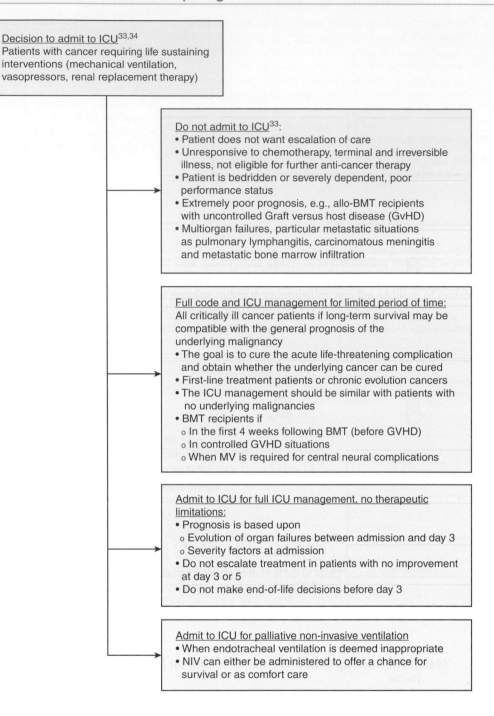

Decision to admit to ICU[33,34]
Patients with cancer requiring life sustaining interventions (mechanical ventilation, vasopressors, renal replacement therapy)

Do not admit to ICU[33]:
• Patient does not want escalation of care
• Unresponsive to chemotherapy, terminal and irreversible illness, not eligible for further anti-cancer therapy
• Patient is bedridden or severely dependent, poor performance status
• Extremely poor prognosis, e.g., allo-BMT recipients with uncontrolled Graft versus host disease (GvHD)
• Multiorgan failures, particular metastatic situations as pulmonary lymphangitis, carcinomatous meningitis and metastatic bone marrow infiltration

Full code and ICU management for limited period of time:
All critically ill cancer patients if long-term survival may be compatible with the general prognosis of the underlying malignancy
• The goal is to cure the acute life-threatening complication and obtain whether the underlying cancer can be cured
• First-line treatment patients or chronic evolution cancers
• The ICU management should be similar with patients with no underlying malignancies
• BMT recipients if
  o In the first 4 weeks following BMT (before GVHD)
  o In controlled GVHD situations
  o When MV is required for central neural complications

Admit to ICU for full ICU management, no therapeutic limitations:
• Prognosis is based upon
  o Evolution of organ failures between admission and day 3
  o Severity factors at admission
• Do not escalate treatment in patients with no improvement at day 3 or 5
• Do not make end-of-life decisions before day 3

Admit to ICU for palliative non-invasive ventilation
• When endotracheal ventilation is deemed inappropriate
• NIV can either be administered to offer a chance for survival or as comfort care

Highlights of Management of Critically Ill Patients With Hematologic Malignancies (HM)

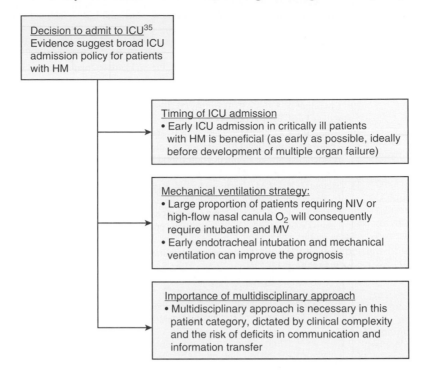

Decision to admit to ICU[35]
Evidence suggest broad ICU admission policy for patients with HM

Timing of ICU admission
• Early ICU admission in critically ill patients with HM is beneficial (as early as possible, ideally before development of multiple organ failure)

Mechanical ventilation strategy:
• Large proportion of patients requiring NIV or high-flow nasal canula O_2 will consequently require intubation and MV
• Early endotracheal intubation and mechanical ventilation can improve the prognosis

Importance of multidisciplinary approach
• Multidisciplinary approach is necessary in this patient category, dictated by clinical complexity and the risk of deficits in communication and information transfer

REFERENCES

1. Lichtin A. Anemia workup: five-step approach. *Cleve Clin J Med*. 1992;59(6):568.
2. Drews RE. Critical issues in hematology: anemia, thrombocytopenia, coagulopathy, and blood product transfusions in critically ill patients. *Clin Chest Med*. 2003;24(4):607–622.
3. Babitt JL, Lin HY. Mechanisms of anemia in CKD. *J Am Soc Nephrol*. 2012;23(10):1631–1634.
4. Peyssonnaux C, Nizet V, Johnson RS. Role of the hypoxia inducible factors in iron metabolism. *Cell Cycle*. 2008;7(1):28–32.
5. Nairz M, Theurl I, Wolf D, Weiss G. Iron deficiency or anemia of inflammation?: differential diagnosis and mechanisms of anemia of inflammation. *Wien Med Wochenschr*. 2016;166(13–14):411–423.
6. Nemeth E, Ganz T. Anemia of inflammation. *Hematol Oncol Clin North Am*. 2014;28(4):671–681.
7. Gallagher PG. Abnormalities of the erythrocyte membrane. *Pediatr Clin North Am*. 2013;60(6):1349–1362.
8. Go RS, Winters JL, Kay NE. How I treat autoimmune hemolytic anemia. *Blood*. 2017;129(22):2971–2979.
9. Dhaliwal G, Cornett PA, Tierney Jr LM. Hemolytic anemia. *Am Fam Physician*. 2004;69(11):2599–2606.
10. Bacigalupo A. How I treat acquired aplastic anemia. *Blood*. 2017;129(11):1428–1436.
11. Gurion R, Gafter-Gvili A, Paul M, et al. Hematopoietic growth factors in aplastic anemia patients treated with immunosuppressive therapy-systematic review and meta-analysis. *Haematologica*. 2009;94(5):712–719.
12. Chonat S, Quinn CT. Current standards of care and long term outcomes for thalassemia and sickle cell disease. *Adv Exp Med Biol*. 2017;1013:59–87.
13. Piel FB, Steinberg MH, Rees DC. Sickle cell disease. *N Engl J Med*. 2017;376(16):1561–1573.
14. Zeidan AM, Faltas B, Douglas Smith B, Gore S. Myelodysplastic syndromes: what do hospitalists need to know? *J Hosp Med*. 2013;8(6):351–357.
15. Gangat N, Patnaik MM, Tefferi A. Myelodysplastic syndromes: contemporary review and how we treat. *Am J Hematol*. 2016;91(1):76–89.
16. Ziman A, Mitri M, Klapper E, Pepkowitz SH, Goldfinger D. Combination vincristine and plasma exchange as initial therapy in patients with thrombotic thrombocytopenic purpura: one institution's experience and review of the literature. *Transfusion*. 2005;45(1):41–49.
17. Go RS, Winters JL, Leung N, et al. Thrombotic microangiopathy care pathway: a consensus statement for the Mayo Clinic Complement Alternative Pathway-Thrombotic Microangiopathy (CAP-TMA) disease-oriented group. *Mayo Clin Proc*. 2016;91(9):1189–1211.
18. Scully M, Hunt BJ, Benjamin S, et al. Guidelines on the diagnosis and management of thrombotic thrombocytopenic purpura and other thrombotic microangiopathies. *Br J Haematol*. 2012;158(3):323–335.
19. Arnold DM, Patriquin CJ, Nazy I. Thrombotic microangiopathies: a general approach to diagnosis and management. *CMAJ (Can Med Assoc J)*. 2017;189(4):E153–E159.
20. Masias C, Vasu S, Cataland SR. None of the above: thrombotic microangiopathy beyond TTP and HUS. *Blood*. 2017;129(21):2857–2863.
21. Greinacher A. Clinical practice. Heparin-induced thrombocytopenia. *N Engl J Med*. 2015;373(3):252–261.
22. Tefferi A, Vannucchi AM, Barbui T. Essential thrombocythemia treatment algorithm 2018. *Blood Cancer J*. 2018;8(1).

23. White GC. Congenital and acquired platelet disorders: current dilemmas and treatment strategies. *Semin Hematol.* 2006;43(suppl 1):S37–S41.

24. Previtali E, Bucciarelli P, Passamonti SM, Martinelli I. Risk factors for venous and arterial thrombosis. *Blood Transfus.* 2011;9(2):120–138.

25. Khan S, Dickerman JD. Hereditary thrombophilia. *Thrombosis J.* 2006;4.

26. Altiok E, Marx N. Orale antikoagulation. *Dtsch Arztebl Int.* 2018;115(46):776–783.

27. Safavi-Naeini P, Saeed M. Target-specific oral anticoagulants: should we switch from warfarin? *Texas Hear Inst J.* 2015;42(3):229–233.

28. Hanley JP. Warfarin reversal. *Am J Clin Pathol.* 2004;57(11):1132–1139.

29. Colantino A, Jaffer AK, Brotman DJ. Resuming anticoagulation after hemorrhage: a practical approach. *Cleve Clin J Med.* 2015;82(4):45–256.

30. Broderick J, Connolly S, Feldmann E, et al. Guidelines for the management of spontaneous intracerebral hemorrhage in adults: 2007 update: a guideline from the American Heart Association/American Stroke Association Stroke Council, High Blood Pressure Research Council, and the quality of care and out. *Stroke.* 2007;38(6):2001–2023.

31. Steiner T, Kaste M, Forsting M, et al. Recommendations for the management of intracranial haemorrhage—part I: spontaneous intracerebral haemorrhage. The European stroke initiative writing committee and the writing committee for the EUSI executive committee. *Cerebrovasc Dis.* 2006;22(4):294–316.

32. Lipinska-Gediga M. Coagulopathy in sepsis—a new look at an old problem. *Anaesthesiol Intensive Ther.* 2016;48(5):352–359.

33. Saillard C, Mokart D, Lemiale V, Azoulay E. Mechanical ventilation in cancer patients. *Minerva Anestesiol.* 2014;80(6):712–725.

34. Kiehl MG, Beutel G, Böll B, et al. Consensus statement for cancer patients requiring intensive care support. *Ann Hematol.* 2018;97(7):1271–1282.

35. Kusadasi N, Muller MCA, van Westerloo DJ, et al. The management of critically ill patients with haematological malignancies. *Neth J Med.* 2017;75(7):265–271.

CHAPTER 9

Rheumatology, Immunology, Allergy
Alexander Goldfarb-Rumyantzev

Rheumatological Causes for Intensive Care Unit (ICU) Admission

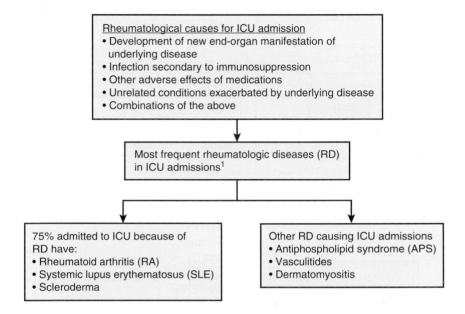

Rheumatological causes for ICU admission
• Development of new end-organ manifestation of underlying disease
• Infection secondary to immunosuppression
• Other adverse effects of medications
• Unrelated conditions exacerbated by underlying disease
• Combinations of the above

Most frequent rheumatologic diseases (RD) in ICU admissions[1]

75% admitted to ICU because of RD have:
• Rheumatoid arthritis (RA)
• Systemic lupus erythematosus (SLE)
• Scleroderma

Other RD causing ICU admissions
• Antiphospholipid syndrome (APS)
• Vasculitides
• Dermatomyositis

Added Complexity of RD in Critically Ill Patients

- Signs of underlying disease flare and sepsis are very similar
- Immunosuppression due to their underlying RD or treatment regimen
  - infection not normally present in immunocompetent host should always be considered (e.g., *Pneumocystis jirovecii* tuberculosis, fungi)

- RDs are frequently multisystem diseases with potential multiorgan failure
- High ICU mortality
- Complicated pharmacotherapy

Additional Facts About Autoimmune Disease in ICU Patients[2]

- Most frequent autoimmune diseases in patients admitted to ICU: SLE, rheumatoid arthritis, systemic vasculitis

- Mortality rate 17%–55% in all autoimmune diseases, but as high as 79% in SLE cases
- Variables associated with mortality: high APACHE score, multiorgan dysfunction, older age, cytopenia

Anaphylaxis

Anaphylaxis is caused by mast cell and/or basophil degranulation triggered by activation of inflammatory pathways (including both immunoglobulin E [IgE]- and non–IgE-dependent pathway).[3]

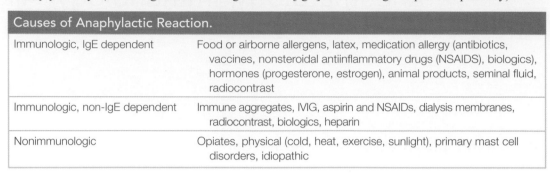

Causes of Anaphylactic Reaction.	
Immunologic, IgE dependent	Food or airborne allergens, latex, medication allergy (antibiotics, vaccines, nonsteroidal antiinflammatory drugs (NSAIDS), biologics), hormones (progesterone, estrogen), animal products, seminal fluid, radiocontrast
Immunologic, non-IgE dependent	Immune aggregates, IVIG, aspirin and NSAIDs, dialysis membranes, radiocontrast, biologics, heparin
Nonimmunologic	Opiates, physical (cold, heat, exercise, sunlight), primary mast cell disorders, idiopathic

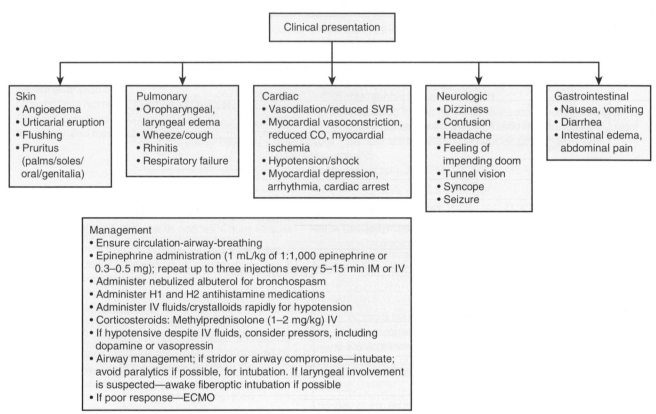

Clinical presentation

Skin
- Angioedema
- Urticarial eruption
- Flushing
- Pruritus (palms/soles/oral/genitalia)

Pulmonary
- Oropharyngeal, laryngeal edema
- Wheeze/cough
- Rhinitis
- Respiratory failure

Cardiac
- Vasodilation/reduced SVR
- Myocardial vasoconstriction, reduced CO, myocardial ischemia
- Hypotension/shock
- Myocardial depression, arrhythmia, cardiac arrest

Neurologic
- Dizziness
- Confusion
- Headache
- Feeling of impending doom
- Tunnel vision
- Syncope
- Seizure

Gastrointestinal
- Nausea, vomiting
- Diarrhea
- Intestinal edema, abdominal pain

Management
- Ensure circulation-airway-breathing
- Epinephrine administration (1 mL/kg of 1:1,000 epinephrine or 0.3–0.5 mg); repeat up to three injections every 5–15 min IM or IV
- Administer nebulized albuterol for bronchospasm
- Administer H1 and H2 antihistamine medications
- Administer IV fluids/crystalloids rapidly for hypotension
- Corticosteroids: Methylprednisolone (1–2 mg/kg) IV
- If hypotensive despite IV fluids, consider pressors, including dopamine or vasopressin
- Airway management; if stridor or airway compromise—intubate; avoid paralytics if possible, for intubation. If laryngeal involvement is suspected—awake fiberoptic intubation if possible
- If poor response—ECMO

Macrophage Activation Syndrome

Macrophage activation syndrome (MAS) is a life-threatening complication of various rheumatic diseases with a mortality rate of 8% to 20%.[1,4]

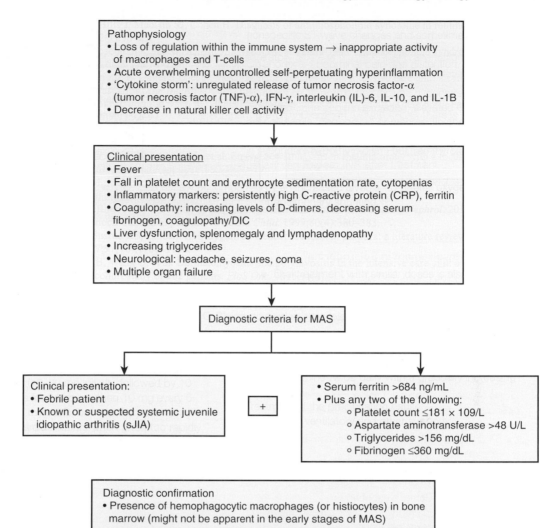

Pathophysiology
• Loss of regulation within the immune system → inappropriate activity of macrophages and T-cells
• Acute overwhelming uncontrolled self-perpetuating hyperinflammation
• 'Cytokine storm': unregulated release of tumor necrosis factor-α (tumor necrosis factor (TNF)-α), IFN-γ, interleukin (IL)-6, IL-10, and IL-1B
• Decrease in natural killer cell activity

Clinical presentation
• Fever
• Fall in platelet count and erythrocyte sedimentation rate, cytopenias
• Inflammatory markers: persistently high C-reactive protein (CRP), ferritin
• Coagulopathy: increasing levels of D-dimers, decreasing serum fibrinogen, coagulopathy/DIC
• Liver dysfunction, splenomegaly and lymphadenopathy
• Increasing triglycerides
• Neurological: headache, seizures, coma
• Multiple organ failure

Diagnostic criteria for MAS

Clinical presentation:
• Febrile patient
• Known or suspected systemic juvenile idiopathic arthritis (sJIA)

+

• Serum ferritin >684 ng/mL
• Plus any two of the following:
  ◦ Platelet count ≤181 × 109/L
  ◦ Aspartate aminotransferase >48 U/L
  ◦ Triglycerides >156 mg/dL
  ◦ Fibrinogen ≤360 mg/dL

Diagnostic confirmation
• Presence of hemophagocytic macrophages (or histiocytes) in bone marrow (might not be apparent in the early stages of MAS)

Treatment[1]

• Early, aggressive supportive therapy
• High-dose corticosteroids
• Additional immune suppression with cyclosporin
• Elimination of known or suspected triggers
• Infection control

Additional Treatment Options in Refractory Cases

• IV immunoglobulin therapy (1 g/kg for 2 days)
• Plasmapheresis
• Biologicals[4]
  • Interleukin(IL)-1–inhibiting agents (anakinra, canakinumab, rilonacept)
  • IL-6–inhibiting agents (tocilizumab)

Scleroderma (Systemic Sclerosis)

Scleroderma (systemic sclerosis) is an autoimmune disease, associated with progressive fibrosis of the skin and various internal organs.[5]

Pathophysiology

• Autoantibody formation
• Abnormalities of cytokine regulation
• Microvascular abnormalities
• Endothelial cell disruption and additional components of vasospasm
• Vascular fibrosis, upregulation of adhesion molecules, disseminated intravascular coagulation, and microangiopathic hemolytic anemia[5]

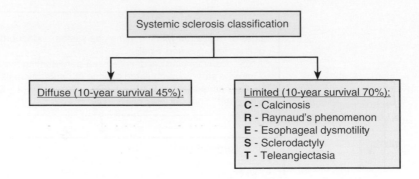

Internal Organ Involvement in Scleroderma[6]

- Pulmonary (leading cause of death in scleroderma)
  - Fibrosing alveolitis/ILD → restrictive lung disease (develops in ~50% of patients with diffuse skin disease and in ~35% of patients with limited disease)
  - Obliterative vasculopathy of medium and small pulmonary vessels → pulmonary arterial hypertension (PAH)
- GI (a major contributor to a poor QOL)
  - Decreased oral aperture
  - Loss of normal amounts of saliva, gum recession and periodontal disease, loosening or loss of teeth
  - Muscle dysfunction
    - Pharyngeal dysfunction → malnutrition and aspiration
    - Esophageal dysfunction → heartburn, regurgitation, dysphagia → esophagitis, bleeding, esophageal strictures, and/or Barrett's esophagus
    - Delayed gastric emptying → early satiety, aggravation of GERD, anorexia, bloating
    - Gastric antral vascular ectasia (GAVE) with significant asymptomatic bleeding
    - Recurrent bouts of pseudo-obstruction
    - Diarrhea secondary to bacterial overgrowth and malabsorption
- Kidney
  - Scleroderma renal crisis
- Heart
  - Immune mediated inflammation (myocarditis), microvascular disease, and/or myocardial fibrosis → pericardial effusions, LV diastolic dysfunction, conduction abnormalities, arrhythmias, right ventricular malfunction
  - Reversible vasospasm of small coronary arteries and arterioles → ischemia reperfusion injury
- Other associated issues
  - Microstomia, xerostomia, Sjogren's syndrome, periodontal disease, audio-vestibular disease, primary biliary cirrhosis, autoimmune hepatitis, bladder dysfunction, erectile dysfunction, thyroid disease, neuropathy

GERD, Gastroesophageal reflux disease; *GI,* gastrointestinal; *ILD,* interstitial lung disease; *LV,* left ventricular; *QOL,* quality of life.

Treatment of Scleroderma[6]

Raynaud's Phenomenon

- Dihydropyridine-type calcium channel blockers (first line)
- If not effective—add another vasodilator (topical nitroglycerin, phosphodiesterase inhibitor, or intermittent infusion of prostacyclin)
- Digital sympathectomy or repair of occlusive macrovascular disease
- Patients with recurrent digital ulcers:
  - Endothelin receptor antagonist or inhibitor of 3-hydroxy-3-methylglutaryl-coenzyme A (HMG-CoA) reductase
  - Antiplatelet and antioxidant agents (e.g., *N*-acetylcysteine)
  - Chronic anticoagulation is not recommended in the absence of a hypercoagulable state

Scleroderma Skin Disease Without Major Organ Disease

- Early, active inflammatory disease—immunosuppressive therapy more effective
- Later fibrotic disease—immunosuppressive therapy might not be very effective

Options:

- Follow with serial observations to define the severity and course
- Traditional low-dose immunosuppressive therapy (e.g., methotrexate, mycophenolate, or cyclophosphamide) ± ATG ± IVIG

- The use of corticosteroids is questionable and potentially dangerous (association with scleroderma renal crisis)
- Novel innovative therapy, including research trials:
  - Biological agents: (rituximab), anticytokines (tocilizumab, anti–TGF-beta), proteasome inhibitors (bortezomib), agents that may alter integrin binding, and blocking lysophosphatidic acid
  - Immunoablation with or without hematopoietic stem cell transplant

ATG, Antithymocyte globulin; *IVIG,* intravenous immunoglobulin; *TGF,* transforming growth factor.

Musculoskeletal

- To improve quality of life
  - Nonsteroidal antiinflammatory, low-dose (<10 mg) corticosteroids, and pain control
- Disease modifying therapy
  - Weekly methotrexate, TNF inhibitors, IVIG
- Physical and occupational intervention early in the course

TNF, Tumor necrosis factor.

Pulmonary

- Interstitial lung disease
  - Treatment is still not fully defined
  - If active alveolitis is present, treatment with immunosuppressive drugs is indicated:
    - Daily oral cyclophosphamide (2 mg/kg) or monthly IV cyclophosphamide or
    - Nother maintenance immunosuppressive drug (e.g., mycophenolate or azathioprine)
    - Steroids are not well supported by evidence and potentially risky

- Pulmonary arterial hypertension (PAH)
  - Oral agents: endothelin receptor antagonists (bosentan, ambrisentan) and phosphodiesterase type 5 inhibitors (sildenafil, tadalafil)
  - Aerosolized prostaglandins (iloprost, treprostinil) for severe PAH
  - Continuous infusion of a prostacyclin analogue (epoprostenol, treprostinil, or iloprost)
  - Disease modifying drugs (e.g., immunosuppression: rituximab, or antifibrotic agents: imatinib)
  - Lung transplantation for selected patients with progressive and severe life-threatening disease

Gastroenteritis

- Treatment of esophageal reflux (proton-pump inhibitors)
- Prokinetic drug, when gastroparesis is present and/or with symptoms of dysphagia and reflux despite effective acid suppression

- Management of lower bowel disease: avoid a constipation-diarrhea cycle (use fiber diet, stool softener, periodic polyethylene glycol, probiotics), the use of cyclic antibiotics
- Octreotide for recurrent pseudo-obstruction
- Total parenteral nutrition if severe scleroderma-related bowel disease without response to other medical therapy

Cardiac

- Vasodilators, particularly the calcium channel blockers (used with caution in severe PAH)

- Conventional treatment of cardiomyopathy or arrhythmias
- Lack of studies re: role of immunosuppression

PAH, Pulmonary arterial hypertension.

Scleroderma Renal Crisis

Risk Factors for Scleroderma Renal Crisis

- Corticosteroid therapy
- Rapidly progressive skin disease
- Diffuse cutaneous systemic sclerosis

Presentation[1,7]

- Acute onset of moderate-to-severe "accelerated" hypertension (new-onset hypertension >150/80)
- In up to 10% of cases, SRC occurs without hypertension (normotensive SRC)
- Renal failure (>30% reduction in eGFR), oliguria
- Left ventricular insufficiency
- Hypertensive encephalopathy
- Rheumatological emergency as rapid diagnosis and treatment may save lives and renal function

eGFR, Estimated glomerular filtration rate; *SRC,* scleroderma renal crisis.

Consider Other Causes of Renal Failure

These might mimic (especially in patients with limited scleroderma who present with abnormal sediment or significant proteinuria)[6]:

- Scleroderma with lupus nephritis
- ANCA-related crescentic glomerulonephritis
- Multiple organ failure

Treatment[7,8]

- Aggressive management of hypertension is required to prevent irreversible renal damage
- The goal is to bring the SBP down by 20 mm Hg per 24 hours and the DBP down by 10 mm Hg per 24 hours until the BP is within normal limits, while avoiding hypotension
- Angiotensin-converting enzyme inhibitors—first line of therapy
- Calcium-channel blockers
- Angiotensin receptor blockers
- Alpha-blockers
- Plasmapheresis for TMA
- Dialysis
- Try to avoid corticosteroids

BP, Blood pressure; *DBP,* diastolic blood pressure; *SBP,* systolic blood pressure; *TMA,* thrombotic microangiopathy.

Antiphospholipid Syndrome

Antiphospholipid syndrome is a diverse family of antibodies that are associated with a hypercoagulable state.

Causes of Antiphospholipid Syndrome (APS)[5]

- SLE or lupus-like disorders, RA, systemic sclerosis, Behçet's disease
- Infections
- Drugs
- Miscellaneous conditions
- In approximately 50% of cases, it occurs in the absence of a defined underlying etiology (primary antiphospholipid antibody syndrome)

Clinical Presentations of Antiphospholipid Syndrome[5]

- Venous thrombosis: DVT ± PE, superficial venous thrombosis, cerebral, retinal, renal, hepatic
- Arterial thrombosis: cerebral, peripheral, coronary, renal, retinal
- Other manifestations:
  - Obstetric: pregnancy loss, intrauterine growth retardation
  - Hematologic: thrombocytopenia, hemolytic anemia
  - Cardiac: myocardial infarction, valvular vegetations, intracardiac thrombus, cardiomyopathy
- Neurologic: coma, seizures, stroke, chorea, transverse myelopathy, complicated migraine, encephalopathy, retinal artery thrombosis
- Pulmonary: pulmonary hypertension, adult respiratory distress syndrome, alveolar hemorrhage, PE
- Renal: malignant hypertension, renal failure
- Gastrointestinal: abdominal pain, visceral ischemia/gangrene/vascular occlusion
- Endocrine: adrenal infarction
- Skin: livedo reticularis, digital ischemia, splinter hemorrhages, ulcerations, superficial gangrene in lower limbs

Catastrophic Antiphospholipid Syndrome

- <1% of APS cases
- Rapid multiorgan failure and over 50% mortality despite treatment
- Microangiopathy of small vessels, resulting in organ failure and SIRS-like state

SIRS, Systemic inflammatory response syndrome.

Precipitating Event/Trigger

- Infection
- Surgical procedures
- Trauma
- Withdrawal of anticoagulation
- May be unknown

Diagnostic Laboratory Tests[9]

- Lupus anticoagulant
- Anti-beta-2-glycoprotein-I
- Anticardiolipin

Specific Therapy[10]

- Anticoagulation: unfractionated heparin; given elevated PTT at baseline, follow additional readouts to monitor heparin infusion rate (e.g., an anti-factor Xa)
- Corticosteroids: intravenous pulse (methylprednisolone 500–1000 mg daily for 1–3 days) or 1–2 mg/kg/day (methylprednisolone equivalent, oral or intravenous)
- Therapeutic plasma exchange or IVIG (0.4 g/kg/day × 5 days) or the combination (IVIG after TPE)
- Cyclophosphamide (when CAPS occurs in a patient with SLE: 500–750 mg/m², adjusted for renal function)
- Rituximab (if TPE is used—use rituximab after TPE course is complete)
- Eculizumab (in CAPS patients who failed to respond to other therapy: 900 mg once weekly for 4 weeks, and 1200 mg every-other-week thereafter)
- Other ICU considerations:
  - Minimize arterial instrumentation when possible (risk of new clots)
  - Lung-protective ventilation
  - Glycemic control
  - Gastric ulcer preventative measures (given high doses of corticosteroids and anticoagulation)

CAPS, Catastrophic antiphospholipid syndrome; *INIG,* intravenous immunoglobin; *PTT,* partial thromboplastin time; *TPE,* therapeutic plasma exchange.

Vasculitides

The natural course of systemic vasculitis may be complicated by acute and life-threatening manifestations that require management in an intensive care unit.[11]

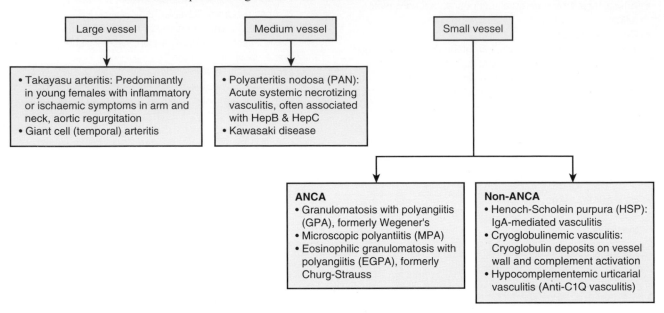

Diagnosis of Vasculitis in ICU[12]

Diagnosis of Vasculitis in ICU.				
	Granulomatosis with polyangiitis (Wegener's)	Microscopic polyangiitis (MPA)	Eosinophilic Granulomatosis With Polyangiitis (Churg-Strauss syndrome)	Polyarteritis nodosa
Frequency	Somewhat rare	Rare	Extremely rare	Rare
Vessels involved	Small-sized blood vessels in the nose, sinuses, ears, lungs, and kidneys	Capillaries	Small-to-medium-sized vessels	Small-to-medium-sized vessels
Frequently affected areas	Upper respiratory tract (sinuses, nose, ears, and trachea), the lungs, and the kidneys	Kidneys, lung, nerves, skin, and joints	Nose, sinuses, lungs, heart, intestines, and nerves	Nerves, intestinal tract, heart, joints, kidneys
Generalized constitutional symptoms	++	++	++	++
Sinusitis	+++	+	+++	+
Asthma	–	–	+++	–
Dyspnea, cough	+++	+	++	+
Skin rash	+	+	++	+
Abdominal pain	+	+	+	++
HTN	+	+	+	++
Proteinuria/hematuria	+++	+++	++	–
CHF/pericarditis	+	+	++	+
Mononeuritis (multiplex)	+	+	++	++
Eosinophilia	Rare	Rare	Present	Not

Diagnosis of Vasculitis in ICU—cont'd				
	Granulomatosis with polyangiitis (Wegener's)	Microscopic polyangiitis (MPA)	Eosinophilic Granulomatosis With Polyangiitis (Churg-Strauss syndrome)	Polyarteritis nodosa
Pulmonary-renal syndrome	Yes	Yes	Usually not, just pulmonary	Usually not, just renal
ANCA positivity	ANCA (typically c-ANCA, with anti-protein kinase-3 [PR-3] antibodies) 90% ANCA positive	ANCA (typically p-ANCA or MPO-ANCA, with anti-myeloperoxidase [MPO] antibodies) 90% ANCA positive	ANCA positive in 30%–60%, typically p-ANCA (with anti-MPO antibodies)	Only ~5% ANCA positive

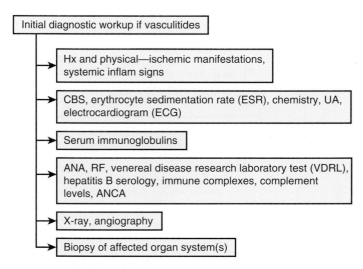

Antineutrophil Cytoplasmic Antibodies (ANCA)-Associated Vasculitides (AAV)

ANCA-Associated Vasculitides (AAV)

- Microscopic polyangiitis (MPA)
- Granulomatosis with polyangiitis (GPA, formerly Wegener's)
- Eosinophilic granulomatosis with polyangiitis (EGPA, formerly Churg–Strauss)
- Single-organ AAV (e.g., renal-limited AAV)

Respiratory Tract and Kidneys Most Commonly Affected by AAV[13]

- Pulmonary involvement is more frequent in GPA (90%) and eosinophillic GPA (EGPA) (70%) and less frequent in MPA (50%). In GPA, all parts of the respiratory tract can be affected from the nasal mucosa to the pleura and pulmonary artery.
- Renal involvement occurs more frequently in MPA (90%) and in GPA (80%) and less frequently in EGPA (45%).

It presents as pauci immune (without deposits of immunoglobulins or complement particles) necrotizing glomerulonephritis with crescents → rapidly progressive glomerulonephritis
- The heart is involved most commonly in EGPA (heart blocks, myocarditis, pericarditis, myocardial infarction)
- GI presentations: bowel perforation (resulting from vasculitic ulceration of the intestine), pancreatic or liver involvement

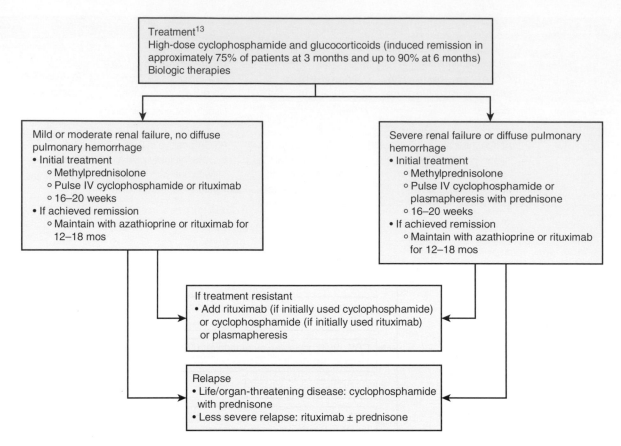

Polyarteritis Nodosa

Polyarteritis nodosa (PAN) is relatively rare and was one of the first described vasculitis affecting small- and medium-sized arteries. It is ANCA Ab positive in less than 5% of cases.[14]

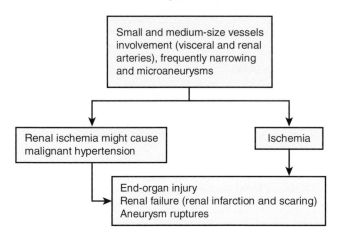

Treatment[15]

- Life-threatening manifestations: high-dose glucocorticoids + cyclophosphamide
- Non–severe disease: glucocorticoids alone

- Hepatitis B virus–associated PAN: add antiviral agent, short-term glucocorticoids and plasma exchanges
- Cutaneous PAN: less aggressive therapy—NSAIDs or other agents (colchicine or dapsone)

IgA Vasculitis (Henoch–Schönlein Purpura)

Henoch-Schönlein purpura (HSP) is an IgA vasculitis (associated with IgA deposits in affected tissues). It is an ANCA-negative, leukocytoclastic vasculitis.[14,16–18] HSP is relatively frequent, involves the small vessels and presents with multiorgan (skin, gastrointestinal tract, kidney, joints) involvement. Kidney signs of HSP are nephritic or nephrotic. The characteristic features of the disease pathology are the mesangial deposits of IgA.

Potential Triggers

- Infection, particularly with β-hemolytic streptococci, viral infections
- Vaccination
- Coagulation disorders

Clinical Presentation

- Skin: non-thrombocytopenic palpable purpura
- Joints: arthritis and arthralgia
- GI: abdominal pain, gastrointestinal hemorrhage
- Kidneys: glomerulonephritis (microscopic or macroscopic hematuria with mild proteinuria, sometimes even nephrotic or nephritic syndrome, mesangial deposits of IgA) → AKI → end-stage kidney disease
- Most cases involve pediatric population

Diagnosis

Diagnostic criteria for Henoch-Schönlein purpura (HSP), as developed byEULAR/PRINTO/PRES[18]:

Mandatory criterion:
- Purpura or petechiae with lower limb
Plus at least one out of the following four:
- Diffuse abdominal pain with acute onset
- Histopathology showing leukocytoclastic vasculitis or proliferative glomerulonephritis, with predominant IgA deposits
- Arthritis or arthralgia of acute onset
- Renal involvement in the form of proteinuria or hematuria
- No specific useful biomarkers
- Skin biopsies are the gold standard for diagnosing any cutaneous vasculitis: IgA-predominant vascular deposits are characteristic for HSP

Treatment[18]

- Frequently a self-limited disease
- Symptomatic treatment, e.g., pain medication, rehydration therapy and surgery for intussusception, wound therapy for ulcerations
- Cyclosporine or other immunosuppression (mycophenolate mofetil), dapsone, rituximab
- Cyclophosphamide, corticosteroids (including pulse steroids) are controversial
- Anticoagulation—not well documented
- Plasmapheresis

Cryoglobulinemic Vasculitis

Cryoglobulinemic vasculitis (CV) affects small vessels with complement activation subsequent to deposition of cryoglobulins on a vessel wall.[11]

Types of Cryoglobulinemia

- Cryoglobulins are immunoglobulins, which reversibly precipitate under cool conditions (<37°C).
- Type I is a monoclonal antibody that does not have rheumatoid factor activity (typical for the monoclonal gammopathies).
- Both types II and III are rheumatoid factors—antibodies that bind to the Fc fragment of IgG. Both types are called mixed cryoglobulins.

- In type II, the rheumatoid factor is monoclonal.
- In type III it is polyclonal (associated with systemic connective tissue disorders, leukemia, hepatobiliary disorders, and infections).
- Close relationship between the mixed type II cryoglobulinemia and hepatitis C virus infection.

Presentation[14]

- Skin purpura with leucoclastic vasculitis, may be accompanied by large ulcerations
- Non-specific symptoms: weakness, fatigue, fever
- Arthralgia

- Raynaud's syndrome
- Peripheral neuropathy (dysesthesia or anesthesia)
- Hepatosplenomegaly may indicate hepatitis C
- Proteinuria and microscopic hematuria, renal insufficiency, nephritic or nephrotic syndrome, hypertension

---

Diagnosis

- Laboratory: presence of the mixed cryoglobulin, low complement components, and positivity of rheumatoid factors.

- Renal biopsy in cases of type II mixed cryoglobulinemia with membranoproliferative glomerulonephritis.

Management[14]

- Avoiding hypothermia, especially in case of extracorporeal circulation use (e.g. hemodialysis, ECMO).
- Address the cause: in case of HCV-related CV, the eradication of HCV infection
- Symptoms control
  - Patients with glomerulonephritis should receive angiotensin-converting enzyme inhibitors or angiotensin II receptor blockers and antihypertensive drugs to achieve the blood pressure and proteinuria targets
- Glucocorticoids
- Immunosuppression: cyclophosphamide, azathioprine, methotrexate, cyclosporine, mycophenolate mofetil, and rituximab

- IV Immunoglobulins
- In cases of granulomatosis with polyangiitis and/or severe (e.g., RPGN), life-threatening (e.g., pulmonary hemorrhage) vasculitis (in critically ill patients)[11]:
  - High-dose steroids (intravenous methylprednisolone pulses of 500–1000 mg/day for 3 days, followed by oral prednisone 1 mg/kg/day)
  - Immunosuppressive drugs—cyclophosphamide (2 mg/kg/day orally or 600 mg/m²/month intravenously for 2–4 months) or rituximab (375 mg/m²/week for 4 weeks)
  - Sometimes plasma exchanges (3 L of plasma per exchange, three times a week for 2–3 weeks); mandatory in patients with hyperviscosity syndrome (replacement fluids for plasma exchange in CV should be warmed before infusion)

ECMO, Extracorporeal membrane oxygenation; *HCV,* hepatitis C virus; *RPGN,* rapidly progressive glomerulonephritis.

Dermatomyositis/Polymyositis

The course of dermatomyositis/polymyositis might have life-threatening complications with ICU admission, and is associated in those cases with poor outcome.[19]

Presentation

- Predominant symptoms are proximal muscle weakness and typical skin finding in dermatomyositis heliotrope rash and Gottron's papules
- May affect esophagus and rarely myocardium

- Pulmonary:
  - Diffuse fibrosing alveolitis → pulmonary fibrosis
  - Respiratory restriction caused by weakness of respiratory muscles
  - Increased risk of aspiration and related aspiration pneumonia

Diagnosis

- Positive antisynthetase antibodies (e.g., anti-Jo)
- Respiratory function test, radiography, high-resolution CT, and bronchoalveolar lavage

- Disease focused tests: serum muscle enzyme levels, electromyography (EMG), muscle biopsy, and immunology

Treatment

- High dose glucocorticoids

- Immunosuppression (azathioprine, methotrexate)
- High-dose polyclonal immunoglobulins, if indicated

Systemic Lupus Erythematosus

Systemic lupus erythematosus (SLE) is a complex, multisystem disease with a number of potential critical presentations, including coronary artery disease, overwhelming sepsis, renal failure, pericarditis, and more rare alveolar hemorrhage and transverse myelitis.[1]

Life-threating complications of SLE[14]

- Cardiac: coronary artery disease, myocarditis, pericarditis, endocarditis
- Hypertensive crisis
- Pulmonary: pneumonitis, pulmonary hemorrhage, ARDS
- Renal: glomerulonephritis, renal failure
- CNS disease (seizures, psychosis, organic brain syndrome, transverse myelitis)
- Cytopenias (thrombocytopenia, hemolytic anemia)
- Infectious complications of treatment; sepsis
- Polyarteritis-like vasculitis of the gut
- Acute pancreatitis

Diagnosis

- Antinuclear autoantibodies (ANA)
- Anti-dsDNA antibodies

- Extractable nuclear antigen (ENA) antibodies
- Antiphospholipid antibodies
- Reduced levels of complement

Treatment of Systemic Lupus Erythematosus[14]

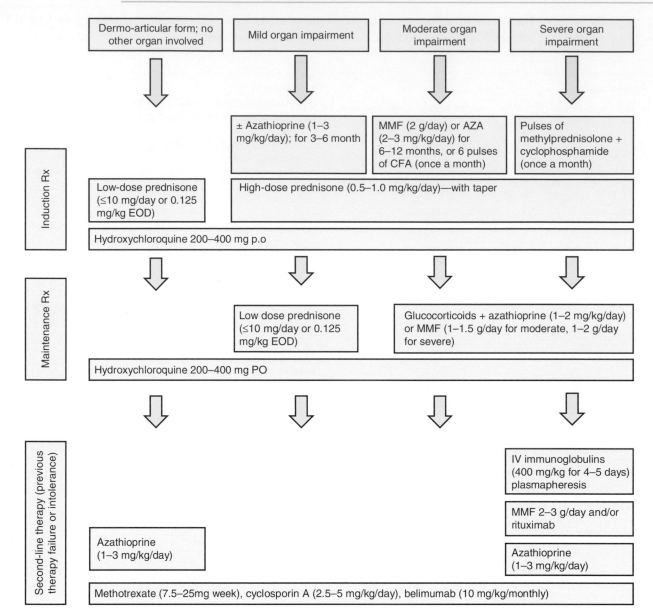

Arthritis

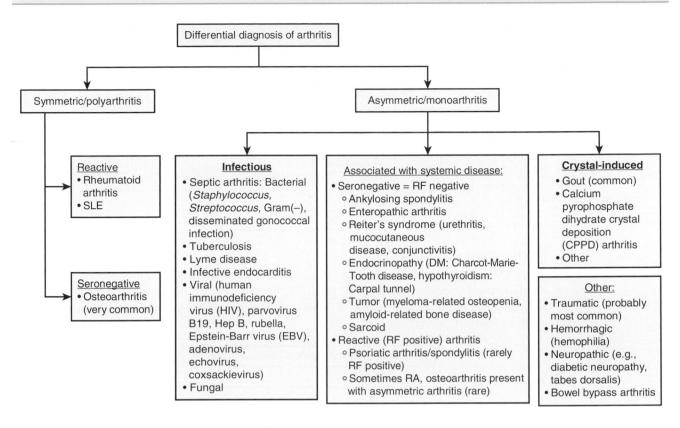

Differential diagnosis of arthritis

Symmetric/polyarthritis

Reactive
- Rheumatoid arthritis
- SLE

Seronegative
- Osteoarthritis (very common)

Asymmetric/monoarthritis

Infectious
- Septic arthritis: Bacterial (*Staphylococcus, Streptococcus,* Gram(−), disseminated gonococcal infection)
- Tuberculosis
- Lyme disease
- Infective endocarditis
- Viral (human immunodeficiency virus (HIV), parvovirus B19, Hep B, rubella, Epstein-Barr virus (EBV), adenovirus, echovirus, coxsackievirus)
- Fungal

Associated with systemic disease:
- Seronegative = RF negative
  ○ Ankylosing spondylitis
  ○ Enteropathic arthritis
  ○ Reiter's syndrome (urethritis, mucocutaneous disease, conjunctivitis)
  ○ Endocrinopathy (DM: Charcot-Marie-Tooth disease, hypothyroidism: Carpal tunnel)
  ○ Tumor (myeloma-related osteopenia, amyloid-related bone disease)
  ○ Sarcoid
- Reactive (RF positive) arthritis
  ○ Psoriatic arthritis/spondylitis (rarely RF positive)
  ○ Sometimes RA, osteoarthritis present with asymmetric arthritis (rare)

Crystal-induced
- Gout (common)
- Calcium pyrophosphate dihydrate crystal deposition (CPPD) arthritis
- Other

Other:
- Traumatic (probably most common)
- Hemorrhagic (hemophilia)
- Neuropathic (e.g., diabetic neuropathy, tabes dorsalis)
- Bowel bypass arthritis

Rule Out Other Medical Emergencies

- Infection
- Compartment syndrome
- Acute myelopathy/neuropathy/radiculopathy

Inflammatory arthritis: stiffness, increased pain with immobility
Noninflammatory (e.g., osteoarthritis, traumatic): increased pain with motion

---

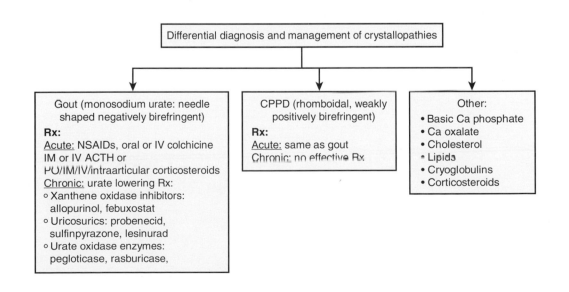

Differential diagnosis and management of crystallopathies

Gout (monosodium urate: needle shaped negatively birefringent)

Rx:
Acute: NSAIDs, oral or IV colchicine IM or IV ACTH or PO/IM/IV/intraarticular corticosteroids
Chronic: urate lowering Rx:
  ○ Xanthene oxidase inhibitors: allopurinol, febuxostat
  ○ Uricosurics: probenecid, sulfinpyrazone, lesinurad
  ○ Urate oxidase enzymes: pegloticase, rasburicase,

CPPD (rhomboidal, weakly positively birefringent)

Rx:
Acute: same as gout
Chronic: no effective Rx

Other:
- Basic Ca phosphate
- Ca oxalate
- Cholesterol
- Lipids
- Cryoglobulins
- Corticosteroids

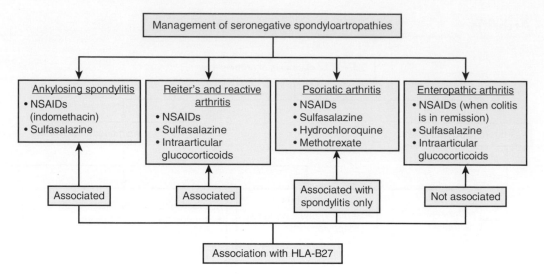

Rheumatoid Arthritis

Patients with rheumatoid arthritis (RA) requiring ICU admission (most common reasons—respiratory failure and infections) demonstrate high mortality (30-day mortality rate of patients with RA who were admitted to the general ICU of a tertiary hospital was 34.9%), with infection being the most common cause of death.[20]

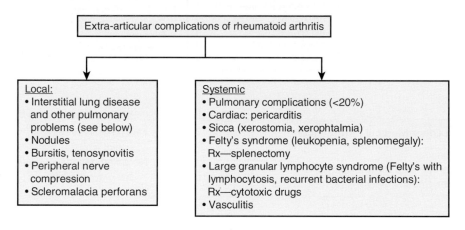

Pulmonary manifestations of rheumatoid arthritis[21]

Interstitial lung disease
- Most common pulmonary manifestation of RA
- Both rheumatoid factor and anti-CCP have been linked to the
- development of interstitial lung disease (ILD)
- Diagnosis
  ○ Restrictive pattern on PFTs with or without decreased DLCO and hypoxemia
  ○ High resolution computed tomography (CT) (HRCT)
  ○ Surgical lung biopsy
- Treatment
  ○ Treatment with antiinflammatory and/or immunosuppression is recommended
    regardless of the pattern of fibrosis
  ○ Corticosteroids are the mainstay of therapy
  ○ Cyclophosphamide, azathioprine, methotrexate—varying success
  ○ Cyclosporine and/or mycophenolate
  ○ Anti-tumor necrosis factor, rituximab—controversial

Pleural disease
- Presentation
  ○ Presents as pleural effusions (mostly unilateral)
  ○ Fever and pleuritic pain are also common
- Diagnosis
  ○ Imaging
  ○ Pleural fluid studies (sterile exudative fluid with low pH (<7.3), low glucose
    (<60 mg/dL) and elevated lactate dehydrogenase (may be >700 IU/L), presence
    of cholesterol crystals, cell count is variable)
- Treatment
  ○ Most improve with treatment of the underlying rheumatoid arthritis
  ○ Therapeutic thoracentesis when indicated

Upper airway disease
- Presentation:
  ○ Nodules on the vocal cords, vasculitis affecting the recurrent laryngeal or vagus nerves → vocal
    cord paralysis; arthritis of the cricoarytenoid joint
  ○ Acute stridor or obstructive respiratory failure may occur from sudden subluxation or
    superimposed airway edema from infection or intubation
- Diagnosis: HRCT of the neck
- Treatment
  ○ Mild symptoms: nonsteroidal anti inflammatory drugs or rheumatoid arthritis-directed therapy
  ○ More severe obstruction: Immediate airway management if necessary + surgical intervention

Lower airway disease
- Presentation
  ○ Bronchial hyperresponsiveness, follicular bronchiolitis, obliterative bronchiolitis, bronchiectasis
- Diagnosis: HRCT
- Treatment
  ○ Follicular bronchiolitis
    ▪ Directed at the underlying rheumatoid arthritis
  ○ Obliterative bronchiolitis
    ▪ Discontinue the offending agent
    ▪ High-dose corticosteroids, azathioprine, cyclophosphamide—unclear benefit
    ▪ Some improvement with anti-TNF therapy
    ▪ Macrolide antibiotics (e.g., erythromycin) may also be effective
    ▪ In severe cases, lung transplant may be necessary
  ○ Bronchiectasis
    ▪ Presence of bronchiectasis complicates the use of immunosuppressive medications, particularly
      anti-TNF agents
    ▪ Therapy is the same as for either condition (RA and bronchiectasis) alone, with bronchodilators,
      antibiotics and bronchial hygiene used to treat bronchiectasis

Pulmonary nodules
- Rheumatoid nodule(s) in the lungs usually located along the interlobular septa or in subpleural regions
- Pathology: central fibrinoid necrosis with palisading mononuclear cells and associated vasculitis
- Symptomatic only if cavitate or rupture → infection, pleural effusion or bronchopleural fistula
- DDx: malignancy
- Diagnosis: positron emission tomography scan (PET) for nodules ≥8 mm (RA-related nodules show little
  or no uptake)
- Treatment: uncomplicated nodules may spontaneously regress or improve with standard RA treatment,
  though might increase with methotrexate

Vascular disease—higher risk for:
- Pulmonary hypertension
- Venous thromboembolism (DVT and PE both)

Drug toxicity
- Methotrexate: acute/subacute hypersensitivity pneumonitis/interstitial lung disease, progressive pulmonary
  fibrosis, rheumatoid nodule formation, small increase in risk of respiratory infections
- Leflunomide: interstitial lung disease
- TNF-α inhibitors: interstitial lung disease: sarcoid-like granulomatous disease, organizing pneumonia and
  exacerbation of pre-existing
- ILD
- Rituximab: controversial data re: organizing pneumonia
- NSAIDs and gold: organizing pneumonia
- Sulfasalazine and penicillamine: obliterative bronchiolitis
- Azathioprine and tacrolimus: exacerbation of pre existing ILD
- Any immune modulating agents: opportunistic lung infections

Diagnostic Antibody Profiles of Rheumatologic and Other Autoimmune Disorders[22]

Autoantibodies In Rheumatic Or Autoimmune Disease	
Rheumatologic or Autoimmune Disorder	**Serum Antibodies**
SLE	ANA—non-specific Anti-dsDNA Anti-Sm (Smith nuclear antigen) Anti-ENA (extractable nuclear antigen) Anti-Ro/SSA, anti-La/SSB (predictor of neonatal lupus in babies) Rheumatoid factor (RF) Antiphospholipid antibodies Antihistone in drug-induced SLE
Drug-induced SLE	Rarely have anti-dsDNA Almost always have antihistone Ab
Antiphospholipid antibody syndrome	Anticardiolipin Ab Lupus anticoagulant Anti-beta-2-glycoprotein-I
Rheumatoid arthritis	ANA, RF, anti-citrullinated protein antibodies (ACPA), anti-Carp, anticyclic citrullinated peptide (CCP)
Polymyositis, dermatomyositis, interstitial lung disease, Raynaud's phenomenon	Myositis-specific: Antisynthetase antibodies: (Jo-1, PL-7, EJ, OJ, PL-12) Nonsynthetase anticytoplasmic antibodies (SRP, KJ) Non-specific: Ribonucleoprotein, Sm, PM-Scl, Ku, Ro/SSA, ANA, RF
Sjögren's syndrome	ANA, anti-Ro/SSA, anti-La/SSB, RF
Systemic sclerosis/scleroderma	Ribonucleoprotein, anti-Scl-70, Ku, RF, ANA, anti-centromere
Polyarteritis nodosa, Churg-Strauss syndrome	ANCA (usually p-ANCA)
Wegener's	ANCA (almost always c-ANCA), RF, ↑IgA
RPGN	Anti-GBM: anti-α3 chain of basement membrane Collagen (type IV collagen) (in Goodpasture) ANCA in vasculitides
Autoimmune hepatitis	Anti-smooth muscle, ANA; autoimmune hepatitis type 2: anti-LKM (anti-liver/kidney microsomal Ab)
Primary biliary cirrhosis	Anti-mitochondrial
Primary sclerosing cholangitis	ANCA
Acanthosis nigricans	Antibody to insulin receptors
Myasthenia gravis	Antibody to acetylcholine receptor
Pernicious anemia/atrophic gastritis	Antibody to parietal cells

REFERENCES

1. Bell A, Tattersall R, Wenham T. Rheumatological conditions in critical care. *BJA Educ.* 2016;16(12):427–433.
2. Quintero OL, Rojas-Villarraga A, Mantilla RD, Anaya JM. Autoimmune diseases in the intensive care unit. An update. *Autoimmun Rev.* 2013;12(3):380–395.
3. LoVerde D, Iweala OI, Eginli A, Krishnaswamy G. Anaphylaxis. *Chest.* 2018;153(2):528–543.
4. Grom AA, Horne A, De Benedetti F. Macrophage activation syndrome in the era of biologic therapy. *Nat Rev Rheumatol.* 2016;12(5):259–268.
5. Schlesinger PA, Leatherman JW. Rheumatology. *Am J Respir Crit Care Med.* 2002;166(9):1161–1165.
6. Shah AA, Wigley FM. My approach to the treatment of scleroderma. *Mayo Clin Proc.* 2013;88(4):377–393.
7. Shanmugam VK, Steen VD. Renal disease in scleroderma: an update on evaluation, risk stratification, pathogenesis and management. *Curr Opin Rheumatol.* 2012;24(6):669–676.
8. Fernández-Codina A, Walker KM, Pope JE. Treatment algorithms for systemic sclerosis according to experts. *Arthritis Rheumatol.* 2018;70(11):1820–1828.

9. Gardiner CK, Hills J, MacHin SJ, Cohen H. Diagnosis of antiphospholipid syndrome in routine clinical practice. *Lupus*. 2013;22(1):18–25.

10. Kazzaz NM, Joseph McCune W, Knight JS. Treatment of catastrophic antiphospholipid syndrome. *Curr Opin Rheumatol*. 2016;28(3):218–227.

11. Zaidan M, Mariotte E, Galicier L, et al. Vasculitic emergencies in the intensive care unit: a special focus on cryo-globulinemic vasculitis. *Ann Intensive Care*. 2012;2(1):31.

12. Semple D, Keogh J, Forni L, Venn R. Clinical review: vasculitis on the intensive care unit - Part 1: diagnosis. *Crit Care*. 2005;9(1):92–97.

13. Jennette JC, Nachman PH. ANCA glomerulonephritis and vasculitis. *Clin J Am Soc Nephrol*. 2017;12(10):1680–1691.

14. Vymetal J, Skacelova M, Smrzova A, et al. Emergency situations in rheumatology with a focus on systemic auto-immune diseases. *Biomed Pap*. 2016;160(1):20–29.

15. de Menthon M, Mahr A. Treating polyarteritis nodosa: current state of the art. *Clin Exp Rheumatol*. 29(1 suppl 64):S110-S116.

16. Brogan P, Eleftheriou D. Vasculitis update: pathogenesis and biomarkers. *Pediatr Nephrol*. 2018;33(2):187–198.

17. Tizard EJ. Henoch-Schonlein purpura. *Arch Dis Child*. 1999;80(4):380–383.

18. Hetland LE, Susrud KS, Lindahl KH, Bygum A. Henoch-Schönlein purpura: a literature review. *Acta Derm Venereol*. 2017;97(10):1160–1166.

19. Peng JM, Du B, Wang Q, et al. Dermatomyositis and polymyositis in the intensive care unit: a single-center retrospective cohort study of 102 patients. *PloS One*. 2016;11(4).

20. Haviv-Yadid Y, Segal Y, Dagan A, et al. Mortality of patients with rheumatoid arthritis requiring intensive care: a single-center retrospective study. *Clin Rheumatol*. 2019;38(11):3015–3023.

21. Shaw M, Collins BF, Ho LA, Raghu G. Rheumatoid arthritis-associated lung disease. *Eur Respir Rev*. 2015;24(135):1–16.

22. Suurmond J, Diamond B. Autoantibodies in systemic autoimmune diseases: specificity and pathogenicity. *J Clin Invest*. 2015;125(6):2194–2202.

CHAPTER 10

Endocrinology Issues in Critical Care

Alexander Goldfarb-Rumyantzev

Critical care endocrinology is a fundamental area of intensive care practice and is rapidly expanding in its knowledge base and therapeutic implications.[1]

Diabetes Mellitus

Diabetes mellitus (DM) is very common and is frequently associated with comorbidities and complications, leading to or exacerbating acute conditions requiring ICU care. Below we discuss diagnostic criteria and treatment approaches to diabetes in general, as well as complicating conditions (i.e., hyperglycemic crises and hypoglycemia).

Diagnostic Criteria of DM and Prediabetes

Fasting plasma glucose (FPG)
Normal: less than 100 mg/dL
Prediabetes: 100 mg/dL to 125 mg/dL
Diabetes: 126 mg/dL (7.0 mmol/L) or higher
Oral glucose tolerance test (OGTT) at 2 hours
Normal: less than 140 mg/dL
Prediabetes: 140 mg/dL to 199 mg/dL

Diabetes: 200 mg/dL (11.1 mmol/L) or higher during a 75-g oral glucose tolerance test
HbA1c
Normal: <5.7%
Prediabetes: ≥5.7%–6.4%
Diabetes: ≥6.5%—point of controversy as a criterion
A random plasma glucose of 200 mg/dL (11.1 mmol/L) or higher in a patient with classic symptoms of hyperglycemia or hyperglycemic crisis

---

Treatment of Diabetes Mellitus

Self-Monitoring Glucose Level[2]

- Type 1 DM
  - Before eating
  - At bedtime
  - Before exercise
  - If hypoglycemia is suspected

  - Until hypoglycemia is corrected
  - Postprandially upon occasion
  - Before critical tasks (i.e., driving)
- Type 2 DM
  - Recommended to monitor, but less specific, might use same recommendations as in type 1 as a guideline

---

General Treatment Goal[2]:

Preprandial blood glucose 80–120 mg/dL

Bedtime blood glucose 100–140 mg/dL
HbA1c <7.0% (or 6.5% in select patients if can be achieved without significant hypoglycemia)

Available Non-Insulin Treatments[2-4]

- Insulin sensitizers
  - Biguanides (metformin)
  - Thiazolidinediones (rosiglitazone, pioglitazone)
- Insulin secretagogues
  - Sulfonylureas (chlorpropamide, glimepiride, glipizide, glyburide, tolazamide)
  - Glinides (nateglinide, repaglinide)
- Alpha-glucosidase inhibitors (acarbose, miglitol)
- Incretins
  - GLP-1 (glucagon-like peptide 1) receptor agonists (SQ injections)
    - Short-acting (4–6 h) (exenatide [Byetta])
    - Intermediate-acting (24 h) (liraglutide [Victoza])
    - Long-acting (7 days) (exenatide ER [Bydureon], albiglutide [Tanzeum], dulaglutide [Trulicity])
  - DPP-4 inhibitors (sitagliptin [Januvia], saxagliptin [Onglyza], linagliptin [Tradjenta], alogliptin [Nesina])
- Others
  - Pramlinitide (Symlin): adjunctive treatment with insulin
  - Rapid-release bromocriptine (Bromocriptine)
  - SGLT-2 (sodium–glucose cotransporter 2) inhibitors (canagliflozin [Invokana], dapagliflozin [Farxiga], empagliflozin [Jardiance])

Available Insulin Formulations

Insulin (Brand)	Onset	Peak	Effective Duration	Variability
Rapid-acting (Aspart [Novolog], Lispro [Humalog], Glulisine [Apidra])	5–15 min	30–90 min	<5 h	Minimal
Short-acting (Regular insulin [HumuLIN R, NovoLIN R])	30–60 min	2–3 h	5–8 h	Moderate
Intermediate-acting, basal (Insulin NPH)	2–4 h	4–10 h	10–16 h	High
Long-acting, basal				
Insulin glargine (Lantus, Toujeo, Basaglar)	2–4 h	No peak	20–24 h	Moderate
Insulin detemir (Levemir)	3–8 h	No peak	6–23 h	
Insulin degludec (Tresiba)	1 h		>25 h	
Premixed				
75% Insulin lispro protamine/25% insulin lispro (Humalog mix 75/25)	5–15 min	Dual	10–16 h	
50% Insulin lispro protamine/50% insulin lispro (Humalog mix 50/50)	5–15 min	Dual	10–16 h	
70% Insulin lispro protamine/30% insulin aspart (Novolog mix 70/30)	5–15 min	Dual	10–16 h	
70% Neutral Protamine Hagedorn (NPH) insulin/30% regular	30–60 min	Dual	10–16 h	
Inhaled: Technosphere insulin inhalation system (Afrezza)				

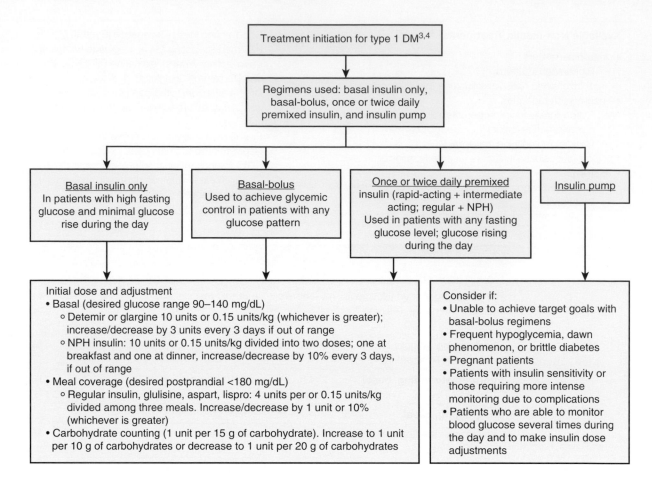

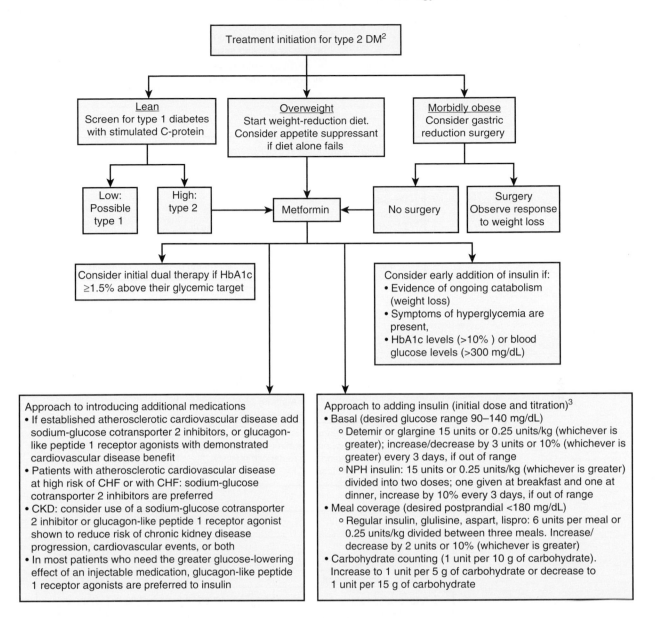

Hyperglycemic Crises in DM: Diabetic Ketoacidosis and Hyperosmolar Hyperglycemic State

Diabetic ketoacidosis (DKA) is caused by insulin deficiency lipolysis leading to acidosis caused by the presence of ketone bodies exceeding the body's buffering capacity.[5] DKA is characterized by ketoacidosis and hyperglycaemia, while hyperosmolar hyperglycaemic state (HHS) usually has more severe hyperglycaemia but no ketoacidosis.

Potential Precipitating Factors of Hyperglycemic Crises in Diabetic Patients

- Infection (most common)
- Cardiovascular disease (e.g., stroke, MI)
- Alcohol abuse
- Pancreatitis

- Trauma
- Discontinuation of insulin or inadequate insulin
- Drugs: steroids, thiazides, sodium-glucose cotransporter-2 inhibitors
- Sometimes no obvious precipitant, e.g., in ketosis-prone diabetes (an atypical form of type 2 diabetes). DKA is the presenting condition

Presentation

- Polyuria
- Polydipsia
- Weight loss

- Nausea and vomiting
- Weakness and lethargy
- Altered mental state
- Kussmaul respiration
- Acetone on breath

Potential precipitating factors of hyperglycemic crises in diabetic patients
- Infection (most common)
- Cardiovascular disease (e.g., stroke, MI)
- Alcohol abuse
- Pancreatitis
- Trauma
- Discontinuation of insulin or inadequate insulin
- Drugs: steroids, thiazides, sodium-glucose cotransporter-2 inhibitors
- Sometimes no obvious precipitant, e.g., in ketosis-prone diabetes
(an atypical form of type 2 diabetes) - DKA is the presenting condition

Presentation
- Polyuria
- Polydipsia
- Weight loss
- Nausea and vomiting
- Weakness and lethargy
- Altered mental state
- Kussmaul respiration
- Acetone on breath

Diagnosis
- Hyperglycemia (might not always be present)
- Anion gap metabolic acidosis
- Ketosis

Diagnostic criteria[8,17]

	DKA			HHS
	Mild	Moderate	Severe	
Plasma glucose (mg/dL)	>250			>600
Arterial blood pH	7.25–7.30	7.00–7.24	<7.00	>7.30
Serum bicarbonate (mEq/L)	15–18	10 to <15	<10	>15
Presence of urine ketones	+	+	+	Small
Serum ketones	+	+	+	Small
Calculated serum osmolarity (mOsm/kg)	Variable			>320
Anion gap	>10	>12		Variable
Mental status	Alert	Alert/drowsy	Stupor/coma	

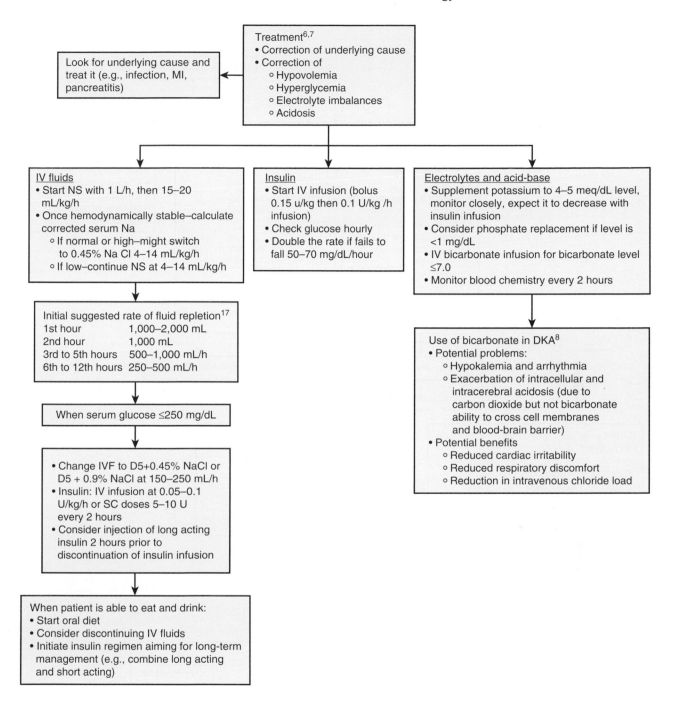

Potential Complications of Hyperglycemic Emergencies

- Cerebral edema (rare)
- Pulmonary edema, hypoxemia
- Complications of treatment

- Hypoglycemia due to overly aggressive correction
- Hypokalemia
- Hypervolemia
- Hyperchloremia due to excessive IV NaCl

Hypoglycemia

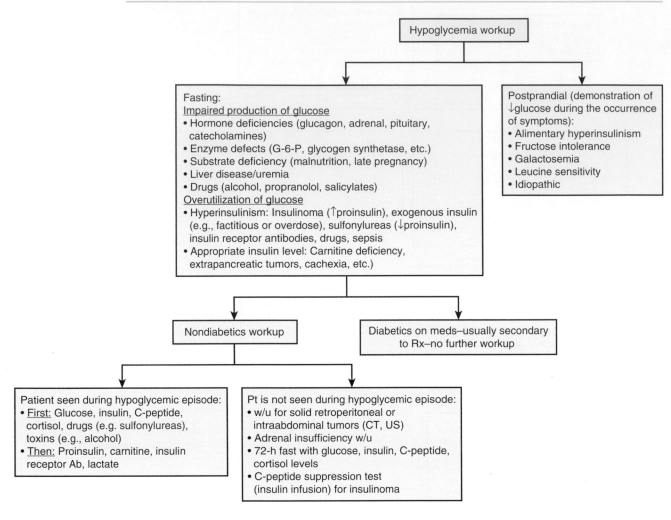

Hypoglycemia workup

Fasting:
Impaired production of glucose
• Hormone deficiencies (glucagon, adrenal, pituitary, catecholamines)
• Enzyme defects (G-6-P, glycogen synthetase, etc.)
• Substrate deficiency (malnutrition, late pregnancy)
• Liver disease/uremia
• Drugs (alcohol, propranolol, salicylates)
Overutilization of glucose
• Hyperinsulinism: Insulinoma (↑proinsulin), exogenous insulin (e.g., factitious or overdose), sulfonylureas (↓proinsulin), insulin receptor antibodies, drugs, sepsis
• Appropriate insulin level: Carnitine deficiency, extrapancreatic tumors, cachexia, etc.)

Postprandial (demonstration of ↓glucose during the occurrence of symptoms):
• Alimentary hyperinsulinism
• Fructose intolerance
• Galactosemia
• Leucine sensitivity
• Idiopathic

Nondiabetics workup

Diabetics on meds–usually secondary to Rx–no further workup

Patient seen during hypoglycemic episode:
• First: Glucose, insulin, C-peptide, cortisol, drugs (e.g. sulfonylureas), toxins (e.g., alcohol)
• Then: Proinsulin, carnitine, insulin receptor Ab, lactate

Pt is not seen during hypoglycemic episode:
• w/u for solid retroperitoneal or intraabdominal tumors (CT, US)
• Adrenal insufficiency w/u
• 72-h fast with glucose, insulin, C-peptide, cortisol levels
• C-peptide suppression test (insulin infusion) for insulinoma

Hypoglycemia in Diabetes[9]

Pathophysiology of hypoglycemia in diabetes.

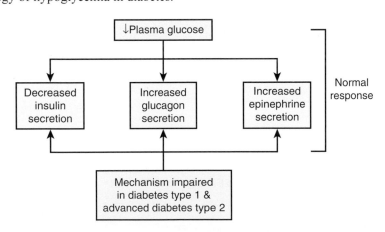

↓Plasma glucose

Decreased insulin secretion

Increased glucagon secretion

Increased epinephrine secretion

Normal response

Mechanism impaired in diabetes type 1 & advanced diabetes type 2

Signs of Hypoglycemia

- Diaphoresis
- Tachycardia, hypertension (HTN)
- Often hypothermia
- Neuroglycopenic symptoms
- Transient focal neurological deficits (e.g., diplopia, hemiparesis)

Treatment

- Ingestion of glucose tablets or carbohydrate in the form of juice, a soft drink, etc.
- Parenteral therapy (when a hypoglycemic patient is unable or unwilling to take carbohydrate orally
- Parenteral glucagon for hypoglycemia in type 1 diabetes (less useful in type 2 diabetes because it stimulates insulin secretion as well as glycogenolysis)
- Intravenous glucose is the preferable treatment of severe hypoglycemia

Adrenal Insufficiency

In the context of critical illness, adrenal insufficiency is defined by inadequate response to synthetic corticotropin stimulation (relative adrenal insufficiency [RAI]) rather than absolute adrenal insufficiency. RAI is associated with increased mortality, specifically in patients with septic shock.[10] However, treatment with hydrocortisone did not seem to improve survival or reversal of shock in those patients.[11]

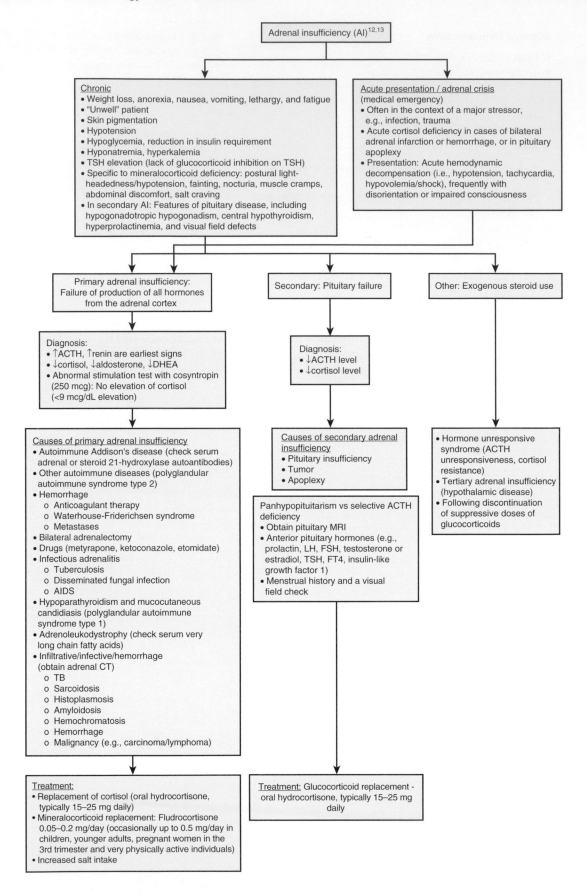

Management of Adrenal Crisis

- Immediate intramuscular or intravenous hydrocortisone 100 mg
- A liter of 0.9% saline IV over 30 minutes
- Continue hydrocortisone as IM injections 50 mg QID or 100 mg TID; or via IV infusion 200 mg/24 h until the patient is hemodynamically stable

- IV fluids as needed per volume status and Na level
- Oral hydrocortisone can be restarted within 12 hours of the admission
- May discharge on a double dose of medication for 48 hours after the precipitating illness is treated and any electrolytes are corrected

Additional Considerations in Patients with Adrenal Insufficiency and Critical Illness

- Usually advised to double or triple glucocorticoids dose for febrile illness
- Usually given at least 200 mg hydrocortisone parenterally on the day of major surgery

- Consider hydrocortisone therapy in patients with septic shock (e.g., if poor response to IV fluid resuscitation and vasopressors, regardless of a random total cortisol level or the response to adrenocorticotropic hormone [ACTH]),[14] although no strong evidence to support it (no short-term mortality benefit)[15]
- Overall, the role of glucocorticoids in recovery from critical illness is not well understood

Summary of Diagnostic Tests for Disorders Associated with Adrenal Insufficiency.

	C-21 pathway products: Cortisol	Pituitary hormones: ACTH, LH, FSH	17 KS pathway products: androgens, DHEA, 17-KS (urine)	Stimulation test with 0.25 mg cosyntropin/ ACTH
Primary adrenal insufficiency	↓	↑ACTH		cortisol rises <10
Secondary adrenal insufficiency	↓	↓ACTH		cortisol rises >10
11 or 21-hydroxylase deficiency	↓	↑ACTH ↑LH/FSH ratio (>2.5–3)	↑	

ACTH, Adrenocorticotropic hormone; *DHEA,* dehydroepiandrosterone; *FSH,* follicle-stimulating hormone; *LH,* luteinizing hormone.

Hyperadrenalism

Although hyperadrenalism probably does not play as important role in critical care as adrenal insufficiency, there are important issues associated with it: insulin resistance, slow wound healing, and predisposition to infections.[16]

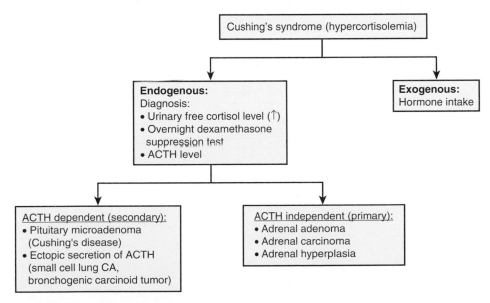

Summary of Diagnostic Tests for Disorders Associated with Hyperadrenalism.

	C-21 pathway products: Cortisol	Pituitary hormones: ACTH, LH, FSH	17 KS pathway products: androgens, DHEA, 17-KS (urine)	Overnight dexamethasone suppression test (DST) (1 mg × 1) or low dose 48 hours DST (0.5 mg Q6 × 8)	High dose 48 hours DST (2 mg Q6 × 8) DST
Normal	Normal or ↑	Normal	Normal	suppressed cortisol level (cortisol level <5)	suppressed
Cushing's disease (pituitary adenoma/carcinoma)	↑	↑ACTH	↑	not suppressed	suppressed
Primary Cushing's syndrome (adrenal adenoma/carcinoma)	↑	↓ACTH	↓ – adenoma ↑ – carcinoma	not suppressed	not suppressed
Ectopic ACTH production (e.g., small cell carcinoma of the lung)	↑	↑		not suppressed	not suppressed
Pituitary carcinoma	↑	↑		not suppressed	not suppressed

ACTH, Adrenocorticotropic hormone; *DHEA,* dehydroepiandrosterone; *FSH,* follicle-stimulating hormone; *LH,* luteinizing hormone.

Mineralocorticoids

Mineralocorticoid regulation (renin-angiotensin-aldosterone system).

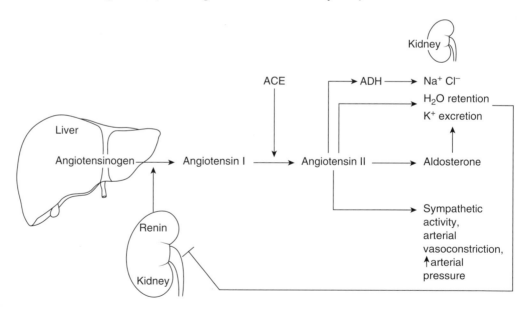

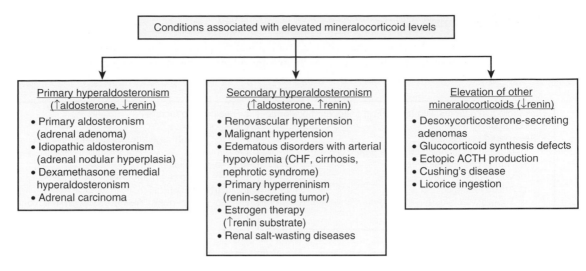

The typical presentation of hyperaldosteronism is a combination of hypertension and hypokalemia. Poorly controlled hypertension in combination with hypokalemia should raise a suspicion of hyperaldosteronism.

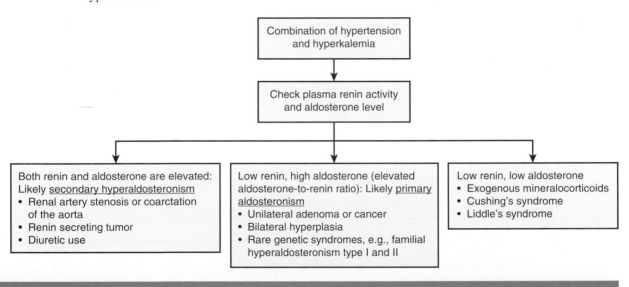

Diagnostic Tests for Disorders Associated with Abnormal Mineralocorticoids.

	Aldosterone	Renin	aldosterone/ renin ratio	Aldosterone suppression: fluid loading test with normal saline	Cortisol stimulation test with 0.25 mg cosyntropin/ACTH	Renin-aldosterone stimulation with furosemide and 3 hours of upright posture (check plasma renin activity and aldosterone concentration)
Primary hyperaldosteronism	↑	↓	↑	aldosterone level does not ↓	N/A	N/A
Secondary hyperaldosteronism	↑	↑	Not elevated	↓ aldosterone level after fluid loading	N/A	N/A
Primary hypoaldosteronism	↓	↑	N/A	N/A	cortisol rises <10	↑ renin, ↓ aldosterone
Secondary hypoaldosteronism	↓	↓	N/A	N/A	cortisol rises >10 (means adrenals work fine)	↓ renin, ↓ aldosterone

Pheochromocytoma Crisis

Pheochromocytoma crisis is a complicating event in the course of pheochromocytoma. It can be prevented if the diagnosis is known and addressed; however, sometimes this hypertensive crisis is the initial manifestation of the disease.[8]

Risk factors in patients with underlying pheochromocytoma:
- Spontaneous
- Associated conditions:
  o Multiple endocrine neoplasia type 2
  o Neurofibromatosis type 1
  o Von Hippel-Lindau syndrome
  o Ataxia telangiectasia
  o Tuberose sclerosis
  o Sturge-Weber syndrome

Precipitating factors
- Spontaneous
  o Hemorrhage into pheochromocytoma
- Other
  o Exercise
  o Pressure on abdomen
  o Urination
  o Drugs: guanethidine, glucagon, naloxone, metoclopramide, ACTH, cytotoxics, tricyclic antidepressants

↓

Action of unopposed high circulating levels of catecholamines acting at adrenoreceptors:
- Alpha-receptors cause a pressor response with increases in blood pressure
- Beta-receptor activation has positive inotropic and chronotropic effects

↓

Presentation
Cardio-vascular: Hypertension, palpitations, myocardial infarction
Autonomic: Sweating, pallor, hyperhidrosis, nausea and vomiting
Psych/neuro: Anxiety and tremulousness, feeling of impending death, altered consciousness (hypertensive encephalopathy), pounding headache, stroke
Abdominal: Pain (tumor hemorrhage), paralytic ileus
Endocrine: Hyperglycemia

↓

Diagnosis
- Urine (acidified bottles) for estimation of 24-hour free catecholamines and metanephrines
- Plasma metanephrines and catecholamines

↓

Treatment
- Do not wait for biochemical confirmation – start treatment
- Monitor in the ICU
- Use noncompetitive alpha-1/alpha-2 antagonist phenoxybenzamine, 10 mg orally three times a day, increasing to a maximum dose of 240 mg/24 h
- Alpha-blockade should precede beta-blockade for 48 hours to avoid exacerbating a crisis through the unopposed action of catecholamines at alpha-receptors
- Longer acting competitive alpha-antagonists (e.g., doxazosin, calcium channel antagonists) not recommended for crisis treatment
- The use of labetalol is not recommended due to relatively greater beta-blocking action compared alpha-blocking action

Thyroid Disease

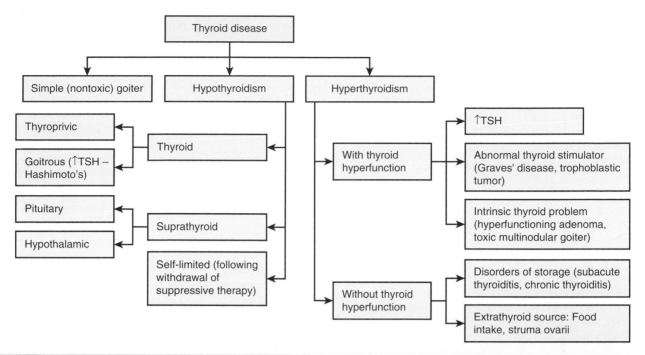

Differential Diagnosis of Thyroid Syndromes

	T_4	T_3RU	T_3	TSH	Free T_4	Antibodies to TSH receptor	ESR	I-131 uptake	Thyroid globulin
Grave's	↑	↑	↑	0	↑	+	N	↑	N
Pregnancy	↑	↓	↑	N	N	–	–	N	N
Exogenous T_4	↑	↑	N – ↓	↓	↑	–	–	↓	↓
Subacute thyroiditis (hyperthyroid)	↑	↑	↑	↓	↑	–	↑	↓	↑
Subacute thyroiditis (hypothyroid)	N – ↓	↓	N – ↓	N – ↑	N – ↓	–	N – ↑	↓	↓
Euthyroid sick syndrome	↑ – ↓	↑	↓	N – ↑	N	–	–	–	N
Iodine deficiency	↓	↓	↓	↑	↓	–	N	↑	

ESR, Erythrocyte sedimentation rate; T_3, triiodothyronine; T_3RU, T_3 resin uptake; T_4, thyroxine; *TSH,* thyroid stimulation hormone.

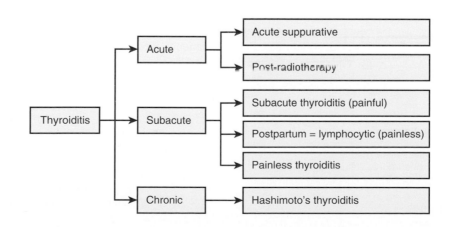

Thyroid Storm

Thyroid storm represents a medical emergency. It is a life-threatening condition that is associated with untreated or undertreated hyperthyroidism and requires prompt recognition and treatment.[8]

Precipitating Factors (in a Patient with Existing Thyrotoxicosis)

- General:
  - Infection
  - Nonthyroidal trauma or surgery
  - Psychosis
  - Parturition
  - Myocardial infarction or other acute medical problems
- Thyroid specific:
  - High doses of iodine-containing compounds (e.g., radiographic contrast media)
  - Discontinuation of antithyroid drug treatment
  - Thyroid injury (palpation, infarction of an adenoma)
  - New institution of amiodarone therapy

Presentation

- Severe fever (>38.5°C)
- GI symptoms (vomiting, diarrhea, occasional jaundice)
- Cardiac: tachycardia, congestive heart failure (particularly in the elderly, and most patients have systolic hypertension)
- Neurological: agitation, confusion, delirium, coma
- Biochemical: hyperglycemia, leukocytosis, mild hypercalcemia, abnormal liver function tests
- Circulating thyroid hormone levels are generally no higher than in patients with uncomplicated thyrotoxicosis, T_3 might be normal (due to impaired deiodination of thyroxine)

Treatment[8,17]

- Rapid inhibition of thyroid hormone synthesis and release
  - IV methimazole 20 mg 4–6 hourly or propylthiouracil 200 mg 4 hourly orally or via nasogastric tube
  - One hour after starting propylthiouracil, iodide (Lugol's iodine 0.3 mL diluted to 50 mL water 8 hourly) or lithium carbonate (to inhibit thyroid hormone release)
  - Alternatively: radiographic contrast media, sodium ipodate or iopanoic acid, loading dose of 2 g followed by 1 g daily
  - Carbimazole
  - Cholestyramine, 4 g every 6–8 hours (binds thyroid hormone in the gut and thus interrupts its modest enterohepatic circulation)
- Inhibition of the peripheral effects of thyroid hormone excess
- High doses of beta-blocker should be given (propranolol 80 mg 8 hourly orally or via nasogastric tube); alternative, calcium channel blocker or digoxin)
- Dexamethasone 4 mg intravenous 6 hourly
- Treatment of underlying causes and supportive care

Myxedema Coma

Myxedema coma, the extreme manifestation of hypothyroidism, is uncommon; however, when it occurs, it represents a potentially lethal condition in patients with hypothyroidism. It usually happens in previously untreated elderly patients, those with inadequate or discontinued treatment (the mean age of patients is around 75 years).[8,18]

Precipitating Factors

- Hypothermia, hypoglycemia
- Infections: pneumonia, influenza, UTI, sepsis
- Myocardial infarction or congestive heart failure
- Stroke
- CO_2 retention
- Surgery
- Respiratory depression due to drugs (for example, anesthetics, sedatives, tranquilizers)
- Other medication: amiodarone, rifampin, phenytoin
- Withdrawal of levothyroxine
- Trauma, burns, or gastrointestinal blood loss

Presentation

- Neurological: altered mental state (poor cognitive function, psychosis, coma)
- Hypothermia (as low as 23°C) or absence of fever with severe infection (prognosis worsens as the core temperature falls)
- Physical signs of hypothyroidism
- Respiratory depression
- Cardiac: hypertrophy, bradycardia, decreased ventricular contractility, hypotension, and ECG changes (low voltage, nonspecific ST-wave changes and sometimes torsades de pointes with a long QT interval)
- GI: anorexia, abdominal pain and distention, and constipation
- Biochemical abnormalities include hyponatremia, normal or increased urine sodium excretion, elevated CPK and LDH, hypoglycemia, normocytic or macrocytic anemia. TSH values may only be modestly raised (and will be normal or low in secondary hypothyroidism) but free thyroxine levels are usually very low

CPK, creatine phosphokinase; *LDH,* lactate dehydrogenase; *TSH,* thyroid stimulating hormone

Treatment

- Rapid institution of thyroid hormone replacement:
  - "High-dose" regimen options:
    - Intravenous thyroxine bolus of 300–500 mg, followed by 50–100 mg daily
    - Oral thyroxine in similar doses (usually by nasogastric tube), but absorption may be impaired
    - Tri-iodothyronine (10–20 mg initially, followed by 10 mg every 4 hours for 24 hours, then 10 mg every 6 hours) instead of thyroxine, but has the potential to cause adverse cardiac effects when given too rapidly
    - Oral treatment with similar doses is also possible
    - Give 200 mg thyroxine with 10 mg tri-iodothyronine initially, and then tri-iodothyronine 10 mg every 12 hours and thyroxine 100 mg every 24 hours, until the patient resumes normal thyroxine orally
  - "Low dose" approach
  - 25 mg of thyroxine daily for a week, or 5 mg of tri-iodothyronine twice daily with a gradually increasing dose
- Treatment of the precipitating cause
- Provision of ventilatory and other support

Hyperparathyroidism

Hyperparathyroidism Mechanisms.	
Type of Hyperparathyroidism	Mechanism
Primary	Primary elevated parathyroid hormone (PTH) production
Secondary	Elevated PTH secondary to other factors (low Ca++ levels, vitamin D deficiency, renal failure) causing ↑PTH
Tertiary	After long-standing secondary hyperparathyroidism with elevated Ca++ (due to prolonged overstimulation of PT gland – sometimes develop adenoma)
Pseudohyperparathyroidism	Elevated PTH with resistance in end-organs

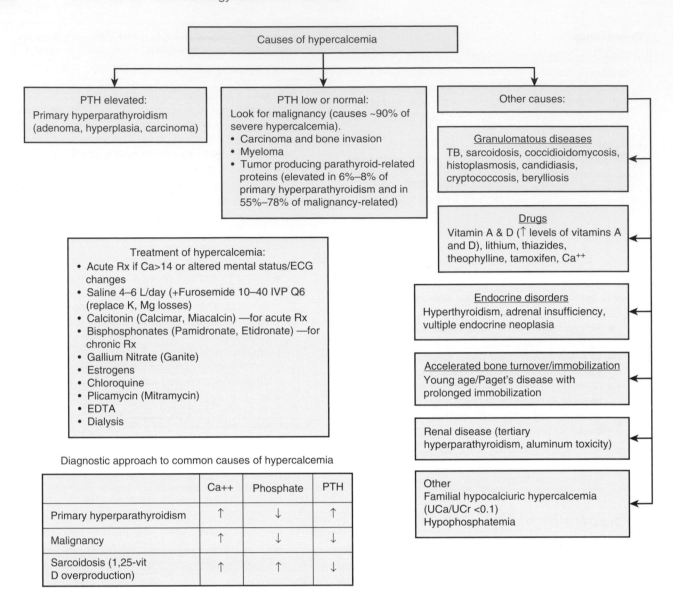

Diagnostic approach to common causes of hypercalcemia

	Ca++	Phosphate	PTH
Primary hyperparathyroidism	↑	↓	↑
Malignancy	↑	↓	↓
Sarcoidosis (1,25-vit D overproduction)	↑	↑	↓

Acute Hypercalcemia

Presentation

- Polyuria, polydipsia, dehydration
- Bone pain
- Confusion, anorexia
- Constipation

Work Up

- PTH
  - Elevated PTH—primary hyperparathyroidism
  - Normal or low PTH—malignancy or other cause
- Serum total protein with electrophoresis of immunoglobulins (for myeloma)
- Other: albumin, phosphate, magnesium, ESR, CBC, ECG, and CXR

PTH, parathyroid hormone; *ESR,* erythrocyte sedimentation rate; *CBC,* complete blood count

Treatment

- Rehydration: 0.9% NaCl 4–6 L/d
- Bisphosphonates IV: zoledronic acid 4mg over 15 mins or pamidronate 30–90mg at 20mg/h
- Second line treatments: calcitonin 4 U/kg, glucocorticoids, calcimimetics, parathyroidectomy

REFERENCES

1. Bellomo R. Preface modern critical care endocrinology and its impact on critical care medicine. *Crit Care Clin.* 2019;35:xiii–xvi.
2. Skugor M. Medical treatment of diabetes mellitus. *Cleve Clin J Med.* 2017;84(7 suppl 1):S57–S61.
3. Skugor M. *Diabetes Mellitus Treatment.* Cleveland Clinic Foundation; 2018.
4. American Diabetes Association. *Standards of Medical Care in Diabetes - 2019.* Diabetes Care; 2019. [Online] Available: https://care.diabetesjournals.org/content/diacare/suppl/2018/12/17/42.Supplement_1.DC1/DC_42_S1_2019_UPDATED.pdf.
5. Misra S, Oliver NS. Diabetic ketoacidosis in adults. *BMJ (Online).* 2015;351:h5660.
6. American Diabetes Association. Hyperglycemic crises in diabetes. *Diabetes Care.* 2004;27(suppl 1):s94–s102.
7. Chaithongdi N, Subauste JS, Koch CA, Geraci SA. Diagnosis and management of hyperglycemic emergencies. *Hormones (Basel).* 2011;10(4):250–260.
8. Savage MW, Mah PM, Weetman AP, Newell-Price J. Endocrine emergencies. *Postgrad Med J.* 2004;80(947):506–515.
9. Cryer PE, Davis SN, Shamoon H. Hypoglycemia in diabetes. *Diabetes Care.* 2003;26(6):1902–1912.
10. Meyer NJ, Hall JB. Relative adrenal insufficiency in the ICU: can we at least make the diagnosis? *Am J Respir Crit Care Med.* 2006;174(12):1282–1284.
11. Sprung CL, Annane D, Keh D, et al. Hydrocortisone therapy for patients with septic shock. *N Engl J Med.* 2008;358(2):111–124.
12. Neary N, Nieman L. Adrenal insufficiency: etiology, diagnosis and treatment. *Curr Opin Endocrinol Diabetes Obes.* 2010;17(3):217–223.
13. Pazderska A, Pearce SHS. Adrenal insufficiency - recognition and management. *Clin Med J R Coll Physicians London.* 2017;17(3):258–262.
14. Marik PE, Pastores SM, Annane D, et al. Recommendations for the diagnosis and management of corticosteroid insufficiency in critically ill adult patients: consensus statements from an international task force by the American College of Critical Care Medicine. *Crit Care Med.* 2008;36(6):1937–1949.
15. Venkatesh B, Finfer S, Cohen J, et al. Adjunctive glucocorticoid therapy in patients with septic shock. *N Engl J Med.* 2018;378(9):797–808.
16. Kem DC, Metcalf JP, Cornea A, Dunnam M, Engelbrecht A, Yu X. Is pseudo-Cushing's syndrome in a critically ill patient 'pseudo'? Hypothesis and supportive case report. *Endocr Pract.* 2007;13(2):153–158.
17. Kearney T, Dang C. Diabetic and endocrine emergencies. *Postgrad Med J.* 2007;83(976):79–86.
18. Wall CR. Myxedema coma: diagnosis and treatment. *Am Fam Physician.* 2000;62(11):2485–2490.

CHAPTER 11

Toxicology Highlights

Alexander Goldfarb-Rumyantzev

General Principles of Management of Poisoned Patients[1,2]

Initial management
- Thorough assessment (intoxication does not rule out other potential medical emergencies, e.g., stroke, acute MI)
- Stabilization (standard "ABC" approach, IV access)
- Supportive care (seizure control, correction of hypoglycemia, correction of hyperthermia)
- Resuscitation antidotes

Diagnosis: Examine patients (look for "toxydromes"), identify symptoms potentially associated with particular intoxications (e.g., hypertherima), ECG (e.g., QT and QRS interval prolongation), laboratory tests (e.g., urine and serum toxicology screen)

Look for toxydromes (toxicologic syndrome)

Syndrome	Clinical presentation
Sympathomimetic	Agitation, mydriasis, tachycardia, hypertension, hyperthermia, diaphoresis
Anticholinergic (similar to sympathomimetic effect except for diaphoresis vs. dry skin)	Altered mental status, sedation, hallucinations, mydriasis, dry skin, dry mucous membranes, decreased bowel sounds, and urinary retention
Cholinergic	Altered mental status, seizures, miosis, lacrimation, diaphoresis, bronchospasm, bronchorrhea, vomiting, diarrhea, bradycardia
Sedative-hypnotic (gamma-aminobutyric acid receptors)	Sedation, normal pupils, decreased respirations
Opioid	Sedation, miosis (except for meperidine), decreased bowel sounds, decreased respirations
Serotonin syndrome	Altered mental status, tachycardia, hypertension, hyperreflexia, clonus, hyperthermia

Toxic effect of several poisons (or drug overdose) and symptoms are easier to understand in the context of response to particular receptor stimulation, which is discussed below

Tissue	Receptor type	End organ response
Heart	β_1 M_2 β_3	Increased inotropism and chronotropism Decreased inotropism and chronotropism Decreased inotropism and chronotropism (cannot be downregulated by catecholamines)
Coronary and pulmonary arterioles, blood vessels to skeletal muscle	α β_2 (predominant) M_2	Constriction Dilatation Dilatation
Other arterioles	α β M_2	Constriction Dilatation Dilatation
Veins	α β_2	Constriction Dilatation
Bronchi	β_2 M_2	Relaxation Constriction
Gastrointestinal tract	α, β M_2	Decreased motility and secretion Increased motility and secretion
Bladder	α, β M_2	Retention Evacuation
Eye	α_1 β M_2	Mydriasis Relaxation of ciliary muscle Miosis, constriction of ciliary muscle

α, β - adrenergic receptors
M_2 - muscarinic acetylcholine receptors

Hyperthermic syndromes
- Sympathomimetic fever (amphetamines and cocaine) due excess serotonin and dopamine. Treatment: Supportive, cooling, ± benzodiazepines
- Uncoupling syndrome, when process of oxidative phosphorylation is disrupted (salicylate). Treatment: Hyperthermia with salicylate poisoning indicates severe intoxication, requires dialysis
- Serotonin syndrome (monoamine oxidase inhibitors + meperidine; serotonergic agents). Treatment: Serotonin antagonist cyproheptadine + benzodiazepines and other supportive treatments (e.g., active cooling)
- Neuroleptic malignant syndrome, due to relative deficiency of dopamine within the central nervous system (dopamine receptor antagonists; withdrawal of dopamine agonists, e.g., levodopa/carbidopa). Treatment: Bromocriptine, amantadine, and dantrolene
- Malignant hyperthermia (depolarizing neuromuscular blocking agents or volatile general anesthetics). Treatment: Removing the inciting agent, supportive care, dantrolene
- Anticholinergic poisonings: Impairment of normal cooling mechanisms such as sweating. Treatment: Cooling and benzodiazepines

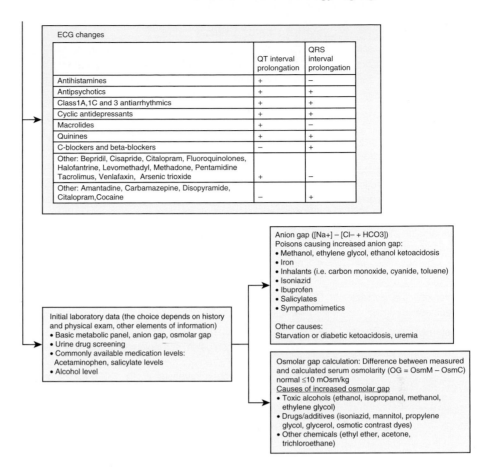

ECG changes		
	QT interval prolongation	QRS interval prolongation
Antihistamines	+	−
Antipsychotics	+	+
Class1A,1C and 3 antiarrhythmics	+	+
Cyclic antidepressants	+	+
Macrolides	+	−
Quinines	+	+
C-blockers and beta-blockers	−	+
Other: Bepridil, Cisapride, Citalopram, Fluoroquinolones, Halofantrine, Levomethadyl, Methadone, Pentamidine Tacrolimus, Venlafaxin, Arsenic trioxide	+	−
Other: Amantadine, Carbamazepine, Disopyramide, Citalopram,Cocaine	−	+

Initial laboratory data (the choice depends on history and physical exam, other elements of information)
• Basic metabolic panel, anion gap, osmolar gap
• Urine drug screening
• Commonly available medication levels: Acetaminophen, salicylate levels
• Alcohol level

Anion gap ([Na+] − [Cl− + HCO3])
Poisons causing increased anion gap:
• Methanol, ethylene glycol, ethanol ketoacidosis
• Iron
• Inhalants (i.e. carbon monoxide, cyanide, toluene)
• Isoniazid
• Ibuprofen
• Salicylates
• Sympathomimetics

Other causes:
Starvation or diabetic ketoacidosis, uremia

Osmolar gap calculation: Difference between measured and calculated serum osmolarity (OG = OsmM − OsmC) normal ≤10 mOsm/kg
Causes of increased osmolar gap
• Toxic alcohols (ethanol, isopropanol, methanol, ethylene glycol)
• Drugs/additives (isoniazid, mannitol, propylene glycol, glycerol, osmotic contrast dyes)
• Other chemicals (ethyl ether, acetone, trichloroethane)

Symptoms of Acute Poisoning and Withdrawal[3]

Symptoms of Toxicity and Withdrawal		
	Symptoms of Toxicity	Symptoms of Withdrawal
Alcohol and barbiturates (acetylcholine-like action)	• Lethargy, stupor • ↓BP, ↓pupils, ↓bowel sounds • Hypothermia • Nystagmus	Alcohol Hallucinosis Auditory hallucinations, no clouding of consciousness Delirium Tremens Tremor, nausea, vomiting, weakness, irritability, depression, anxiety, autonomous hyperreactivity (tachycardia, fever), hyperreflexia, hypoglycemia
Opioids (morphine, heroin, meperidine, codeine) (Acetylcholine-like action through dopamine and morphine receptors)	• Sleepiness, lethargy, or coma • Euphoria, dysphoria, or apathy • ↓BP, ↓↓pupils, ↓bowel sounds, ↓heart rate • Hyperventilation or apnea • With severe respiratory depression, hypoxemia, hypercarbia, respiratory acidosis, rhythm disturbances, pulmonary edema	• Insomnia, fatigue, anxiety, nausea • Fever, chills, sweating, yawning, diarrhea, lacrimation, rhinorrhea, piloerection • ↑BP, ↑pupils, ↑heart rate
Antimuscarinic (Atropine)	• Seizures • ↑pupils, ↑heart rate, ↓bowel sounds, hot, dry skin • ↑BP	

	Symptoms of Toxicity	Symptoms of Withdrawal
Tricyclic antidepressants Epinephrine-like action	• TCA – ↓BP, 3C's: **c**oma, **c**onvulsions, **c**ardiac problems • CNS excitability, confusion, blurred vision, dry mouth, fever, mydriasis, seizures, coma, arrhythmias, hypotension, tachycardia, respiratory depression; physical condition can rapidly change. • ECG findings of increased QRS interval >0.10 seconds, sinus tachycardia, conduction abnormalities	
Stimulants (amphetamines, cocaine, PCP) Epinephrine-like action Work through dopamine receptors	• Seizures, agitation, psychosis • ↑BP, ↑heart rate, ↑pupils • Hyperactivity of ANS: fever, warm sweaty skin, ↑muscle tone, arrhythmias • PCP—horizontal and vertical nystagmus	• Depressed mood • Disturbed sleep • Increased dreaming
Cannabis (marijuana) Psychotomimetic (LSD)	• Euphoria or apathy, hallucinations, psychosis, slowed time sensation, intensification of perception • ↑heart rate, ↑appetite, dry mouth • conjunctival injection	
Antianxiety (benzodiazepines)	Drowsiness, lethargy, dysarthria, ataxia, hypotension, hypothermia, coma, respiratory depression with severe overdoses	• Tremor • Restlessness
Acetaminophen (Tylenol)	• Nausea, vomiting, malaise, right upper quadrant abdominal pain, jaundice, confusion, somnolence; coma may develop later • Labs: After 24 hours, increased AST (>1,000 IU/L is characteristic), increased ALT, increased bilirubin, PT may increase	
Salicylates	• Nausea, vomiting, hyperpnea, tinnitus, fever, disorientation, lethargy, coma, seizures, diaphoresis, abdominal pain. • Laboratory tests: Respiratory alkalosis with progressive anion-gap metabolic acidosis, hyperglycemia/hypoglycemia, hypernatremia/hyponatremia, hypokalemia	
Calcium channel blockers	• Drowsiness, confusion, chest pain, hypotension, bradycardia, peripheral cyanosis, coma, seizures, respiratory distress. • ECG findings of first-, second- or third-degree heart block, metabolic acidosis, hyperglycemia, pulmonary edema	

ALT, Alanine aminotransferase; *ANS,* autonomic nervous system; *AST,* aspartate aminotransferase; *BP,* blood pressure; *CNS,* central nervous system; *PT,* prothrombin time; *TCA,* tricarboxylic acid cycle.

Principles of Treatment[1,4,3]

Treatment approach
- Decontamination
- Antidotes
- Enhancement of clearance

Decontamination
- Induce emesis (syrup of ipecac, intramuscularly administered apomorphine)
- Activated charcoal; although metals, ions and alcohols do not bind to charcoal (contraindicated in caustic ingestions). Dose of activate charcoal = 1 g/kg of body weight
- Gastric lavage with large bore orogastric tube (36–40 French) to eliminate pill fragments
- Whole bowel irrigation: laxative agent, e.g., polyethylene glycol to fully flush the bowel of stool (contraindicated in ileus, bowel obstruction or perforation, and in patients with hemodynamic instability)
- For corrosive substances ingestion (e.g., acids or bases) – rapid irrigation of the mucous membranes. Induced vomiting and the use of activated charcoal are contraindicated

Antidotes

Toxin	Antidote
Acetaminophen	N-acetylcysteine
Anticholinergics	Physostigmine
β-blocker	Glucagon
Benzodiazepine	Flumazenil
Ca^{++} channel blocker	Calcium and glucagon
Carbon monoxide	Oxygen
Crotalid envenomation	Crotalidae polyvalent immune Fab
Cyanide	Hydroxocobalamin, amyl nitrite, sodium nitrite, sodium thiosulfate
Digitalis	Digoxin-specific Ab fragment (digoxin immune Fab), avoid Ca^{++}, atropine for bradycardias
Ethylene glycol,	Fomepizole, ethanol (inhibition of alcohol dehydrogenase)
Iron	Deferoxamine mesylate
Isoniazid	Pyridoxine
Lead	Succimer, dimercaprol, calcium ethylenediamine tetra-acetic acid
Local anesthetics	Lipid emulsions
Methanol	Fomepizole (4-methylpyrazole), ethanol (inhibition of alcohol dehydrogenase)
Methemoglobinemia	Methylene blue
Monomethylhydrazine Mushrooms	Pyridoxime
Nitrites	Methylene blue
Opioids	Naloxone
Organophosphates/carbamates	Atropine, pralidoxime
Sulfonylurea	Glucose, octreotide
Tricyclic antidepressant	Sodium bicarbonate

Empiric treatment with naloxone (narcan), dextrose and thiamine should be considered in patients with altered mental status

Enhancement of clearance
- Urine alkalization for agents that are excreted as weak acids in the urine (IV sodium bicarbonate): Chlorpropamide, 2, 4-dichlorophenoxyacetic acid diflunisal, fluoride, methylchlorophenoxypropionic acid, methotrexate, phenobarbital and salicylates
- Dialysis for poisons that are amenable to filtration across dialysis membranes (low molecular weight, low volume of distribution, and low protein binding): Salicylates, lithium, methylxanthines, and the toxic alcohols
- Repeated administration of activated charcoal
- Hemoperfusion

Distribution volume of toxin = amount ingested / plasma concentration

Acetaminophen Toxicity[5,6]

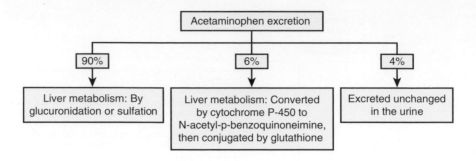

Toxic dose: 7.5 g in adults and 150 mg/kg in children

Treatment

- Gut decontamination: single dose of activated charcoal (50%–90% of binding of acetaminophen to activated charcoal during PO administration, 10%–50% binding of acetylcysteine to charcoal)

- Acetylcysteine administration
- Cytochrome P-450 inhibitors (cimetidine)—no advantage over acetylcysteine alone
- Hemoperfusion and high-flux hemodialysis—questionable advantage over acetylcysteine alone

Criteria for Listing for/Considering Liver Transplantation[6]

- Arterial pH <7.3 after adequate fluid resuscitation
- Arterial blood lactate concentration >3.5 mmol/L after early fluid resuscitation

- All three of the following are true within a 24-hour period:
  o Creatinine >3.4 mg/dL
  o PT >100 s (INR >6.5)
  o Grade III/IV encephalopathy

REFERENCES

1. Boyle JS, Bechtel LK, Holstege CP. Management of the critically poisoned patient. *Scand J Trauma Resusc Emerg Med.* 2009;17(1):29.
2. Daly FFS, Little M, Murray L. A risk assessment based approach to the management of acute poisoning. *Emerg Med J.* 2006;23(5):396–399.
3. Larsen LC, Cummings DM. Oral poisonings: guidelines for initial evaluation and treatment. *Am Fam Physician.* 1998;57(1):85–92.
4. Müller D, Desel H. Ursachen, diagnostik und therapie häufiger vergiftungen. *Dtsch Arztebl Int.* 2013;110(41): 690–700.
5. Zed PJ, Krenzelok EP. Treatment of acetaminophen overdose. *Am J Health Syst Pharm.* 1999;56(11):1081–1093.
6. Dargan PI, Jones AL. Acetaminophen poisoning: an update for the intensivist. *Crit Care.* 2002;6(2):108–110.

CHAPTER 12

Neurology Aspects of Critical Care

Alexander Goldfarb-Rumyantzev

Neurological Examination

Neurological examination
1. Mental status (time, place, person)
2. Cranial nerves
3. Sensory (light touch, pinprick, positional sense)
4. Motor
- Muscle tone (passive movements: Clasp-knife rigidity–upper motor neuron, cogwheel–basal ganglia)
- Involuntary movements
- Muscle strength
- Reflexes (DTR: ↑ in upper motor neuron, ↓ in lower motor neuron)
5. Cerebellar
- Coordination
- Stance
- Gait
- Romberg test
6. Pathological reflexes
- Babinski, clonus (upper motor neuron), snout, grasp, sucking, (palmar-mental)
- Meningeal (Kernig, Brudzinski, neck stiffness)

In comatose patients, also check brainstem reflexes:
- "Doll's eye" (oculocephalic)
- Ciliospinal (↑ of pupils in response to pain)
- Corneal, gag, cough, blink

Questions to answer during neuro history and exam

- Is there a nervous system damage?
- Localize (muscle, nerve, spinal cord, brain)

Localization of Spinal Segments Involved in a Specific Neurological Deficit

C5	Deltoid muscle, biceps tendon reflex	L3	Quadriceps muscle
C6	Biceps/thumb muscle, biceps tendon reflex	L4	Patella reflex
C7	Affects triceps muscle, triceps reflex, grip strength, sensation index/middle fingers	L5	Great toe dorsiflexion, sensation at web of great and first toes
C8	Intrinsic hand muscle	S1	Achilles reflex, gastrocnemius muscle and plantar flexors

Headache

Headache is probably one of the most common symptoms and can be caused by a variety of factors with a wide spectrum of seriousness, from relatively benign muscle tension headache to real emergencies, e.g., subarachnoid hemorrhage. The diagram below is designed to help understand the most frequent cases of headache and help to choose the next diagnostic step.[1]

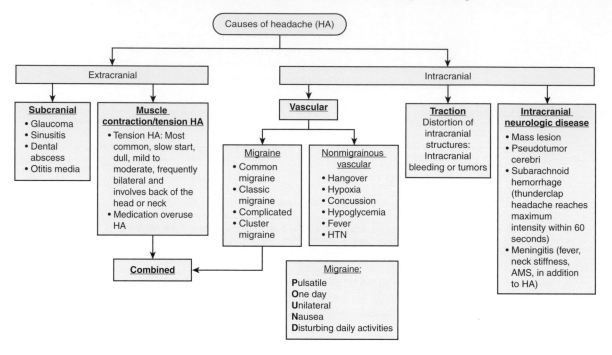

Tremor

Tremor is another frequent neurological symptom. Although a general understanding of the types of tremor is helpful, when chronic, it is usually not very pertinent to critical care practice.

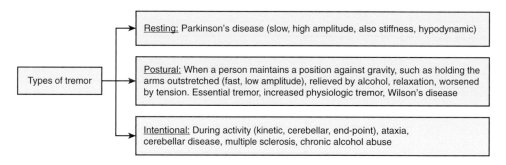

Dizziness

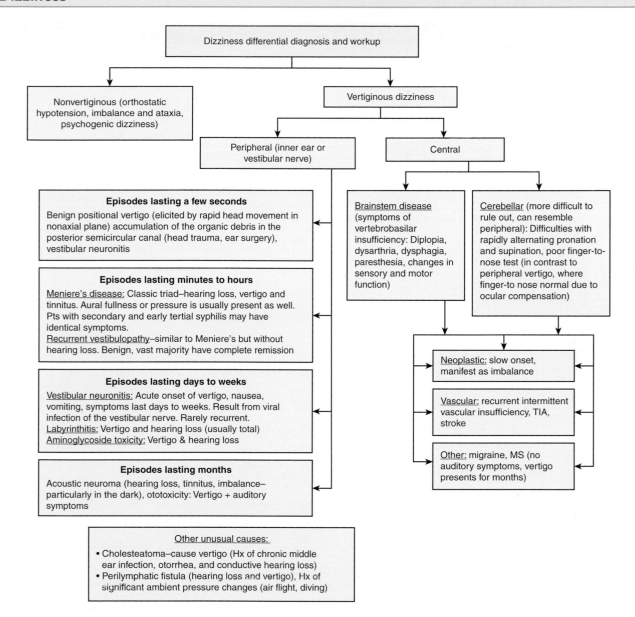

Other Unusual Causes

• Cholesteatoma – causes vertigo (Hx of chronic middle ear infection, otorrhea, and conductive hearing loss)

• Perilymphatic fistula (hearing loss and vertigo), Hx of significant ambient pressure changes (air flight, diving)

Aphasia

Type, Site, and Presentation of Aphasia		
Type	**Localization**	**Presentation**
Conductive	Dominant supramarginal gyrus	Deficit in repetition Normal fluency Normal comprehension
Sensory (Wernicke's)	Posterior and superior lobe	Deficit in repetition Normal fluency Deficit comprehension
Motor (Broca's)	Dominant frontal lobe	Deficit in repetition Deficit in fluency Normal comprehension
Transcortical (motor and sensory)		Normal repetition Deficit in fluency Deficit in comprehension

ICU Management of Ischemic Stroke

Intensive care management of stroke is focused on reducing the deficit caused by stroke, restoring circulation, minimizing complications of reperfusion (e.g., hemorrhagic transformation), and avoiding secondary brain injury, including brain edema and progressive stroke.[2]

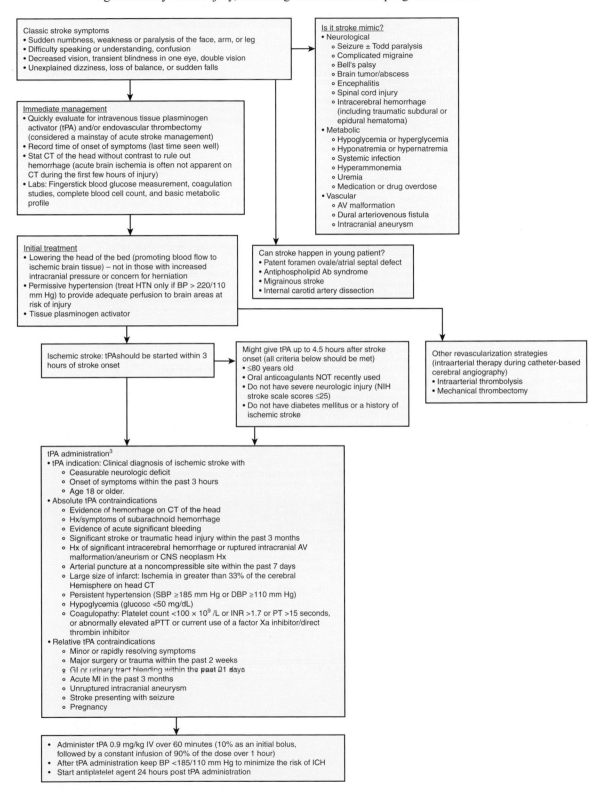

Classic stroke symptoms
- Sudden numbness, weakness or paralysis of the face, arm, or leg
- Difficulty speaking or understanding, confusion
- Decreased vision, transient blindness in one eye, double vision
- Unexplained dizziness, loss of balance, or sudden falls

Is it stroke mimic?
- Neurological
  - Seizure ± Todd paralysis
  - Complicated migraine
  - Bell's palsy
  - Brain tumor/abscess
  - Encephalitis
  - Spinal cord injury
  - Intracerebral hemorrhage (including traumatic subdural or epidural hematoma)
- Metabolic
  - Hypoglycemia or hyperglycemia
  - Hyponatremia or hypernatremia
  - Systemic infection
  - Hyperammonemia
  - Uremia
  - Medication or drug overdose
- Vascular
  - AV malformation
  - Dural arteriovenous fistula
  - Intracranial aneurysm

Immediate management
- Quickly evaluate for intravenous tissue plasminogen activator (tPA) and/or endovascular thrombectomy (considered a mainstay of acute stroke management)
- Record time of onset of symptoms (last time seen well)
- Stat CT of the head without contrast to rule out hemorrhage (acute brain ischemia is often not apparent on CT during the first few hours of injury)
- Labs: Fingerstick blood glucose measurement, coagulation studies, complete blood cell count, and basic metabolic profile

Initial treatment
- Lowering the head of the bed (promoting blood flow to ischemic brain tissue) – not in those with increased intracranial pressure or concern for herniation
- Permissive hypertension (treat HTN only if BP > 220/110 mm Hg) to provide adequate perfusion to brain areas at risk of injury
- Tissue plasminogen activator

Can stroke happen in young patient?
- Patent foramen ovale/atrial septal defect
- Antiphospholipid Ab syndrome
- Migrainous stroke
- Internal carotid artery dissection

Ischemic stroke: tPA should be started within 3 hours of stroke onset

Might give tPA up to 4.5 hours after stroke onset (all criteria below should be met)
- ≤80 years old
- Oral anticoagulants NOT recently used
- Do not have severe neurologic injury (NIH stroke scale scores ≤25)
- Do not have diabetes mellitus or a history of ischemic stroke

Other revascularization strategies (intraarterial therapy during catheter-based cerebral angiography)
- Intraarterial thrombolysis
- Mechanical thrombectomy

tPA administration[3]
- tPA indication: Clinical diagnosis of ischemic stroke with
  - Ceasurable neurologic deficit
  - Onset of symptoms within the past 3 hours
  - Age 18 or older.
- Absolute tPA contraindications
  - Evidence of hemorrhage on CT of the head
  - Hx/symptoms of subarachnoid hemorrhage
  - Evidence of acute significant bleeding
  - Significant stroke or traumatic head injury within the past 3 months
  - Hx of significant intracerebral hemorrhage or ruptured intracranial AV malformation/aneurism or CNS neoplasm Hx
  - Arterial puncture at a noncompressible site within the past 7 days
  - Large size of infarct: Ischemia in greater than 33% of the cerebral Hemisphere on head CT
  - Persistent hypertension (SBP ≥185 mm Hg or DBP ≥110 mm Hg)
  - Hypoglycemia (glucose <50 mg/dL)
  - Coagulopathy: Platelet count <100 × 10⁹/L or INR >1.7 or PT >15 seconds, or abnormally elevated aPTT or current use of a factor Xa inhibitor/direct thrombin inhibitor
- Relative tPA contraindications
  - Minor or rapidly resolving symptoms
  - Major surgery or trauma within the past 2 weeks
  - GI or urinary tract bleeding within the past 21 days
  - Acute MI in the past 3 months
  - Unruptured intracranial aneurysm
  - Stroke presenting with seizure
  - Pregnancy

- Administer tPA 0.9 mg/kg IV over 60 minutes (10% as an initial bolus, followed by a constant infusion of 90% of the dose over 1 hour)
- After tPA administration keep BP <185/110 mm Hg to minimize the risk of ICH
- Start antiplatelet agent 24 hours post tPA administration

Other acute treatments of stroke patient

Respiratory complications
- Indications for endotracheal intubation (similar to other patient populations):
  o Respiratory failure (hypoxemic or hypercarbic)
  o Failure to protect the airway
    ▪ Reduced level of consciousness (Glasgow coma scale (GCS) <8)
    ▪ Impaired oropharyngeal function due to the stroke injury itself
      (common with cerebellar, brainstem, and large hemispheric strokes)
- Management of aspiration
  o Nothing by mouth until a swallow screening can be performed
  o Head of bed elevated 15–30 degrees
  o Antibiotics for aspiration pneumonia
Extubation vs tracheostomy placement
- Limiting factor in extubation is oropharyngeal control and the timing and pace of
  neurological recovery
- Predictors of successful extubation
  o GCS ≥8 (in large hemispheric middle cerebral artery stroke)
  o GCS >6 at the time of intubation + mechanical ventilation time of less than 7
    days (in posterior fossa stroke)
  o Ability to follow four separate commands
- Tracheostomy indications
  o Extubation failure
  o Low chance to recover oropharyngeal function for a prolonged period of time

Hemodynamic issues
- HTN is common in the acute phase
- Low BP as well as high BP in the acute phase are associated with negative
  outcome, avoid extremes, allow for autoregulation in the initial 24 hours after the stroke.
- Target SBP <220 mm Hg, but a lower goal (<180 mm Hg) is appropriate (especially if signs of
  cardiac strain or comorbid conditions, i.e., acute myocardial infarction, heart failure or aortic
  dissection)
- Induced hypertension may be appropriate in some cases
- Maintain SBP <180/105 mm Hg post tPA or endovascular thrombectomy to minimize the risk of
  hemorrhagic conversion

Treat/prevent cerebral edema
- Hyperosmolar therapy[4]
  o Maintain eunatremia (135–145 mmol/L); evidence for clinical efficacy of
    hypernatremia is lacking
  o Intermittent administration of hyperosmolar agents:
    ▪ Mannitol 25% (osmolarity 1,098): At a dose of 1g/kg body weight every
      6 hours; monitor anion gap, if >10 – hold the dose
    ▪ Mannitol 25% (osmolarity 1,375)
    ▪ 3% sodium chloride (osmolarity 1,026)
    ▪ 23.4% sodium chloride (osmolarity 8,008) bolus of 30 mL every 6
      hours
  o If severe, refractory edema, mannitol and hypertonic saline can be given in an
    alternating regimen
  o Taper treatment by spacing doses of hyperosmolar agents to every 8 or 12 hours
    before tapering off
- Decompressive craniectomy
  o Hemicraniectomy within 24–48 hours of presentation in patients up to age 60
    with large (>2/3 of MCA territory) hemispheric infarction and a decreased level
    of consciousness
  o For patients between the ages of 60–80, hemicraniectomy remains a life-saving
    procedure, only to be done if the patient's goals of care include likelihood of
    living with severe disability
  o Consider suboccipital craniectomy for any large cerebellar infarct: Cerebellar
    stroke in patients with development of
    ▪ New cranial nerve findings
    ▪ Reduced level of consciousness
    ▪ Evidence of brainstem compression
    ▪ Hydrocephalus
    ▪ And/or with lesions >3cm in diameter

Management of hemorrhagic transformation[2]
- Predictors: Large infarct size is a risk factor, high level of matrix metalloproteinase 9 (especially after tPA)
- Reverse coagulopathy
  - Hemorrhage in the first 24 hours after tPA–administer either cryoprecipitate or concentrated fibrinogen (use fibrinogen levels to guide therapy, if <100 mg/dL, give 0.15 units/kg of cryoprecipitate, repeat an hour later if bleeding persists
  - Bleeding in the setting of elevated INR from warfarin–resh frozen plasma or prothrombin complex concentrate (PCC)
  - Newer oral anticoagulants
    - Coagulopathy due to dabigatran–specific reversal agent idarucizumab.
    - Reverse factor Xa inhibitors using 4-factor prothrombin complex concentrate[5]
    - In all cases of severe bleeding–non specific strategies (early administration of activated charcoal, hemodialysis (for dabigatran), or use of an anti-fibrinolytic agent (e.g., tranexamic acid or aminocaproic acid)
- Control blood pressure
  - To maintain adequate perfusion pressure immediately following ischemic stroke, maintain SBP <180 mmHg following hemorrhagic transformation, unless large or expanding hematoma, then risk balance may favor a lower BP target
  - Intensive (SBP <140 mm Hg) BP control after ICH is achievable and safe, associated with less hematoma growth
- Surgical clot evacuation
  - Not routinely recommended
  - May be isolated cases where the volume of hematoma and resulting mass effect is significant

Prevention of early recurrence/progression
- Antiplatelet therapy: ASA; combined aspirin and clopidogrel if already on ASA or in substantial intracranial arterial atherosclerosis
- An antiplatelet agent should be started quickly in patients who do not receive tPA
- Indications for potential acute anticoagulation
  - Embolization from carotid disease (artery-to-artery) or from cardiogenic source
  - Patients who have or at high risk of ongoing embolization
  - Anticoagulation as a bridge to carotid endarterectomy in patients where the stroke volume is low
- Delayed endovascular therapy: Angioplasty
  - Intracranial stenting showed no benefit over medical therapy
  - Theoretical benefit in those with intracranial stenosis and recurrent stroke or blood pressure dependence
  - Clot retrieval is sometimes considered up to 24 hours after onset for basilar disease
  - Delayed angioplasty considered in those with vertebrobasilar stenosis with recurrent infarct or fluctuating symptoms

Other issues
- Hyperthermia post ischemic stroke is associated with increased mortality
  - Identify potential infectious sources of fever
  - Maintain normothermia with antipyretic medications and mechanical cooling if necessary
- Hyperglycemia is correlated with poor outcome
  - Target of <180 mm Hg is suggested

Predictors of Ischemic Cerebral Edema

- Young age
- NIH Stroke Scale/Score (NIHSS) ≥20 for dominant hemisphere or ≥15 for non–dominant hemisphere lesions
- Nausea/vomiting within 24 hours
- Systolic BP >180 mm Hg within 12 hours
- Early decrease in level of alertness
- Head CT within 6 hours with hypodensity in >50% of the middle cerebral artery (MCA) territory
- Involvement of multiple vascular territories
- Presence of a diffusion weighted imaging (DWI) lesion of >82 cm^3 within 6 hours of symptom onset alongside known vessel occlusion

Overview of the Role of Anticoagulation in Stroke and Carotid Stenosis

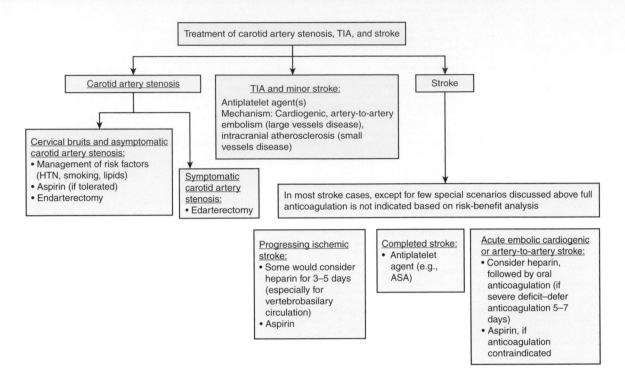

Acute Hemorrhagic Stroke/Intracerebral Hemorrhage[3,6]

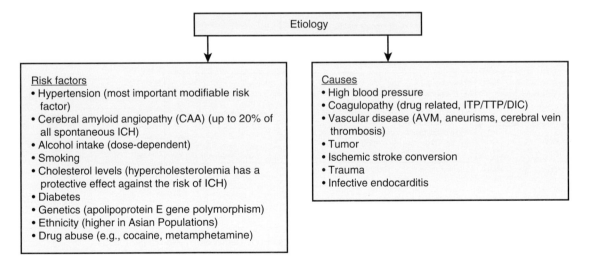

Diagnosis and Evaluation

- Labs: complete blood count, electrolytes and creatinine, glucose and coagulation
- Noncontrast CT: to diagnose acute intracerebral hemorrhage (ICH)

- CT Angiography (CTA) to identify vascular abnormalities as causes of ICH
- MRI sensitivity for ICH is equivalent to noncontrast CT; use MRI to detect underlying causes of ICH (e.g., neoplastic lesions or hemorrhagic transformation of ischemic stroke)
- Magnetic resonance angiography (MRA) in patients with kidney disease when contrast study is contraindicated

Treatment
- Airway protection and cardiovascular support
- BP control: systolic blood pressure goal less than 140 mm Hg within the first hour (no permissive hypertension)
- Treat coagulopathy
  - Reverse warfarin with FFP, vitamin K
  - Reverse dabigatran with idarucizumab
  - For other TSOA: FFP, prothrombin complex concentrate, consider hemodialysis
  - Platelet transfusion in patients with thrombocytopenia (suggested thresholds for transfusion between 50,000/mcL and 100,000/mcL)
  - To reverse IV heparin or LMW heparin -protamine sulfate 1 mg per 100 units of heparin (max rate: 5 mg/min), max dose 50 mg and the infusion must be slow
  - Post-tPA bleed: immediate discontinuation of rtPA and administration of cryoprecipitate 10 U, followed by further administration until normalization of fibrinogen level; alternative option: antifibrinolytic aminocaproic acid 5 g IV bolus over 15–30 minutes
- Watch for elevated intracranial pressure (acute decline in mental status)

Reversal strategy for warfarin-associated ICH
- Stop warfarin
- Obtain INR and CBC
- Infuse 10 mg of Vitamin K IV over 10 minutes
- Administer 4-factor prothrombin complex concentrates (PCC) as below:
  - 20 IU/kg if INR<2.0
  - 30 IU/kg if INR 2.0–3.0
  - 50 IU/kg if INR>3.0
- Alternatively, administer FFP 10–20 mL/kg
- Repeat INR after treatment

Manage complications
- Intracranial pressure
  - ICP monitoring in patients with coma, significant intraventricular hemorrhage (IVH) with hydrocephalus and evidence of transtentorial herniation (cerebral perfusion pressure target of 50 to 70 mm Hg)
  - Elevation of the head to 30 degrees, sedation, avoidance of hyponatremia
  - Hyperosmolar therapy (mannitol or hypertonic saline) in patients at risk of transtentorial herniation
- Seizure
  - Prophylactic administration of antiepileptic therapy is not recommended
  - Treat if clinical or EEG evidence of seizures
  - Continuous EEG monitoring if impaired mental status disproportionate to the degree of brain damage
- Blood glucose management
- Maintain normal body temperature
- Surgical options
  - IVH management: external ventricular drain (EVD) placement ± thrombolytic drugs for patients with hydrocephalus, coma, and significant IVH
  - Surgical hematoma evacuation is controversial except is indicated in cerebellar hematomas with signs of hydrocephalus and/or brainstem compression
  - Decompressive craniotomy with or without hematoma evacuation in those with coma, large hematoma with significant midline shift, or elevated ICP not medically controlled
  - Vinimally invasive surgery: endoscopic treatment of IVH, parenchymal hematoma evacuation with or without tPA

Subarachnoid Hemorrhage[3]

Presentation
- Blood collects mainly in the cerebral spinal fluid-containing spaces → hydrocephalus from impaired drainage of cerebro-spinal fluid
- "Worse headache of my life"
- Causes: trauma, rupture of an intracranial aneurysm

Diagnosis

- CT of the brain (noncontrast)
- Lumbar puncture (xanthochromia)

- Once diagnosed, look for underlying vascular malformation:
  ○ CT angiography
  ○ Magnetic resonance angiography
  ○ The gold standard test—catheter-based cerebral angiography

Treatment

- Similar to those for intracranial hemorrhage

- Aneurysms are treated (or "secured") either by surgical clipping or by endovascular coiling

Seizures

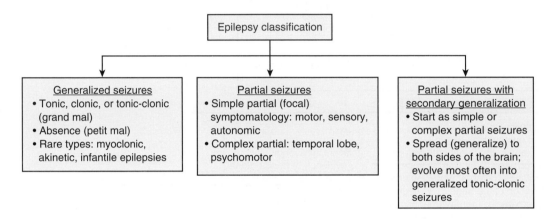

Status Epilepticus

Status epilepticus is associated with significant morbidity and mortality and considered a medical emergence and has to be promptly treated.[3,7,8]

```
┌─────────────────────────────────────────────────────────────┐
│ Presentation                                                  │
│ continuous unremitting seizure >5 minutes or recurrent        │
│ seizure activity in a patient who does not regain             │
│ consciousness between seizures                                │
└─────────────────────────────────────────────────────────────┘
                              │
                              ▼
┌─────────────────────────────────────────────────────────────┐
│ Initial management                                            │
│ • ABCs of emergency stabilization: airway protection,         │
│   hemodynamic resuscitation, and intravenous access           │
│ • Establish reliable vascular access                          │
│ • Stat labs: CBC, DMP, UA, toxicology screen, and             │
│   antiepileptic drug levels                                   │
│ • Choice of drug is based on advantages and side effects in   │
│   the context of individual patient (no good comparative data)│
│ • Start with benzodiazepine or barbiturate                    │
│     ○ Lorazepam in 2-mg IV boluses until seizures resolve     │
│       (maximum dose 0.1 mg/kg) or continuous infusion 2 mg/min│
│     ○ Diazepam 0.15 mg/kg IV up to 10 mg per dose every 5     │
│       minutes or continuous infusion 5 mg/min                 │
│     ○ Midazolam 0.2–0.4 mg/kg IV every 5 minutes, maximum     │
│       dose: 2 mg/kg                                           │
│     ○ Propofol 2 mg/kg IV every 5 minutes maximum dose:       │
│       10 mg/kg                                                │
│     ○ Phentobarbital 5 mg/kg IV up to 50 mg/min every 5       │
│       minutes, maximum loading dose of 15 mg/kg               │
│ • Give thiamine 100 mg IV, followed by 1 ampule of dextrose   │
│   50% in water                                                │
└─────────────────────────────────────────────────────────────┘
                              │
                              ▼
┌─────────────────────────────────────────────────────────────┐
│ If continues to seize (after 20–30 minutes)                   │
│ • Give anticonvulsant                                         │
│     ○ Phenytoin loading 15–20 mg/kg IV, 5–10 mg/kg 10 minutes │
│       after loading, or infusion at 50 mg/min                 │
│     ○ Fosphenytoin 15–20 mg phenytoin equivalents/kg IV bolus │
│     ○ Valproic acid loading 20–40 mg/kg IV, then 20 mg/kg in  │
│       10 minutes after loading or infusion at 3–6 mg/kg/min   │
│     ○ Levetiracetam 1000–3000 mg IV or infusion 2–5 mg/kg     │
└─────────────────────────────────────────────────────────────┘
                              │
                              ▼
┌─────────────────────────────────────────────────────────────┐
│ If continues to seize (after 1–2 hours after onset)           │
│ • Intubate (if not intubated yet)                             │
│ • Continuous IV sedation with propofol or midazolam           │
│ • Connect patient to video electroencephalographic monitoring │
└─────────────────────────────────────────────────────────────┘
                              │
                              ▼
┌─────────────────────────────────────────────────────────────┐
│ Once seizure controlled additional studies are ordered:       │
│ • Head CT with contrast or MRI (look for any structural        │
│   abnormality that may explain seizures)                      │
│ • Labs: toxicology screening, metabolic panel                 │
│ • Fever or possible signs of meningitis: cerebrospinal fluid  │
│   analysis                                                    │
└─────────────────────────────────────────────────────────────┘
```

Neuromuscular Diseases Potentially Causing Respiratory Compromise[3]

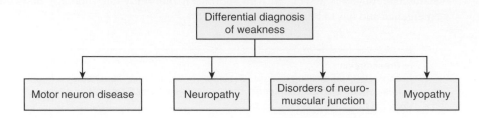

Motor Neuron Disease and Neuropathy

- Peripheral nerve involvement
  - Acute inflammatory demyelinating polyneuropathy (Guillain-Barré syndrome)
  - Chronic inflammatory demyelinating polyneuropathy

- Central/Motor neuron disease
  - Amyotrophic lateral sclerosis
  - Progressive bulbar palsy

Neuromuscular Diseases Potentially Causing Respiratory Compromise

	Etiology/Mechanism	Symptoms	Diagnosis
Multiple sclerosis	Autoimmune disease of CNS, viral trigger	Diversified symptoms: sensory, motor, visual, cognitive	• MRI: areas of demyelination • Evoked potential • CSF: pleocytosis, ↑ γ-globulin, oligoclonal bands
Parkinsonism	↓ Dopamine in basal ganglia	Muscular stiffness, bradykinesia, masked face, resting tremor, abnormal gait, soft speech	
Amyotrophic lateral sclerosis	Anterior horn cell degeneration	Weakness and wasting of muscles. Fasciculation of involved muscles. Both upper and lower motor neurons signs	• Clinical: combination of diffuse muscle atrophy, fasciculation, and retained reflexes, sensory changes are absent • EMG
Alzheimer's	Unknown	Recent memory loss, subtle emotional changes	Pathologically: neurofibrillary tangles and senile plaques
Peripheral neuropathy	Inherited, DM, uremia, alcohol, drugs/toxins, nutrition, etc.		• EMG • Serum chemistry (DM, uremia, B_{12}, etc.) • Urinalysis for toxins

CNS, Central nervous system; *CSF*, cerebrospinal fluid; *DM*, diabetes mellitus; *EMG*, electromyography; *MRI*, magnetic resonance imaging.

Disorders of Neuromuscular Junction and Myopathies

- Neuromuscular junction
  - Myasthenia gravis
  - Lambert-Eaton syndrome
  - Botulism

- Muscle
  - Polymyositis/Dermatomyositis
  - Spinal muscular atrophy
  - Muscular dystrophy

Neuromuscular Diseases Potentially Causing Respiratory Compromise (cont'd).

	Etiology/Mechanism	Symptoms	Diagnosis
Myasthenia gravis (differentiate from Eaton-Lambert)	Ab against acetylcholine receptor	Fatigue of effort, double vision, swallowing difficulties, muscle weakness. 4 D's: dysphagia, dysarthria, dyspnea, diplopia	• Anti-AChR level • Improvement upon injection of anticholinesterase drugs (edrophonium) • Repetitive nerve stimulation • Single-fiber EMG
Inflammatory myopathies	Polymyositis/ Dermatomyositis	Peripheral muscle weakness, rash	• CPK • Serology • EMG • Muscle biopsy
Noninflammatory myopathies	Metabolic disorders, endocrinopathies (hypothyroidism, corticosteroids use)		• CPK • EMG • Muscle biopsy
Myotonic dystrophy	Autosomal dominant	Muscle stiffness	Associated with heart block, testicular atrophy, premature balding, cataract
Muscular dystrophy	Genetic group of diseases	Duchenne's disease in young males. Muscles slowly deteriorate	

Ab, Antibody; *AChR*, acetylcholine receptor; *CPK*, creatine phosphokinase; *EMG*, electromyography.

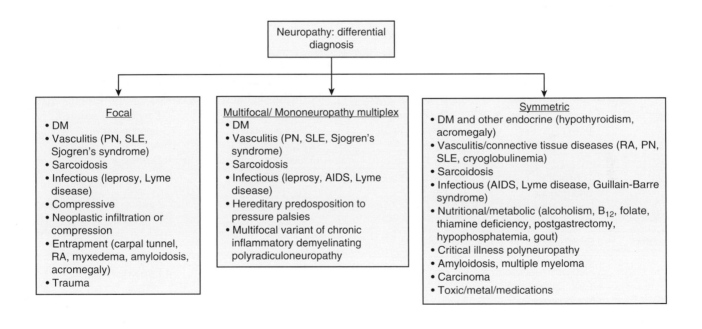

Neuropathy: differential diagnosis

Focal
• DM
• Vasculitis (PN, SLE, Sjogren's syndrome)
• Sarcoidosis
• Infectious (leprosy, Lyme disease)
• Compressive
• Neoplastic infiltration or compression
• Entrapment (carpal tunnel, RA, myxedema, amyloidosis, acromegaly)
• Trauma

Multifocal/ Mononeuropathy multiplex
• DM
• Vasculitis (PN, SLE, Sjogren's syndrome)
• Sarcoidosis
• Infectious (leprosy, AIDS, Lyme disease)
• Hereditary predosposition to pressure palsies
• Multifocal variant of chronic inflammatory demyelinating polyradiculoneuropathy

Symmetric
• DM and other endocrine (hypothyroidism, acromegaly)
• Vasculitis/connective tissue diseases (RA, PN, SLE, cryoglobulinemia)
• Sarcoidosis
• Infectious (AIDS, Lyme disease, Guillain-Barre syndrome)
• Nutritional/metabolic (alcoholism, B_{12}, folate, thiamine deficiency, postgastrectomy, hypophosphatemia, gout)
• Critical illness polyneuropathy
• Amyloidosis, multiple myeloma
• Carcinoma
• Toxic/metal/medications

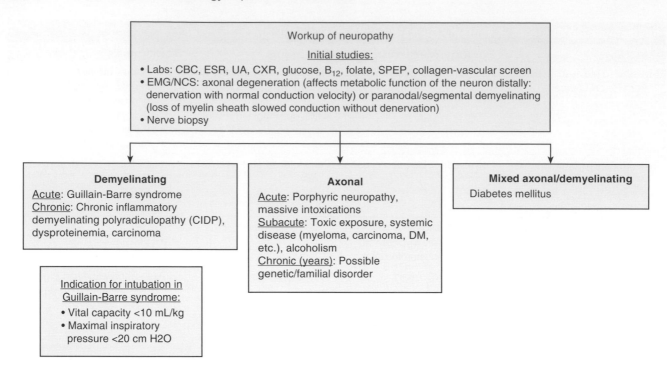

Workup of neuropathy

Initial studies:
- Labs: CBC, ESR, UA, CXR, glucose, B_{12}, folate, SPEP, collagen-vascular screen
- EMG/NCS: axonal degeneration (affects metabolic function of the neuron distally: denervation with normal conduction velocity) or paranodal/segmental demyelinating (loss of myelin sheath slowed conduction without denervation)
- Nerve biopsy

Demyelinating
Acute: Guillain-Barre syndrome
Chronic: Chronic inflammatory demyelinating polyradiculopathy (CIDP), dysproteinemia, carcinoma

Axonal
Acute: Porphyric neuropathy, massive intoxications
Subacute: Toxic exposure, systemic disease (myeloma, carcinoma, DM, etc.), alcoholism
Chronic (years): Possible genetic/familial disorder

Mixed axonal/demyelinating
Diabetes mellitus

Indication for intubation in Guillain-Barre syndrome:
- Vital capacity <10 mL/kg
- Maximal inspiratory pressure <20 cm H2O

Sedation[9–11]

Sedation Scales

	Ramsay Scale	Sedation–Agitation Scale	Richmond Agitation–Sedation Scale (RASS)	Motor Activity Assessment Scale
Agitated	1 Anxious, agitated, or both	7 Dangerously agitated 6 Very agitated 5 Agitated	+4 Combative +3 Very agitated +2 Agitated +1 Restless	6 Dangerously agitated, uncooperative 5 Agitated 4 Restless and cooperative
Calm	2 Cooperative, oriented, and tranquil 3 Patient responds to commands only	4 Calm and cooperative	0 Alert and calm	3 Calm and cooperative
Sedated	4 Brisk response to a light glabellar tap 5 Sluggish response to a light glabellar tap 6 No response	3 Sedated 2 Very sedated 1 Unarousable	−1 Drowsy −2 Light sedation −3 Moderate −4 Deep sedation −5 Unarousable	2 Responsive to touch, name, or both 1 Responsive only to noxious stimuli 0 Unresponsive
Source	Ramsey et al.[12]	Riker et al.[13]	Sessler et al.[14]	Devlin et al.[15]

Choice of Medications Used for Sedation.

	Onset after loading dose /Half life	Dose	Active metabolites (prolong effect, especially in renal failure)	Respiratory depression	Hypotension	Other adverse effects
Midazolam (benzodiazepine, acts through GABAA receptors)	2–5 min/3–11 h	Load with 0.01–0.05 mg/kg over several minutes then 0.02–0.1 mg/kg/h	+	+	+	
Lorazepam (benzodiazepine, acts through GABAA receptors)	15–20 min/8–15 h	Load with 0.02–0.04 mg/kg (≤2 mg), then 0.02–0.06 mg/kg q 2–6 h prn or 0.01–0.1 mg/kg/h (≤10 mg/h)	–	+	+	Propylene glycol-related acidosis, nephrotoxicity
Diazepam (benzodiazepine, acts through GABAA receptors)	2–5 min/20–120 h	Load with 5–10 mg, then 0.03–0.1 mg/kg q 0.5–6 h prn	+	+	+	phlebitis
Propofol (sedative-hypnotic, in part acts through GABAA receptors)	1–2 min/3–12 h if short-term use, up to >50 h if long-term use	Load with 5 µg/kg/min over 5 min, then 5–50 µg/kg/min	–	+	+	Hypertriglyceridemia, pancreatitis, propofol-related infusion syndrome
Dexmedetomidine (α2-adrenoceptor agonist)	5–10 min/1.8–3.5 h	Load with 1 µg/kg over 10 min, then 0.2–0.7 µg/kg/h	–	–	+	Bradycardia, loss of airway reflexes, hypertension
Remifentanil (µ-opioid receptor agonist)	1–3 min/3–10 min	Loading with 0.4–1.5 µg/kg, then 0.5–15 µg/kg/min	–	+		Bradycardia, nausea, constipation

Pain Management[10,16]

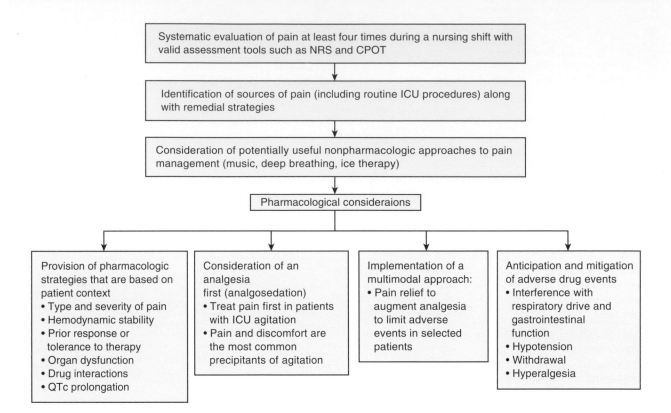

Choices in Analgesics

Choice of Analgesics.		
	Onset/Half life	Adverse Effect
Opiates		
Fentanyl	1–2 min/2–4 h	Accumulation with hepatic impairment
Hydromorphone	5–15 min/2–3 h	Accumulation with hepatic/renal impairment
Morphine	5–10 min/3–4 h	Accumulation with hepatic/renal impairment. Histamine release.
Methadone	1–3 d/15–60 h	Unpredictable pharmacokinetics; unpredictable pharmacodynamics in opiate naïve patients. Monitor QTc
Remifentanil	1–3 min/3–10 min	No accumulation in hepatic/renal failure
Non-Opiates		
Ketamine (IV)	30–40 sec/2–3 h	Hallucinations and other psychological disturbances
Acetaminophen (PO/PR)	30–60 min/2–4 h	Potentially contraindicated in patients with significant hepatic dysfunction
Acetaminophen (IV)	5–10 min/2 h	
Ketorolac (IM/IV)	10 min/2.4–8.6 h	Avoid in renal dysfunction; gastrointestinal bleeding; platelet abnormality; concomitant ACEI, CHF, cirrhosis, asthma. Contraindicated for perioperative pain in CABG
Ibuprofen (IV)	NA/2.2–2.4 h	
Ibuprofen (PO)	25 min/1.8–2.5 h	
Gabapentin (PO)	NA/5–7 h	Sedation, confusion, dizziness, ataxia; withdrawal syndrome: seizures
Carbamazepine immediate release (PO)	4–5 h/25–65 h initially, then 12–17 h	Nystagmus, dizziness, diplopia, lightheadedness, lethargy, toxic epidermal necrolysis with HLA-B1502 gene, multiple drug interactions due to hepatic enzyme induction

ACEI, Angiotensin-converting-enzyme inhibitors; *CABG,* coronary artery bypass grafting; *CHF,* congestive heart failure; *IM,* intramuscular; *IV,* intravenous; *PO,* per os (by mouth); *PR,* per rectum.

Neuromuscular Blockade[17-19]

Indications
- Facilitation of mechanical ventilation and to aid oxygenation (e.g., in ARDS):
    - Improving chest wall compliance
    - Reducing peak airway pressure
    - Preventing asynchrony with ventilator
    - Reduced oxygen consumption
    - Improved PaO_2
    - Prevention of respiratory movements
    - Prone ventilation
    - Lung recruitment
    - Reduced inflammatory-mediator release
    - Reduced dynamic hyperinflation
- Control of increases in intracranial pressure, e.g., after head injury, neurosurgery
- Tetanus
- Neuroleptic malignant syndrome
- Status epilepticus
- Facilitation of procedures and tests (endotracheal intubation, bronchoscopy, tracheostomy, MRI, CT)
- Patient transport

Depolarizing neuromuscular blockers: (depolarize muscle cells)
Suxamethonium or succinylcholine
- Rapid onset and rapid recovery
- Adverse reactions
    - Myalgia
    - Hypertension
    - Bradycardia or transient cardiac arrest (atropine before the second dose of suxamethonium)
    - Small increase in plasma potassium
    - Spasm of the jaw or contracture of extra-ocular muscles

Nondepolarizing neuromuscular blockers
- Classified by duration of action
    - Long-acting: doxacurium, pipecuronium, metocurine, pancuronium
    - Intermediate/long-acting: vecuronium, atracurium, and cisatracurium
    - Intermediate-acting: rocuronium
    - Short-acting:mivacurium, rapacuronium
- Adverse reactions: histamine release, tachycardia, hypotension

Potential clinical consequences of widespread muscular paralysis
- Cephalad displacement of the diaphragm
- Inability to increase minute ventilation in response to need for increased carbon dioxide removal (i.e., excessive caloric intake)
- Airway closure
- VTE
- Compromised skin integrity
- Corneal ulcers
- Nerve compression
- Impaired communication
- Patient awareness and pain while paralyzed
- Impaired cough
- Elimination of protective reflexes
- Protracted weakness
- Unrecognized patient-ventilator disconnection

REFERENCES

1. Chinthapalli K, Logan AM, Raj R, Nirmalananthan N. Assessment of acute headache in adults - what the general physician needs to know. *Clin Med J R Coll Physicians London*. 2018;18(5):422–427.
2. Bevers MB, Kimberly WT. Critical care management of acute ischemic stroke. *Curr Treat Options Cardiovasc Med*. 2017;19(6):41.
3. Kottapally M, Josephson SA. Common neurologic emergencies for nonneurologists: when minutes count. *Cleve Clin J Med*. 2016;83(2):116–126.
4. Peters NA, Farrell LB, Smith JP. Hyperosmolar therapy for the treatment of cerebral edema. *US Pharm*. 2018;43(1):HS-8-HS-11.
5. Jehan F, Aziz H, O'Keeffe T, et al. The role of four-factor prothrombin complex concentrate in coagulopathy of trauma: a propensity matched analysis. *J Trauma Acute Care Surg*. 2018;85(1):18–24.
6. Morotti A, Goldstein JN. Diagnosis and management of acute intracerebral hemorrhage. *Emerg Med Clin*. 2016;34(4):883–899.
7. Tsai LK, Liou HH. Current treatment for generalized convulsive status epilepticus in adults. *Acta Neurol Taiwan*. 2015;24(4):108–115.
8. Rai S, Drislane FW. Treatment of refractory and super-refractory status epilepticus. *Neurotherapeutics*. 2018;15(3):97–712.
9. Pun BT, Dunn J. The sedation of critically ill adults: part 1: assessment. The first in a two-part series focuses on assessing sedated patients in the ICU. *Am J Nurs*. 2007;107(7):40–48, quiz 49.
10. Barr J, Fraser GL, Puntillo K, et al. Clinical practice guidelines for the management of pain, agitation, and delirium in adult patients in the Intensive Care Unit: executive summary. *Am J Health Syst Pharm*. 2013;70(1):53–58.
11. Pun BT, Dunn J. The sedation of critically ill adults: part 2: management. *Am J Nurs*. 2007;107(8):40–49, quiz 50.
12. Ramsay MA, Savege TM, Simpson BR, Goodwin R. Controlled sedation with alphaxalone-alphadolone. *Br Med J*. 1974;2(5920):656–659.
13. Riker RR, Fraser GL, Cox PM. Continuous infusion of haloperidol controls agitation in critically ill patients. *Crit Care Med*. 1994;22(3):433–440.
14. Sessler CN, Gosnell MS, Grap MJ, et al. The Richmond Agitation-Sedation Scale: validity and reliability in adult intensive care unit patients. *Am J Respir Crit Care Med*. 2002;166(10):1338–1344.
15. Devlin JW, Boleski G, Mlynarek M, et al. Motor Activity Assessment Scale: a valid and reliable sedation scale for use with mechanically ventilated patients in an adult surgical intensive care unit. *Crit Care Med*. 1999;27(7):1271–1275.
16. Pandharipande PP, Patel MB, Barr J. Management of pain, agitation, and delirium in critically ill patients. *Pol Arch Med Wewn*. 2014;124(3):114–123. Medycyna Praktyczna.
17. Craig RG, Hunter JM. Neuromuscular blocking drugs and their antagonists in patients with organ disease. *Anaesthesia*. 2009;64(suppl 1):55–65.
18. Bennett S, Hurford WE. When should sedation or neuromuscular blockade be used during mechanical ventilation? *Respir Care*. 2011;56(2):168–180.
19. Tripathi S, Hunter J. Neuromuscular blocking drugs in the critically ill. *Contin Educ Anaesth Crit Care Pain*. 2006;6(3):119–123.

CHAPTER 13

COVID-19 and Critical Care

Alexander Goldfarb-Rumyantzev and Robert Stephen Brown

Since critical care units will be treating many patients with Coronavirus Disease 2019 (COVID-19), this chapter is devoted to the coronavirus pandemic. However, certain aspects are applicable to other severe viral illnesses, such as earlier coronaviruses (CoVs) or even severe influenza, and cases of acute respiratory distress syndromes.

Pearls to Consider

- Early antiviral treatment (e.g., anti-SARS-CoV-2 monoclonal antibodies (casirivimab plus imdevimab, bamlanivimab plus etesevimab, sotrovimab), or perhaps convalescent plasma, remdesivir, favipiravir, or baricitinib) during initial viral replication is more useful than treatment after end-organ damage has occurred. There may be no reason to treat with antivirals later on, as active virus replication does not seem to play a role at this stage of the illness when multiorgan system failure (MOSF) has occurred. We suggest using a prediction model[1,2] to identify those that will have a severe course and treat them early and aggressively.
- Patients might remain stable for some time, but deteriorate quickly as there is a disconnection between low O_2 saturation and symptoms.
- Oxygenation drops after intubation so in many patients, prolonged proning, if tolerated, should be utilized.

- Pneumothorax is common due to high PEEP, and pneumomediastinum and subcutaneous emphysema may occur.
- Intubated patients with respiratory failure are at high risk of mortality and those with acute respiratory distress syndrome (ARDS) and requiring mechanical ventilation may remain on the ventilator for long periods of time.
- Increased peak pressure frequently indicates endotracheal tube obstruction with thick secretion may have occurred.
- Patients frequently present leukopenic, and then develop leukocytosis (which might signify secondary bacterial infection).
- Serum albumin level often become very low.

SARS-CoV-2[3,4]

- CoVs: highly diverse, enveloped, positive-sense, and single-stranded RNA viruses of the order Nidovirales.
- There are seven different CoVs able to infect human cells causing illnesses ranging from mild upper respiratory symptoms to a potentially fatal disease.
- SARS-CoV-2 is a lineage of B-betacoronavirus.
- The receptor-binding domain has a high affinity to the extracellular domain of human ACE2 receptor (expressed in most of human organs):
  o The highest activity of ACE2 is in ileum and kidney
  o Followed by type I and type II pneumocytes, adipocytes, heart, brainstem, small intestine enterocytes, stomach, liver, vasculature, and nasal and oral mucosa

Epidemiology

- The major route of transmission of COVID-19 is by aerosolized droplets or less likely, on surfaces from close contact with an infected person.
- There is a higher proportion of COVID-19 in men (about 55% to 70%; perhaps because men have higher ACE2 levels in their alveolar cells).[5,6]

- COVID-19 appears to be more frequent in patients taking ACE inhibitors and ARBs because of its higher prevalence in those with cardiovascular disease or hypertension, but ACE inhibitors or ARBs do not appear to affect the risk of a severe or fatal outcome.[7,8]
- Transmission rate for the alpha variant is 2.2 to 3.58 per patient, whereas the delta and other variants are about 2 times more contagious and reported to cause more severe illness than the alpha variant.[8a,8b,9,10]
- The mean incubation period is about 5 days (range 1–14 days; 95% of patients are likely to become symptomatic within 12.5 days of contact).[10]
- Although most COVID-19 patients are between 30 and 79 years of age[11] (median age 49–59 years), the severity of illness is greatest in those over 80 years of age.
- In progressive disease the median duration period from illness onset to dyspnea is 8.0 days, and to mechanical ventilation is 10.5 days.[10]
- Between 16% and 25% of symptomatic COVID-19 cases are severe or critical, with up to 25% requiring ICU care for ARDS,[5] with about a 60% mortality in this group after 4 weeks.[12,13]
- Of ICU patients, up to 75% have or develop acute kidney injury (AKI), with half of those requiring renal replacement therapy (RRT) and there is a mortality rate of 30%-70% in those with AKI.[12,13,13a,]
- The current reported mortality for COVID-19 is approximately 3.41% compared to 10% for SARS and 35% for MERS.[10] However, the case fatality rate differs between studies from 2.8% to 15%.[5] The mortality rate of hospitalized patients with COVID-19 has been improving over time as treatment improves,[14] such as the use of proning rather than intubation and the addition of corticosteroids for severely ill patients. While fully vaccinated people get breakthrough infections, they are less severe than in unvaccinated people and most vaccines have been effective against both the alpha and delta variant.[8a]

Symptoms of COVID-19[15]:

Generalized Symptoms	Localized Symptoms
Fever 88%	Headache 14%
Fatigue 38%	Nasal congestion 5%
Chills 11%	Sore throat 14%
	Dry cough 68%
	Productive cough 33%
	Dyspnea 19%
	Nausea/emesis 5%
	Diarrhea 4%–14%
	Myalgias 15%
	Anosmia and ageusia (loss of smell or taste) occurs in 15%–68% with predominance in young females[16,17]
	Neurologic symptoms 36% total[18]

Diagnostic criteria[19,20]

Initial diagnostic tests to be ordered for admitted patients with suspected COVID-19[15]

Diagnostic Tests	Details and Interpretation of Results
SARS-CoV-2 viral test, usually of nasopharyngeal sample	Nucleic acid amplification tests (NAATs) detect the virus' genetic material and are generally more accurate Antigen tests detect viral proteins and are generally not as sensitive as NAATs but are more rapid
Complete blood count (CBC) with differential (lymphocyte and neutrophil counts)	Leukopenia and lymphopenia at the initial stage of the disease (absolute count of peripheral lymphocytes may be less than 0.8 × 10/L, or the count of CD4 and CD8 T cells decreases significantly) However, 25%–30% of patients presented with leukocytosis
Initial biochemical tests	• Basic metabolic panel including electrolytes and creatinine to identify acute kidney injury (AKI), electrolyte, and acid–base disorders • Lactic acid levels

Diagnostic Tests	Details and Interpretation of Results
Inflammatory markers	• Elevated C-reactive protein (CRP), erythrocyte sedimentation rate (ESR), ferritin—acute phase reactants • Inflammatory cytokines (such as interleukin-6 [IL-6], IL-10, and tumor necrosis factor [TNF]-α), T- and B-lymphocyte subsets, and complement can be tested as appropriate
Enzymes	• Increased transaminases: AST, ALT • Elevated creatine phosphokinase (CPK), lactate dehydrogenase (LDH), myoglobin, troponin
Coagulopathy labs	• Partial thromboplastin time/international normalized ratio (PTT/INR) may be mildly elevated. • PTT/INR should be measured for a baseline when anticoagulation is to be prescribed • D-dimer—markedly elevated in many patients with COVID-19
Other labs to rule out alternative causes of respiratory symptoms	• N-terminal-pro hormone BNP (NT-proBNP) to differentiate pulmonary infiltrates from congestive heart failure (CHF) and pulmonary edema • Procalcitonin levels remain normal in many cases (as opposed to bacterial pneumonia) • Viral tests for influenza, respiratory syncytial virus (RSV), other viral causes, Legionella
Chest x-ray (CXR), computerized tomography (CT) scan of the chest, electrocardiogram (ECG)	• Pneumonia with characteristic lesions (bilateral peripheral infiltrates, frequently extensive) • Early stage: multiple small patchy shadows and interstitial changes, multiple bilateral ground-glass opacities and infiltrations • Consolidation in severe cases

Specific diagnostic tests[21]

- Tests based on detecting the genetic material
  - Real-time reverse-transcriptase–polymerase-chain reaction (rRT-PCR): SARS-CoV-2 nucleic acid positive in samples of sputum, nasopharynx swabs, secretions of lower respiratory tract
  - The positive rate of rRT-PCR for throat swab samples was reported to be about 60% in the early stage of COVID-19[10]
  - If negative with high clinical suspicion, repeating of rRT-PCR should be considered after 24 hours
  - SARS-CoV-2 viral genome sequencing to detect new mutant strains done for research or public health studies (may be treated differently in the future)
- Tests based on detecting antibodies to SARS-CoV-2 (IgM and IgG) to detect past infection or late infection (may be affected by prior vaccine immunization)
- Cell culture is NOT recommended for diagnostic purposes
- Chest CT scan
  - The sensitivity of chest CT in suspected patients was 97% based on positive RT-PCR results and 75% based on negative RT-PCR results and lung ultrasound correlates closely with chest CT to diagnose and monitor interstitial pneumonitis.[10,10a,10b]

Severity levels[10,22]

Severity Level	Symptoms	Disposition
Mild type	No pneumonia or mild pneumonia	Do not need to be admitted
Severe type	Dyspnea, respiratory frequency ≥30/min, blood oxygen saturation <93%, partial pressure of arterial oxygen-to-fraction of inspired oxygen ratio (PaO$_2$/FiO$_2$) <300 mm Hg, and/or lung infiltrates >50% within 24/48 hours	Hospitalize but not necessarily to the ICU
Critical type	Respiratory failure (PaO$_2$/FiO$_2$ <200 mm Hg = ARDS), septic shock, and/or multiple organ dysfunction or failure	Admit to ICU

Stages based on CT scan findings[19]

Ultra-early stage	• Single or diffuse foci of clouding • Enlarged lymph nodes in the middle sections of the lungs, often surrounded by circular opacities • Consolidations may occur • Air bronchograms
Early stage	1–3 days after the onset of symptoms • Interstitial edema
Third stage	Rapid progression of changes; 3–7 days from the onset of symptoms • Increased alveolar and interstitial edema • Merging consolidations with air bronchograms
Fourth stage	• Consolidation lesions as a result of fibrin deposition in the lumen of the alveoli and in the lung interstitium
Fifth stage	The changes evolve to the following: • Consolidation, interlobular septal thickening, and striped densities, spreading along the bronchi

Predictors of the occurrence of critical illness

Ten variables were independent predictive factors[1]:
- Chest radiographic abnormality (OR, 3.39; 95% CI, 2.14–5.38)
- Age (OR, 1.03; 95% CI, 1.01–1.05)
- Hemoptysis (OR, 4.53; 95% CI, 1.36–15.15)
- Dyspnea (OR, 1.88; 95% CI, 1.18–3.01)
- Unconsciousness (OR, 4.71; 95% CI, 1.39–15.98)
- Number of comorbidities (OR, 1.60; 95% CI, 1.27–2.00)
- Cancer history (OR, 4.07; 95% CI, 1.23–13.43)
- Neutrophil-to-lymphocyte ratio (OR, 1.06; 95% CI, 1.02–1.10)
- Lactate dehydrogenase level (OR, 1.002; 95% CI, 1.001–1.004)
- Direct bilirubin level (OR, 1.15; 95% CI, 1.06–1.24)

Comorbidities associated with worse clinical outcome: Diabetes, hypertension, coronary heart disease, COPD, cerebrovascular disease, and kidney disease.[23]

An alternative risk stratification prediction model utilizes the following variables: age, sex, number of comorbidities, respiratory rate, percent oxygen saturation, Glasgow coma scale score, blood urea, and CRP.[2]

ICU admission

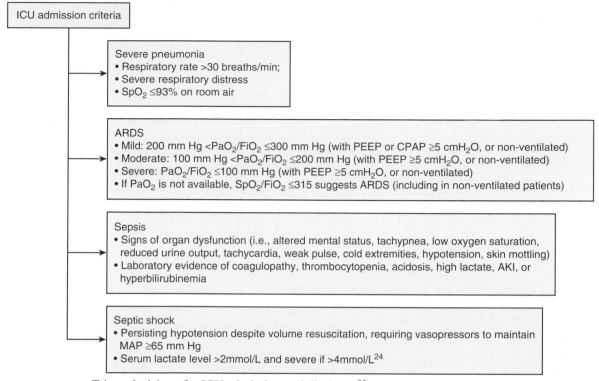

Triage decisions for ICU admission and discharge[25]

	Prior to ICU Admission	Patients Already Admitted to ICU
Stage A (ICU beds available but capacity is limited)	**Inclusion criteria:** Requirement for invasive ventilatory support or hemodynamic support with vasoactive agents **Some of the relative exclusion criteria:** Patient's wishes, cardiac arrest, advanced cancer, severe dementia, COPD GOLD 4, NYHA class 4 heart failure, liver cirrhosis Child–Pugh score >8, estimated survival <12 months	**Criteria to be discharged from ICU:** • Stabilization and improvement • Little or no benefit with ICU treatment: occurrence of cardiac arrest during ICU stay with morbid sequelae following resuscitation; persistence or development of significant triple organ failure
Stage B (very few or no ICU beds available)	**Some of the relative exclusion criteria:** Severe trauma, severe burns, severe cerebral deficit, NYHA class 3 or 4 heart failure, age >75–85 years, liver cirrhosis with refractory ascites or encephalopathy, moderate dementia, and estimated survival <24 months	**Criteria to be discharged from ICU:** • Stabilization and improvement • Little or no benefit with ICU treatment: no improvement in respiratory or hemodynamic status, or in the underlying organ dysfunction; occurrence of cardiac arrest during ICU stay; persistence or development of a significant dual organ failure

Pathophysiology of clinical syndromes in COVID-19

Common mechanisms of end-organ damage:

- Direct viral invasion[26,27]
- Cytokine storm[28]
- Ischemia due to micro-thromboses, endothelial damage, thrombotic microangiopathy (TMA), and/or hypoxemia[29,30]

Pathophysiological mechanisms are described in the following figure and in more detail in the subsequent table.

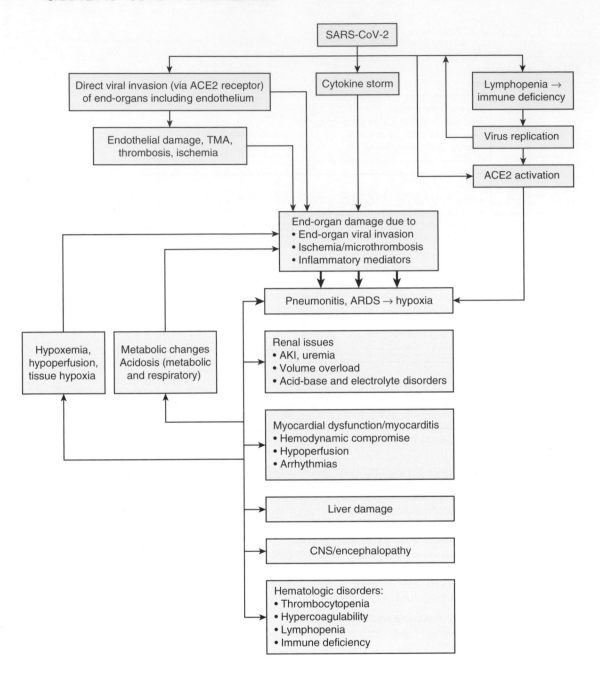

Pathophysiology and Manifestations of COVID-19 by Organ System

Impairment of the respiratory system	**Specific features:** • COVID-19 pneumonia presents as hypoxemic respiratory failure with ARDS-like presentation on imaging. • In one large study, about 6% of COVID-19 patients required admission to an ICU with the percentage of ARDS varying widely from less than half to almost all, but mechanical ventilation being needed for most patients with ARDS and associated with high mortality.[31] • Mechanism of ARDS is likely to be different than "pre-COVID era": In COVID ARDS, there is a dissociation between the severity of the hypoxemia and the maintenance of relatively good respiratory mechanics (compliance). This phenomenon was called "silent hypoxemia" and is characterized by low arterial oxygen content with few or no other respiratory symptoms.[32,33] • Patients do not exhibit increased lung stiffness. • Hypoxemia with COVID-19 is usually accompanied by an increased alveolar-to-arterial oxygen gradient, signifying either ventilation–perfusion mismatch or intrapulmonary shunting.[33] • Hypoventilation is uncommon with COVID-19.[33] • Patients tend to deteriorate quickly and they stay on mechanical ventilation longer than other patients with ARDS, leading to possible (and probably) secondary reinfection, case fatality once intubated is high among the oldest.[22] • Patients do not present with dramatic dyspnea, even in the presence of profound hypoxemia (i.e., arterial blood oxygen levels lower than that seen normally in mixed venous blood). • Urgent intubation and mechanical ventilation with high inflation pressures and raised inhaled oxygen concentration seem to be unhelpful or have worse outcomes.[34] **Mechanism of pulmonary damage:** • Direct viral invasion through ACE2 receptors: alveolar viral damage • ARDS is ascribed to the excessive activation of RAS caused by SARS-CoV-2[35] • Endothelial damage, microvascular thrombosis, and hemorrhage to arrow--> -> extensive alveolar and interstitial inflammation similar to macrophage activation syndrome (MAS)[36,37] • Local inflammatory reaction, cytokine storm/hyperimmune reaction of the host causing additional pulmonary damage[37] • A loss of lung perfusion regulation and hypoxic vasoconstriction, V/Q imbalances, shunting[38] • Fluid overload and "third-spacing" → pulmonary edema
AKI/acute renal failure	• A significant number of patients with COVID-19 pneumonia have renal involvement on admission (75% by some reports[39]) and about one-third overall, most of them with prerenal failure and/or acute tubular necrosis (ATN).[30,40] • Renal abnormalities associated with COVID-19 include proteinuria, hematuria, and AKI.[3] • Proteinuria, hematuria, and AKI often resolve within 3 weeks after the onset of symptoms with renal complications in COVID-19. • Renal abnormalities are associated with higher mortality.[39,41] • About one-third of hospitalized COVID patients had reduced kidney function 6 months later, including 13% who did not have diagnosed AKI[41a] **Mechanism of renal damage:** • Direct renal invasion. SARS-CoV-2 may include kidney tropism; human kidney is a specific target for SARS-CoV-2 infection[26,42]: SARS-CoV-2 can infect podocytes and tubular epithelial cells[3] • Initial proteinuria might be transient and related to fever rather than actual renal damage • Organ ischemia[43] • Micro-thrombosis/TMA[29,30] • Glomerulonephritis of various types, including collapsing glomerulopathy in Blacks with the high risk APOL1 genotype[30,44,45]
Cardiomyopathy/ myocarditis	• Almost 12% of patients without known CVD had elevated troponin levels or cardiac arrest during hospitalization for COVID.[46] **Mechanism of cardiac damage:** • Elevated troponin associated with cytokine storm or secondary hemophagocytic lymphohistiocytosis more than isolated myocardial injury[15] • Some patients present with predominantly cardiac symptoms: potentially viral myocarditis or stress cardiomyopathy possibly by direct myocardial involvement mediated by ACE2 receptors[15] • COVID-19 might destabilize coronary plaques • Aggravated by hypoxia[47]
Encephalopathy and other neurological complications	**CNS involvement may be mediated by the following mechanisms[48]:** • Direct viral invasion (through blood circulation or neuronal pathway, e.g., through the olfactory nerve and the olfactory bulb): ACE2 receptors are expressed in the nervous system. Presence of SARS-CoV-2 in the cerebrospinal fluid confirms the presence of viral encephalitis.[49] • Infectious toxic encephalopathy, also known as acute toxic encephalitis • Acute cerebrovascular events • Immune system response (SIRS and also virus can activate glial cells and cause inflammatory response with production of IL-6, IL-12, IL-15, and TNF-α) • Hypoxia injury leading to cerebral edema, intracranial hypertension, ischemia and congestion, increased risk of acute ischemic stroke

Continued

cont'd	
Vasculitis, endothelial damage, TMA	**Mechanism of endothelial cell damage:** • Direct viral invasion: viral inclusion structures in endothelial cells • Accumulation of inflammatory cells associated with endothelium, as well as apoptotic bodies, in the heart, small bowel, and lung • An accumulation of mononuclear cells was found in the lung, and most small lung vessels appeared congested[50] • TMA: signs and symptoms of severe COVID-19 infection resemble complement–mediated TMA, rather than sepsis–induced coagulopathy or DIC (i.e., the combination of microangiopathic hemolytic anemia, thrombocytopenia, and organ damage: neurological, renal, and cardiac dysfunction)[51]
Coagulation dysfunction, hypercoagulability, thrombotic events: elevated D-dimer, LDH, total bilirubin, decreased platelets	**Coagulopathy:** • The incidence of thrombotic complications is between 16% and 49% in patients with COVID-19 admitted to intensive care. Clinical markers of coagulopathy in patients severely ill with COVID-19 are associated with a higher risk of death.[52] **Potential mechanisms:** • Consequence of severe inflammation (cytokine storm) • Specific effect mediated by the virus (virus directly or indirectly interferes with coagulation pathways causing systemic thrombosis) • Presence of antiphospholipid antibodies reported in up to 45% of the patients[53,54] • Coagulation profile manifestations are consistent with the diagnosis of the hypercoagulable phase of DIC leading to severe hypercoagulability[55] **Thrombocytopenia mechanism[56]:** • Cytokine storm → bone marrow progenitor cell destruction • Direct infection of hematopoietic and bone marrow stromal cells • Increase autoantibodies and immune complexes leading to platelet destruction • Lung injury leading to increased platelet activation and platelet aggregation leading to increased consumption

Immune system: cytokine storm, lymphopenia	• Lymphopenia predicts disease severity. Mechanism of lymphopenia is not completely clear
	• Leukopenia is not uncommon; some patients develop leukocytosis (which might signify secondary bacterial infection)
	• Early-response proinflammatory cytokines such as IL-6, IL-1, and TNF-α, leads to a cytokine storm
	Cytokine release syndrome (CRS)[57]
	• Systemic inflammatory response caused by infection, some drugs and other factors
	• Sharp increase in the level of a large number of proinflammatory cytokines
	• SARS-CoV-2 binds to alveolar epithelial cells leading to activation of innate and adaptive immune system resulting in:
	  ○ Release of a large number of cytokines (e.g., IL-6)
	  ○ Increased vascular permeability → fluid and blood cells accumulating in the alveoli

Liver damage	• Presents as different degrees of abnormal liver biochemical tests (mostly transaminases: AST elevation is more common than ALT[58]) **Mechanism:** • Direct pathogenic effect by the virus • Systemic inflammation • Toxicity from commonly used drugs[59]

Skeletal muscle injury	• Rhabdomyolysis can be an initial presentation of COVID-19 or may present at any time of the disease course[60]
	Mechanism:
	  ○ ACE2 receptors are expressed in skeletal muscles[48]; direct viral invasion can lead to rhabdomyolysis
	  ○ Robust immune response to viruses resulting in cytokine storms and damaging muscle tissues
	  ○ Circulating viral toxins may directly destroy muscle cell membranes[60]

Acid–base disorders	• Acid–base disorders are common and complex and include anion gap metabolic acidosis (due to renal failure and, in some cases, lactic acidosis and newly diagnosed diabetic ketoacidosis[61,62]), non-gap metabolic acidosis, respiratory alkalosis due to hyperventilation caused by hypoxemia, severe respiratory acidosis (due to hypoventilation when we limit tidal volume), metabolic alkalosis

Treatment[19,20,22,63,64]:

Treatment of infection	**Antivirals**[22]
	• Currently, there is little evidence to support the effectiveness of existing antiviral drugs against SARS-CoV-2
	• Viral RNA-dependent RNA polymerase inhibitors
	  ○ Remdesivir—in various trials,[76,77] preliminary report demonstrated benefit by shortening the time to recovery in a placebo-controlled study but has not been shown to decrease mortality[78a,78b]
	  ○ Baricitinib, a Janus kinase inhibitor, either with remdesivir or alone appears to reduce recovery time and decrease mortality[78c,78d,78e]
	  ○ Favipiravir—in trials, shortening the time to recovery and is considerably less expensive than Remdesivir[77,78b,79]
	• Protease inhibitors
	  ○ The combination protease inhibitor lopinavir/ritonavir used to treat HIV infection was demonstrated to have in vitro activity against SARS-CoV and improved clinical outcomes when used in combination with ribavirin for SARS. It can be used when appropriate, two tablets, twice daily for 14 days. When using SCCM guidelines, lopinavir/ritonavir is recommended[63] but the first randomized, controlled trial did not demonstrate statistically significant benefit among hospitalized patients with COVID-19[79]
	  ○ Darunavir or lopinavir in combination with ritonavir and oseltamivir and hydroxychloroquine[80]
	• Other antiviral drugs
	  ○ Ribavirin (± interferon) —unclear benefit, might further reduce Hb
	  ○ Abidol —undergoing trials and may be effective in reducing in-hospital mortality[77,78f,81]
	• Chloroquine and hydroxychloroquine block SARS-CoV-2 cell entry in vitro at similar concentrations that are achieved with treatment for rheumatoid arthritis and although exhibiting a promising inhibitory effect on the virus in vivo[19,22,82,83], *but* did not prevent symptomatic illness in clinical trials and should play no role in therapy[84,85,86]
	• Interferon (IFN β-1a or IFN β-1b) in combination with antivirals may be of benefit[87,88]
	Immunoglobulins
	• Monoclonal antibody treatment using casirivimab plus imdevimab or sotrovimab preferably to bamlanivimab plus etesevimab (because of variant resistance) when given IV in early infection (during the first 10 days of symptomatic infection) are reported to be effective and have received emergency use authorization in the United States. At this time, monoclonal antibodies should be considered to treat early infection in high risk patients[91,92,93,93a,93b]
	• Early intravenous infusion of human immunoglobulin is recommended for critically ill patients, based on their clinical condition, at 0.25–0.5 g/kg per day, for 3–5 days[20]
	• As per SCCM guidelines, no standard intravenous immunoglobulins (IVIG) or convalescent plasma is currently recommended[63] though convalescent plasma therapy may be effective[89,90]
	Empiric antibiotics
	• No preventive antibiotic treatment should be given without microbiologically confirmed bacterial superinfection[19]
	• When there is evidence of bacterial infection—second-generation cephalosporins or fluoroquinolones[20]
	• In patients without risk factors for methicillin-resistant *Staphylococcus aureus* (MRSA) or *Pseudomonas* (i.e., community acquired), and no prior multidrug resistant organism (MDRO) infection, start with ceftriaxone + azithromycin
	• In patients with risk factors for MRSA or *Pseudomonas* (i.e., chronic hospitalization, prior MDRO infection), start with vancomycin + cefepime and consider ciprofloxacin if high concern for *Pseudomonas*

Hemodynamics[63]	• Conservative fluid therapy, prefer buffered/balanced crystalloids over colloids
	• Vasopressors:
	  ○ Goal MAP 60–65 mm Hg
	  ○ Start with norepinephrine
	  ○ If not available — vasopressin or epinephrine
	  ○ Second agent — vasopressin, but if evidence of cardiac dysfunction, persistent hypoperfusion, use dobutamine
	• Shock refractory to vasopressors—might administer corticosteroids:
	  ○ Patients with severe disease could receive glucocorticoid at early stage, e.g., intravenous methylprednisolone 40–80 mg, once daily for 5 days or 50–200 mg intravenous hydrocortisone every 6 h

Continued

cont'd	

Respiratory failure	• Start O_2 supplementation if O_2 Sat <90%–92%, maintain >96%
	• Choice of O_2 therapy:
	  ○ Patients with mild hypoxemia should be put on nasal cannula, 5 L/min
	  ○ If the patient is getting worse, high-flow nasal cannula should be considered, starting with 20 L/min and increasing to 50–60 L/min gradually
	  ○ Trial of nasal intermittent positive pressure ventilation (NIPPV using helmet BiPAP or CPAP)

Intubation and ventilation[19,22,63]	• Hypoxemia with COVID-19 is usually accompanied by ventilation–perfusion mismatch or intrapulmonary shunting[33]
	  ○ If a patient's PaO_2 increases with supplemental oxygen, this signifies the presence of ventilation-perfusion mismatch, and likely does not need intubation
	  ○ If a patient's PaO_2 does not increase with supplemental oxygen, this signifies the presence of an intrapulmonary shunt; likely to progress to earlier invasive ventilator assistance
	• In addition to usual indications for intubation and mechanical ventilation, there are specific to COVID-19 approaches
	  ○ If venturi mask FiO_2 = 60% or SpO_2 <92% (or for hypercapnia or work of breathing), pre-oxygenate with non-rebreather and intubate
	  ○ Rapid sequence induction, avoiding bagging
	  ○ Intubation by even the most experienced airway provider using a video laryngoscope when proning (see below) is often unsuccessful
	Ventilator regimen
	• The strategy is to "buy time" while causing minimal additional damage, by maintaining the lowest possible PEEP and gentle ventilation[38]
	• Controversy re: high PEEP
	  ○ Pro: higher PEEP recommended by some (>10 cm H_2O, usually 13–24 cm H_2O)—extrapolated from ARDS treatment approaches prior to COVID-19 epidemic
	  ○ Con: high PEEP in a poorly recruitable lung tends to result in severe hemodynamic impairment and fluid retention[38]
	• Ventilator settings: either pressure control ventilation (PCV) or volume control ventilation (VCV)
	  ○ VCV: tidal volume (TV): 4–8 mL/kg of predicted body weight
	  ○ PCV/VCV: keep Pplat (plateau pressure) <30 cm H_2O

Early intubation vs delayed intubation	The role of early intubation and mechanical ventilation is not clear.[38] While some guidelines recommend early intubation, there is no supportive outcome evidence.[65] Early intubation might be reserved for deteriorating patients particularly those with underlying cardiopulmonary disease or altered mental status, to reduce the risk of severe hypoxemia.

		Early intubation	Delayed intubation
	Pro	• In patients on continuous positive airway pressure or noninvasive ventilation and clinical signs of excessive inspiratory efforts, intubation might help to avoid excessive intrathoracic negative pressures and self-inflicted lung injury (SILI)[38] • Many patients deteriorate precipitously, and they may be more safely intubated at an earlier stage in a controlled environment with less staff exposure • Maintaining adequate oxygenation	• See Con reasons of Early Intubation • Noninvasive ventilation, high-flow nasal cannula, and other means of O_2 delivery cause aerosolization of virus • Usual ARDS paradigm might not be applicable to COVID-19[38]: patients have normal-to-high compliance and seem to tolerate lower O_2 saturation levels and do reasonably well with Sat <90% • Other strategies are available: high-flow nasal cannula, awake proning (see later), care plan for dying patient, patients will spend less time on ventilators

	Con	• While SILI is not a well-demonstrated phenomenon, endotracheal tube placement and mechanical ventilation are prone to complications, which include the following:
		  ○ Ventilator induced lung injury (VILI)
		  ○ Ventilator-associated pneumonia
		  ○ Hemodynamic disturbances
		  ○ Complications related to sedation and immobilization and risk of encephalopathy and neuropathy
		• Each day of mechanical ventilation exposes patients to complications and increases mortality[66]
			• Prolonged exposure to hypoxia and potential end-organ (heart, liver, kidneys, brain) ischemia
			• Potential risk for crash intubation
			• Staff exposure to COVID-19 during emergency intubation

cont'd	
Prone positioning for nonintubated patients	• Prone position for as long as tolerated up to 24 h/day, for awake, spontaneously breathing COVID-19 patients with severe hypoxemic respiratory failure was associated with improved oxygenation and, if SpO_2 was ≥95% after 1 h prone, a lower rate of intubation[67] • Prone positioning could be maintained for at least 3 h in 84% of patients with substantial improvement in oxygenation (PaO_2/FiO_2 ratio 181 mm Hg supine vs 286 mm Hg prone) and after resupination, improved oxygenation was maintained in 50%. However, 30% of responders required intubation eventually[68] • In another study of COVID-19 hypoxemic respiratory failure managed outside the ICU, only 63% were able to tolerate prone positioning for >3 h and oxygenation increased in only 25% and sustained in only 50% of those after resupination[69]
Prone positioning for intubated patients	• Prone ventilation ~12 h/day (though prone positioning of patients with relatively high compliance provides only a modest benefit at the cost of a high demand for stressed human resources[32]) • However, to avoid delays in cardiopulmonary resuscitation (CPR) for cardiopulmonary arrest, it is advised to try prone CPR first (which has been shown to be successful)[70] since turning patients can require up to six personnel and may lead to dislodging of endotracheal tubes and lines[71]
Additional maneuvers for hypoxemia in mechanically ventilated patients[19,22,63]	• Neuromuscular blocking agents (intermittent unless persistent dyssynchrony, then continuous drip); should be limited exclusively to cases of: ○ Significant patient–ventilator dyssynchrony preventing the achievement of the set tidal volumes or ○ Rapidly progressing hypoxemia or hypercapnia • Trial of inhaled pulmonary vasodilators (as a rescue Rx)[72] • Recruitment maneuvers (but not incremental PEEP) • Diuresis • ECMO: initial reports from China showed poor outcome with 94% mortality[73] but later data suggested a benefit of ECMO with lower mortality (<40%) compared to those who did not receive ECMO[74,75] • If ARDS—systemic corticosteroids (see below)[63]
Cytokine release syndrome (CRS) treatment	• Interleukin-6 receptor (IL-6R) antagonist[57]: tocilizumab, sarilumab for patients who display elements of cytokine storm or secondary hemophagocytic lymphohistiocytosis with markedly elevated IL-6, ferritin, D-dimer, and hs-cTnI levels[15] • A proinflammatory syndrome with features of Kawasaki disease or toxic shock syndrome, but distinct from both, has been described to occur rarely, mainly in children and young adults, that appears to be related to COVID-19 and treated with IVIG, glucocorticoids, and/or IL-6 or IL-1 (1RA) inhibitors[94,95]

Anticoagulation	• Regularly monitoring of D-dimers, prothrombin time, and platelet count and prophylactic use of anticoagulation, e.g., low-molecular-weight heparin (LMWH) in all hospitalized patients, unless there are contraindications. LMWH has both anticoagulant and antiinflammatory effects and lowers mortality[52,96]
	• High-risk patients are identified by abnormal platelet count, prothrombin time, fibrinogen, fibrinogen-degradation products, D-dimer, and/or hypercoagulable thromboelastographic (TEG) parameters[97]
	• Systemic anticoagulation: Life-threatening thrombotic complications are not uncommon in patients with ARDS secondary to COVID-19 even with anticoagulation, suggesting the need for higher anticoagulation targets[98]:
	 ○ An alternative approach is to anticoagulate only those who have specific indications:
	  ■ Therapeutic anticoagulation should be strongly considered in patients at high risk for coagulopathy demonstrating signs of microthrombi-induced organ dysfunction, or with documented or strongly suspected macro-thromboembolism
	  ■ Use LMWH in patients with sepsis-induced coagulopathy (SIC) or DIC (elevated D-dimers). Early anticoagulant therapy (mainly LMWH) is associated with better prognosis in severe COVID-19 patients meeting SIC criteria or with markedly elevated D-dimer[55,96]
	 ○ Note: elevation of D-dimer levels may be associated with other disorders (e.g., infection, severe COVID-19 infection) rather than a blood clot[99]
	• Aspirin should be considered in cases with elevated troponin and cardiac dysfunction, particularly with elevated maximal amplitude on TEG[100]
	• DVT prophylaxis
	 ○ If CrCl >30: enoxaparin 40 mg SC daily
	 ○ If CrCl <30 or AKI: heparin 5000 units SC TID
	 ○ Hold if platelets <30,000 or bleeding, start thromboembolism deterrent (TED) stockings and /or sequential compression device (SCD)

Continued

cont'd	
TMA	• Complement activation plays a central role in the pathophysiology of TMA. Complement-mediated TMA is described by a two–hit disease model. There are two FDA–approved complement inhibitors to treat TMA: eculizumab and ravulizumab[51]
Steroids	• For early disease: little evidence of systemic corticosteroid benefit in the early acute phase of infection with conflicting evidence of risk/benefit from the World Health Organization[101,102] • Dexamethasone (6 mg/day) resulted in lower 28-day mortality among those receiving either mechanical ventilation or oxygen alone but not among those receiving no respiratory support[103,104,104a,104b] • No benefit of inhaled steroids[105] • Potential use in severe cases of ARDS and hemodynamic instability as discussed earlier
AKI with renal failure	• About 5%–35% of ICU patients require dialysis, usually occurring during the second week of COVID-19 with high mortality rates[14,106,107] • All forms of dialysis have been utilized, including intermittent hemodialysis, continuous renal replacement therapy (CRRT), or slow low efficiency dialysis. The latter two modalities, particularly continuous veno-venous hemofiltration (CVVH)[107], and even some peritoneal dialysis were preferred in patients with hemo-dynamics unsuitable for intermittent hemodialysis[107a,107b] • Use of niacinamide 1g/day orally for 7 days appeared to lower the risk of needing dialysis or death in patients with severe COVID-19-related AKI[107c]
GI bleeding (GIB) prophylaxis	• Prior to initiation of anticoagulation, patients at high-risk for GIB should be considered for proton-pump inhibitor (PPI) therapy and *Helicobacter pylori* testing[108] • Famotidine 20 mg IV BID in intubated patients; pantoprazole 20–40 mg IV daily if high risk or history of gastroesophageal reflux disease (GERD) or GIB
Other/supportive care	• Acetaminophen/paracetamol for control of fever • Stress ulcer prophylaxis as described above • Vitamin D supplementation to achieve high normal levels as prophylaxis[109] • Melatonin considered as adjuvant therapy to help sleep/sedation[110] • Blood purification techniques have been tried: either high-volume or high-molecular-weight cutoff hemo-filtration CRRT, blood/plasma perfusion, absorption, continuous plasma filtration absorption or plasma exchange[111]—no clinical evidentiary data to support use
Nutrition	• Enteral nutrition (e.g., osmolite 1.5 @ 10 mL/h, advance by 20 mL Q6h to goal 50 mL/h) • Tube feeding, if patient is prone—trickle tube feeding • Total parenteral nutrition (TPN) if tube feeding is insufficient and course will be prolonged[111a]

Criteria for transfer out of ICU/discharge

Patients could be discharged from the hospital or transferred from the ICU to other departments for comorbidities, when

• The body temperature has returned to normal for more than 3 days
• The respiratory symptoms are significantly improved
• The pulmonary lesions have markedly cleared
• Respiratory nucleic acid is tested negative for SARS-CoV-2 for two consecutive times at least 1 day apart (if viral exposure to others must be avoided).[20]

In addition, ICU patients should be evaluated daily for discharge when ICU beds are in short supply. ICU discharge criteria may also include no improvement and/or deterioration in condition, for example, cardiac arrest during ICU stay or significant organ failure, with consideration of palliative care following ICU discharge (see Table under ICU admission).[112]

REFERENCES

1. Liang W, Liang H, Ou L, et al. Development and validation of a clinical risk score to predict the occurrence of critical illness in hospitalized patients with COVID-19. *JAMA Intern Med.* 2020;180(8):1081–1089.
2. Knight SR, Ho A, Pius R, et al. Risk stratification of patients admitted to hospital with covid-19 using the ISARIC WHO Clinical Characterisation Protocol: development and validation of the 4C Mortality Score [published correction appears in BMJ. 2020 Nov 13;371:m4334]. *BMJ.* 2020;370:m3339.
3. Martínez-Rojas MA, Vega-Vega O, Bobadilla NA. Is the kidney a target of SARS-CoV-2? *Am J Physiol Renal Physiol.* 2020;318(6):F1454–F1462.

4. Chan JF, Kok KH, Zhu Z, et al. Genomic characterization of the 2019 novel human-pathogenic coronavirus isolated from a patient with atypical pneumonia after visiting Wuhan. *Emerg Microbes Infect.* 2020;9(1):221–236.

5. Sun P, Lu X, Xu C, Sun W, Pan B. Understanding of COVID-19 based on current evidence. *J Med Virol.* 2020;92(6):548–551.

6. Abate BB, Kassie AM, Kassaw MW, Aragie TG, Masresha SA. Sex difference in coronavirus disease (COVID-19): a systematic review and meta-analysis. *BMJ Open.* 2020;10(10):e040129.

7. Mancia G, Rea F, Ludergnani M, Apolone G, Corrao G. Renin–angiotensin–aldosterone system blockers and the risk of Covid-19. *N Engl J Med.* 2020;382(25):2431–2440.

8. Reynolds HR, Adhikari S, Pulgarin C, et al. Renin–angiotensin–aldosterone system inhibitors and risk of Covid-19. *N Engl J Med.* 2020;382(25):2441–2448.

8a. Center for Disease Control and Prevention. Delta Variant: What We Know about the Science. Accessed September 10, 2021 at https://www.cdc.gov/coronavirus/2019-ncov/variants/delta-variant.html?s_cid=11511:covid%20delta%20variant%20transmission:sem.ga:p:RG:GM:gen:PTN:FY21.

8b. Center for Disease Control and Prevention. SARS-CoV-2 Variant Classifications and Definitions. Accessed September 11, 2021 at https://www.cdc.gov/coronavirus/2019-ncov/variants/variant-info.html.

9. Rothan HA, Byrareddy SN. The epidemiology and pathogenesis of coronavirus disease (COVID-19) outbreak. *J Autoimmun.* 2020;109:102433.

10. He F, Deng Y, Li W. Coronavirus disease 2019: what we know? *J Med Virol.* 2020;92(7):719–725.

10a. Allinovi M, Parise A, Giacalone M, et al. Lung ultrasound may support diagnosis and monitoring of COVID-19 pneumonia. *Ultrasound Med Biol.* 2020;46(11):2908–2917. https://doi.org/10.1016/j.ultrasmedbio.2020.07.018.

10b. Wang M, Luo X, Wang L, et al. A comparison of lung ultrasound and computed tomography in the diagnosis of patients with COVID-19: a systematic review and meta-analysis. *Diagnostics (Basel).* 2021;11(8):1351. https://doi.org/10.3390/diagnostics11081351.

11. Wu Z, McGoogan JM. Characteristics of and important lessons from the coronavirus disease 2019 (COVID-19) outbreak in China: summary of a report of 72 314 cases from the Chinese Center for Disease Control and Prevention. *J Am Med Assoc.* 2020;323(13):1239–1242.

12. Huang C, Wang Y, Li X, et al. Clinical features of patients infected with 2019 novel coronavirus in Wuhan, China. *Lancet.* 2020;395(10223):497–506.

13. Yang X, Yu Y, Xu J, et al. Clinical course and outcomes of critically ill patients with SARS-CoV-2 pneumonia in Wuhan, China: a single-centered, retrospective, observational study. *Lancet Respir Med.* 2020;8(5):475–481.

13a. Ng JH, Hirsch JS, Hazzan A, et al. Outcomes among patients hospitalized with COVID-19 and acute kidney injury. *Am J Kidney Dis.* 2021;77(2):204–215.e1. https://doi.org/10.1053/j.ajkd.2020.09.002.

14. Thakkar J, Chand S, Aboodi MS, et al. Characteristics, outcomes and 60-day hospital mortality of ICU patients with Covid-19 and acute kidney injury. *Kidney360.* 2020;1(12):1339–1344.

15. Clerkin KJ, Fried JA, Raikhelkar J, et al. Coronavirus disease 2019 (COVID-19) and cardiovascular disease. *Circulation.* 2020;141(20):1648–1655.

16. Meng X, Deng Y, Dai Z, Meng Z. COVID-19 and anosmia: a review based on up-to-date knowledge. *Am J Otolaryngol.* 2020;41(5):102581.

17. Lee Y, Min P, Lee S, Kim SW. Prevalence and duration of acute loss of smell or taste in COVID-19 patients. *J Korean Med Sci.* 2020;35(18):e174.

18. Mao L, Jin H, Wang M, et al. Neurologic manifestations of hospitalized patients with coronavirus disease 2019 in Wuhan, China. *JAMA Neurol.* 2020;77(6):683–690.

19. Wujtewicz M, Dylczyk-Sommer A, Aszkiełowicz A, Zdanowski S, Piwowarczyk S, Owczuk R. COVID-19—what should anaethesiologists and intensivists know about it? *Anaesthesiol Intensive Ther.* 2020;52(1):34–41.

20. Li T. Diagnosis and clinical management of severe acute respiratory syndrome coronavirus 2 (SARS-CoV-2) infection: an operational recommendation of Peking Union Medical College Hospital (V2.0): working group of 2019 novel coronavirus, Peking Union Medical College Hospital. *Emerg Microbes Infect.* 2020;9(1):582–585.

21. Tang YW, Schmitz JE, Persing DH, Stratton CW. Laboratory diagnosis of COVID-19: current issues and challenges. *J Clin Microbiol.* 2020;58(6):e00512–e00520.

22. Coronavirus (COVID-19) update: critical care. YouTube. https://www.youtube.com/watch?v=c7s3fS6RTlQ&feature=youtu.be%3Futm_source%3Dsilverchair&utm_medium=email&utm_campaign=article_alert-jama&utm_content=olf&utm_term=032320.

23. Matthay MA, Aldrich JM, Gotts JE. Treatment for severe acute respiratory distress syndrome from COVID-19. *Lancet Resp Med.* 2020;8(5):433–434.

24. Lee SM, An WS. New clinical criteria for septic shock: serum lactate level as new emerging vital sign. *J Thorac Dis.* 2016;8(7):1388–1390.

25. Swiss Academy of Medical Sciences. COVID-19 pandemic: triage for intensive-care treatment under resource scarcity. *Swiss Med Wkly.* 2020;150:w20229.

26. Khan S, Chen L, Yang C-R, Raghuram V, Khundmiri SJ, Knepper MA. Does SARS-CoV-2 infect the kidney? *J Am Soc Nephrol.* 2020;31(12):2746–2748.

27. Farkash EA, Wilson AM, Jentzen JM. Ultrastructural evidence for direct renal infection with SARS-CoV-2. *J Am Soc Nephrol.* 2020;31(8):1683–1687.

28. Martinez-Rojas MA, Vega-Vega O, Bobadilla NA. Is the kidney a target of SARS-CoV-2? *Am J Physiol Renal Physiol.* 2020;318(6):F1454–F1462.

29. Helms J, Tacquard C, Severac F, et al. High risk of thrombosis in patients with severe SARS-CoV-2 infection: a multicenter prospective cohort study. *Intensive Care Med.* 2020;46(6):1089–1098.

30. Sharma P, Uppal NN, Wanchoo R, et al. COVID-19–associated kidney injury: a case series of kidney biopsy findings. *J Am Soc Nephrol.* 2020;31(9):1948–1958.

31. Grasselli G, Greco M, Zanella A, et al. Risk factors associated with mortality among patients with COVID-19 in intensive care units in Lombardy, Italy. *JAMA Intern Med*. 2020;180(10):1345–1355.

32. Gattinoni L, Chiumello D, Rossi S. COVID-19 pneumonia: ARDS or not? *Crit Care*. 2020;24(1):154.

33. Tobin MJ. Basing respiratory management of COVID-19 on physiological principles. *Am J Respir Crit Care Med*. 2020;201(11):1319–1320.

34. Fisher HK. Hypoxemia in COVID-19 patients: an hypothesis. *Med Hypotheses*. 2020;143:110022.

35. Zhang X, Zhang X, Li S, Niu S. ACE2 and COVID-19 and the resulting ARDS. *Postgrad Med J*. 2020;96(1137):403–407.

36. McGonagle D, O'Donnell JS, Sharif K, Emery P, Bridgewood C. Immune mechanisms of pulmonary intravascular coagulopathy in COVID-19 pneumonia. *Lancet Rheumatol*. 2020;2(7):e437–e445.

37. Ciceri F, Beretta L, Scandroglio AM, et al. Microvascular COVID-19 lung vessels obstructive thromboinflammatory syndrome (MicroCLOTS): an atypical acute respiratory distress syndrome working hypothesis. *Crit Care Resusc*. 2020;22(2):95–97.

38. Gattinoni L, Coppola S, Cressoni M, Busana M, Chiumello D. COVID-19 does not lead to a "typical" acute respiratory distress syndrome. *Am J Respir Crit Care Med*. 2020;201(10):1299–1300.

39. Pei G, Zhang Z, Peng J, et al. Renal involvement and early prognosis in patients with COVID-19 pneumonia. *J Am Soc Nephrol*. 2020;31(6):1157–1165.

40. Hirsch JS, Ng JH, Ross DW, et al. Acute kidney injury in patients hospitalized with COVID-19. *Kidney Int*. 2020;98(1):209–218.

41. Cheng Y, Luo R, Wang K, et al. Kidney disease is associated with in-hospital death of patients with COVID-19. *Kidney Int*. 2020;97(5):829–838.

41a. Yende S, Parikh CR. Long COVID and kidney disease. *Nat Rev Nephrol*. 2021:1–2. https://doi.org/10.1038/s41581-021-00487-3.

42. Farkash EA, Wilson AM, Jentzen JM. Ultrastructural evidence for direct renal infection with SARS-CoV-2. *J Am Soc Nephrol*. 2020;31(8):1683–1687.

43. Ronco C, Reis T, Husain-Syed F. Management of acute kidney injury in patients with COVID-19. *Lancet Respir Med*. 2020;8(7):738–742.

44. Kudose S, Batal I, Santoriello D, et al. Kidney biopsy findings in patients with COVID-19. *J Am Soc Nephrol*. 2020;31(9):1959–1968.

45. Wu H, Larsen CP, Hernandez-Arroyo CF, et al. AKI and collapsing glomerulopathy associated with COVID-19 and APOL1 high-risk genotype. *J Am Soc Nephrol*. 2020;31(8):1688–1695.

46. Zheng YY, Ma YT, Zhang JY, Xie X. COVID-19 and the cardiovascular system. *Nat Rev Cardiol*. 2020;17(5):259–260.

47. Campbell CM, Kahwash R. Will complement inhibition be the new target in treating COVID-19-related systemic thrombosis? *Circulation*. 2020;141(22):1739–1741.

48. Wu Y, Xu X, Chen Z, et al. Nervous system involvement after infection with COVID-19 and other coronaviruses. *Brain Behav Immun*. 2020;87:18–22.

49. Ye M, Ren Y, Lv T. Encephalitis as a clinical manifestation of COVID-19. *Brain Behav Immun*. 2020;88:945–946.

50. Varga Z, Flammer AJ, Steiger P, et al. Endothelial cell infection and endotheliitis in COVID-19. *Lancet*. 2020;395(10234):1417–1418.

51. Gavriilaki E, Brodsky RA. Severe COVID-19 infection and thrombotic microangiopathy: success does not come easily. *Br J Haematol*. 2020;189(6):e227–e230.

52. The Lancet Haematology. COVID-19 coagulopathy: an evolving story. *Lancet Haematol*. 2020;7(6):e425.

53. Zhang Y, Xiao M, Zhang S, et al. Coagulopathy and antiphospholipid antibodies in patients with Covid-19. *N Engl J Med*. 2020;382(17):e38.

54. Harzallah I, Debliquis A, Drénou B. Lupus anticoagulant is frequent in patients with Covid−19. *J Thromb Haemost*. 2020;18(8):2064–2065.

55. Li T, Lu H, Zhang W. Clinical observation and management of COVID-19 patients. *Emerg Microbes Infect*. 2020;9(1):687–690.

56. Xu P, Zhou Q, Xu J. Mechanism of thrombocytopenia in COVID-19 patients. *Ann Hematol*. 2020;99(6):1205–1208.

57. Zhang C, Wu Z, Li JW, Zhao H, Wang GQ. The cytokine release syndrome (CRS) of severe COVID-19 and interleukin-6 receptor (IL-6R) antagonist tocilizumab may be the key to reduce the mortality. *Int J Antimicrob Agents*. 2020;55(5):105954.

58. Su TH, Kao JH. The clinical manifestations and management of COVID-19-related liver injury. *J Formos Med Assoc*. 2020;119(6):1016–1018.

59. Garrido I, Liberal R, Macedo G. Review article: COVID-19 and liver disease—what we know on 1st May 2020. *Aliment Pharmacol Ther*. 2020;52(2):267–275.

60. Suwanwongse K, Shabarek N. Rhabdomyolysis as a presentation of 2019 novel coronavirus disease. *Cureus*. 2020;12(4):e7561.

61. Li J, Wang X, Chen J, Zuo X, Zhang H, Deng A. COVID-19 infection may cause ketosis and ketoacidosis. *Diabetes Obes Metab*. 2020;22(10):1935–1941.

62. Sathish T, Kapoor N, Cao Y, Tapp RJ, Zimmet P. Proportion of newly diagnosed diabetes in COVID-19 patients: a systematic review and meta-analysis. *Diabetes Obes Metab*. 2021;23(3):870–874.

63. Alhazzani W, Møller MH, Arabi YM, et al. Surviving sepsis campaign: guidelines on the management of critically ill adults with coronavirus disease 2019 (COVID-19). *Intensive Care Med*. 2020;48(6):e440–e469.

64. Brigham and Women's Hospital COVID-19 Critical Care Clinical Guidelines. https://www.covidprotocols.org/. Accessed September 14, 2021.
65. Brewster DJ, Chrimes N, Do TB, et al. Consensus statement: Safe Airway Society principles of airway management and tracheal intubation specific to the COVID-19 adult patient group. *Med J Aust*. 2020;212(10):472–481.
66. Tobin MJ, Laghi F, Jubran A. Caution about early intubation and mechanical ventilation in COVID-19. *Ann Intensive Care*. 2020;10(1):78.
67. Thompson AE, Ranard BL, Wei Y, Jelic S. Prone positioning in awake, nonintubated patients with COVID-19 hypoxemic respiratory failure. *JAMA Intern Med*. 2020;180(11):1537–1539.
68. Coppo A, Bellani G, Winterton D, et al. Feasibility and physiological effects of prone positioning in non-intubated patients with acute respiratory failure due to COVID-19 (PRON-COVID): a prospective cohort study. *Lancet Respir Med*. 2020;8(8):765–774.
69. Elharrar X, Trigui Y, Dols AM, et al. Use of prone positioning in nonintubated patients with COVID-19 and hypoxemic acute respiratory failure. *J Am Med Assoc*. 2020;323(22):2336–2338.
70. Douma MJ, MacKenzie E, Loch T, et al. Prone cardiopulmonary resuscitation: a scoping and expanded grey literature review for the COVID-19 pandemic. *Resuscitation*. 2020;155:103–111.
71. Barker J, Koeckerling D, West R. A need for prone position CPR guidance for intubated and non-intubated patients during the COVID-19 pandemic. *Resuscitation*. 2020;151:135–136.
72. Wright BJ. Inhaled pulmonary vasodilators in refractory hypoxemia. *Clin Exp Emerg Med*. 2015;2(3):184–187.
73. Henry BM, Lippi G. Poor survival with extracorporeal membrane oxygenation in acute respiratory distress syndrome (ARDS) due to coronavirus disease 2019 (COVID-19): pooled analysis of early reports. *J Crit Care*. 2020;58:27–28.
74. Barbaro RP, MacLaren G, Boonstra PS, et al. Extracorporeal membrane oxygenation support in COVID-19: an international cohort study of the Extracorporeal Life Support Organization registry. *Lancet*. 2020;396(10257):1071–1078.
75. Shaefi S, Brenner SK, Gupta S, et al. Extracorporeal membrane oxygenation in patients with severe respiratory failure from COVID-19. *Intensive Care Med*. 2021;47(2):208–221.
76. Grein J, Ohmagari N, Shin N, et al. Compassionate use of remdesivir for patients with severe Covid-19. *N Engl J Med*. 2020;382(24):2327–2336.
77. Dong L, Hu S, Gao J. Discovering drugs to treat coronavirus disease 2019 (COVID-19). *Drug Discov Ther*. 2020;14(1):58–60.
78. Beigel JH, Tomashek KM, Dodd LE, et al. Remdesivir for the treatment of Covid-19—preliminary report. *N Engl J Med*. 2020;383(19):1813–1826.
78a. Ansems K, Grundeis F, Dahms K, et al. Remdesivir for the treatment of COVID-19. *Cochrane Database Syst Rev*. 2021;8:CD014962. https://doi.org/10.1002/14651858.CD014962.
78b. Reddy DOS, Lai DW. Tackling COVID−19 using remdesivir and favipiravir as therapeutic options. *Chembiochem*. 2021;22(6):939–948. https://doi.org/10.1002/CBIC.202000595.
78c. Chen C-Y, Chen W-C, Hsu C-K, Chao C-M, Lai C-C. Clinical efficacy and safety of Janus kinase inhibitors for COVID-19: a systematic review and meta-analysis of randomized controlled trials. *Int Immunopharmacol*. 2021;99:108027. https://doi.org/10.1016/j.intimp.2021.108027.
78d. Wijaya I, Andhika R, Huang I, et al. The use of Janus Kinase inhibitors in hospitalized patients with COVID-19: systematic review and meta-analysis. *Clin Epidemiol Glob Heal*. 2021;11:100755. https://doi.org/10.1016/j.cegh.2021.100755.
78e. Kalil AC, Patterson TF, Mehta AK, et al. Baricitinib plus remdesivir for hospitalized adults with covid-19. *N Engl J Med*. 2021;384(9):795–807. https://doi.org/10.1056/NEJMOA2031994.
78f. Antiviral Abidol Is Associated with the Reduction of In-Hosp... : Cardiology Discovery. https://journals.lww.com/cd/Fulltext/2021/03000/Antiviral_Abidol_is_Associated_with_the_Reduction.13.aspx. Accessed September 14, 2021.
79. Agrawal U, Raju R, Udwadia ZF. Favipiravir: a new and emerging antiviral option in COVID-19. *Med J Armed Forces India*. 2020;76(4):370–376.
80. Cao B, Wang Y, Wen D, et al. A trial of lopinavir–ritonavir in adults hospitalized with severe Covid-19. *N Engl J Med*. 2020;382(19):1787–1799.
81. Agrawal S, Goel AD, Gupta N. Emerging prophylaxis strategies against COVID-19. *Monaldi Arch Chest Dis*. 2020;90(1):1289.
82. Zhu S, Guo X, Geary K, Zhang D. Emerging therapeutic strategies for COVID-19 patients. *Discoveries*. 2020;8(1):e105.
83. Colson P, Rolain JM, Lagier JC, Brouqui P, Raoult D. Chloroquine and hydroxychloroquine as available weapons to fight COVID-19. *Int J Antimicrob Agents*. 2020;55(4):105932.
84. Fung KL, Chan PL. Comment on: COVID-19: a recommendation to examine the effect of hydroxychloroquine in preventing infection and progression. *J Antimicrob Chemother*. 2020;75(7):2016–2017.
85. Boulware DR, Pullen MF, Bangdiwala AS, et al. A randomized trial of hydroxychloroquine as postexposure prophylaxis for Covid-19. *N Engl J Med*. 2020;383(6):517–525.
86. Skipper CP, Pastick KA, Engen NW, et al. Hydroxychloroquine in nonhospitalized adults with early COVID-19 : a randomized trial. *Ann Intern Med*. 2020;173(8):623–631.
87. Davoudi-Monfared E, Rahmani H, Khalili H, et al. A randomized clinical trial of the efficacy and safety of interferon β-1a in treatment of severe COVID-19. *Antimicrob Agents Chemother*. 2020;64(9): e01061-20.
88. Rahmani H, Davoudi-Monfared E, Nourian A, et al. Interferon β-1b in treatment of severe COVID-19: a randomized clinical trial. *Int Immunopharmacol*. 2020;88:106903.

89. Roback JD, Guarner J. Convalescent plasma to treat COVID-19: possibilities and challenges. *J Am Med Assoc.* 2020;323(16):1561–1562.

90. Duan K, Liu B, Li C, et al. Effectiveness of convalescent plasma therapy in severe COVID-19 patients. *Proc Natl Acad Sci USA.* 2020;117(17):9490–9496.

91. An EUA for casirivimab and imdevimab for COVID-19. *Med Lett Drugs Ther.* 2020;62(1614):201–202.

92. An EUA for bamlanivimab—a monoclonal antibody for COVID-19. *Med Lett Drugs Ther.* 2020;62(1612):185–186.

93. An EUA for baricitinib (Olumiant) for COVID-19. *Med Lett Drugs Ther.* 2020;62(1614):202–203.

93a. Anti-SARS-CoV-2 Monoclonal Antibodies | COVID-19 Treatment Guidelines. https://www.covid19treatmentguidelines.nih.gov/therapies/anti-sars-cov-2-antibody-products/anti-sars-cov-2-monoclonal-antibodies/. Accessed September 14, 2021.

93b. NIH. The COVID-19 Treatment Guidelines Panel's Statement on the Emergency Use Authorization of Casirivimab Plus Imdevimab as Post-Exposure Prophylaxis for SARS-CoV-2 Infection. https://www.covid19treatmentguidelines.nih.gov/therapies/statement-on-the-prioritization-of-anti-sars-cov-2-monoclonal-antibodies/. Accessed September 14, 2021.

94. Cheung EW, Zachariah P, Gorelik M, et al. Multisystem inflammatory syndrome related to COVID-19 in previously healthy children and adolescents in New York City. *J Am Med Assoc.* 2020;324(3):294–296.

95. Feldstein LR, Rose EB, Horwitz SM, et al. Multisystem inflammatory syndrome in U.S. children and adolescents. *N Engl J Med.* 2020;383(4):334–346.

96. Tang N, Bai H, Chen X, Gong J, Li D, Sun Z. Anticoagulant treatment is associated with decreased mortality in severe coronavirus disease 2019 patients with coagulopathy. *J Thromb Haemost.* 2020;18(5):1094–1099.

97. Mortus JR, Manek SE, Brubaker LS, et al. Thromboelastographic results and hypercoagulability syndrome in patients with coronavirus disease 2019 who are critically ill. *JAMA Netw Open.* 2020;3(6):e2011192.

98. Helms J, Tacquard C, Severac F, et al. High risk of thrombosis in patients with severe SARS-CoV-2 infection: a multicenter prospective cohort study. *Intensive Care Med.* 2020;46(6):1089–1098.

99. World Thrombosis Day. Covid-19 and Thrombosis. https://www.worldthrombosisday.org/news/post/covid-19-thrombosis/. Accessed September 14, 2021.

100. Parker BM, Do VJH, Rattan R. Coagulopathy in covid-19: review and recommendations. https://www.facs.org/-/media/files/covid19/umiami_study_uses_of_coagulopathy.ashx. Accessed September 14, 2021.

101. WHO welcomes preliminary results about dexamethasone use in treating critically ill COVID-19 patients. https://www.who.int/news-room/detail/16-06-2020-who-welcomes-preliminary-results-about-dexamethasone-use-in-treating-critically-ill-covid-19-patients. Accessed September 14, 2021.

102. Russell B, Moss C, Rigg A, Van Hemelrijck M. COVID-19 and treatment with NSAIDs and corticosteroids: should we be limiting their use in the clinical setting? *Ecancermedicalscience.* 2020;14:1023.

103. RECOVERY Collaborative Group, Horby P, Lim WS, et al. Dexamethasone in hospitalized patients with Covid-19—preliminary report. *N Engl J Med.* 2020;384(8):693–704.

104. Wiersinga WJ, Rhodes A, Cheng AC, Peacock SJ, Prescott HC. Pathophysiology, transmission, diagnosis, and treatment of coronavirus disease 2019 (COVID-19): a review. *J Am Med Assoc.* 2020;324(8):782–793.

104a. Noreen S, Maqbool I, Madni A. Dexamethasone: therapeutic potential, risks, and future projection during COVID-19 pandemic. *Eur J Pharmacol.* 2021:894. https://doi.org/10.1016/J.EJPHAR.2021.173854.

104b. Alexaki VI, Henneicke H. The role of glucocorticoids in the management of COVID-19. *Horm Metab Res.* 2021;53(1):9–15. https://doi.org/10.1055/A-1300-2550.

105. Halpin DMG, Singh D, Hadfield RM. Inhaled corticosteroids and COVID-19: a systematic review and clinical perspective. *Eur Respir J.* 2020;55(5):2001009.

106. Durvasula R, Wellington T, McNamara E, Watnick S. COVID-19 and kidney failure in the acute care setting: our experience from Seattle. *Am J Kidney Dis.* 2020;76(1):4–6.

107. Gupta S, Coca SG, Chan L, et al. AKI treated with renal replacement therapy in critically ill patients with COVID-19. *J Am Soc Nephrol.* 2021;32(1):161–176.

107a. Shamy O El, Patel N, Abdelbaset MH, et al. Acute start peritoneal dialysis during the COVID-19 pandemic: outcomes and experiences. *J Am Soc Nephrol.* 2020;31(8):1680. https://doi.org/10.1681/ASN.2020050599.

107b. Chen W, Caplin N, El Shamy O, et al. Use of peritoneal dialysis for acute kidney injury during the COVID-19 pandemic in New York City: a multicenter observational study. *Kidney Int.* 2021;100(1):2–5. https://doi.org/10.1016/j.kint.2021.04.017.

107c. Raines NH, Ganatra S, Nissaisorakarn P, et al. Niacinamide may be associated with improved outcomes in COVID-19-related acute kidney injury: an observational study. *Kidney360.* 2021;2(1):33–41. https://doi.org/10.34067/KID.0006452020.

108. Patel P, Sengupta N. PPIs and beyond: a framework for managing anticoagulation-related gastrointestinal bleeding in the era of COVID-19. *Dig Dis Sci.* 2020;65(8):2181–2186.

109. Grant WB, Lahore H, McDonnell SL, et al. Evidence that vitamin D supplementation could reduce risk of influenza and COVID-19 infections and deaths. *Nutrients.* 2020;12(4):988.

110. Zhang R, Wang X, Ni L, et al. COVID-19: melatonin as a potential adjuvant treatment. *Life Sci.* 2020;250:117583.

111. Yang XH, Sun RH, Zhao MY, et al. Expert recommendations on blood purification treatment protocol for patients with severe COVID-19: recommendation and consensus. *Chronic Dis Transl Med.* 2020;6(2):106–114.

111a. Mechanick JI, Carbone S, Dickerson RN, et al. Clinical nutrition research and the COVID-19 pandemic: a scoping review of the aspen covid-19 task force on nutrition research. *JPEN J Parenter Enteral Nutr.* 2021;45(1):13. https://doi.org/10.1002/JPEN.2036.

112. Tyrrell CSB, Mytton OT, Gentry SV, et al. Managing intensive care admissions when there are not enough beds during the COVID-19 pandemic: a systematic review. *Thorax.* 2020:1–11.

CHAPTER 14

Useful Formulae and Abbreviations

Alexander Goldfarb-Rumyantzev

Water-Electrolyte and Acid-Base Disorders

Anion gap $= (Na^+) - (HCO_3^- + Cl^-)$

Na deficit $= (Na_{normal} - Na_{measured}) \times 0.6 \times$ total body weight

Bicarbonate deficit $= (0.4 \times$ total body weight$) \times ($bicarbonate desired $-$ bicarbonate measured$)$

SubstanceX deficit $=$ Substance*X* Volume of distribution $\times$ (Normal value $-$ real value)

Water deficit $= [(Na_{measured}/Na_{normal})] - 1) \times 0.6 \times$ total body weight

The formula is derived as follows:

TBNa – total body Na

C_{Na0} – concentration of sodium in baseline state

C_{Nai} – concentration of sodium at time i

W – total body water

BW – body weight

Water $=$ TBNa $/ C_{Na}$

TBNa $= C_{Na} \times 0.6 \times$ BW

Water Deficit $= (TBNa/C_{Na0}) - (TBNa/C_{Nai})$

Water Deficit $= (C_{Nai} \times 0.6 \times BW_i/C_{Na0}) - (C_{Nai} \times 0.6 \times BW_i/C_{Nai}) = 0.6 \times BW_i \times [(C_{Nai} - C_{Na0}) -1]$

Corrected Na $=$ Measured Na $+ [1.5 ($Glucose $- 150)/100]$ (or for each 100 of glucose above normal $+1.6$ of Na)

(e.g., Na is 148, glucose 700: corrected Na 148 + [6 × 1.6] = 157.6)

Ca corrected for albumin level $=$ Measured Ca $+ [($Normal albumin $-$ Patient's albumin$) 0.8$ (or 0.7)]

Dilantin level corrected for albumin $= 0.1 + ($Measured Dilantin$/ [$albumin level $\times 0.2])$

Fractional Excretion of Na $= (Na_U/Na_P)/(Cr_U/Cr_P) \times 100\%$ (inverse indicator of the level of reabsorption: $>1\%$ – ATN, $<1\%$ – prerenal)

Osmolality $= 2(Na^+ + K^+) +$ Glucose$/18 +$ BUN$/2.8$

Osmolality $= 2Na^+ + 10$ (if K^+, Glucose, and BUN are normal)

Cr Clearance $= (Cr_{urine}/Cr_{plasma}) \times 24$ h urine volume

Cr Clearance (male) $= [$TBWeight $\times (140 -$ age$)]/[$Serum Cr $\times 72]$

Cr Clearance (female) $= 0.85$ (Cr Clearance male)

pH correction for $pCO_2 =$ for each 10 of $pCO_2 - 0.08$ (acute) or 0.04 (chronic) of pH

Normal Compensation Response in Metabolic Acidosis:

(pH 7.3–7.4): last $pCO_2 = 2$ digits of pH

$pCO_2 = ($bicarbonate $\times 1.5) + 8$

Normal Compensation Response in Metabolic Alkalosis:

$pCO_2 = +6$ for each ↑10 of bicarbonate

$pCO_2 = ($bicarbonate $\times 0.9) + 15$

Nutrition in Hospitalized Patient

Maintenance fluids rate $= 1.3$ mL/kg/h

Daily caloric requirements (kcal): $25 \times$ body weight (kg) if on TPN: $32 \div 40 \times$ body weight

Protein intake (g/day): $0.8 \times$ body weight (kg)

Body mass index $=$ weight in kg/(height in m)^2

>28 associated with four times higher risk of morbidity of stroke, angina, DM

Daily Energy Requirements for Patients with Acute Renal Failure

$BMR = (391.6 + 18.56 \times BW) \times 1.25$

or, if patient is paralyzed or heavily sedated:

$BMR = 391.6 + 18.56 \times BW$

$ER = BMR \times SF$

BW – Body weight (kg)	ER – Energy Requirements (kcal/day)
BMR – Basal Metabolic Rate (kcal)	SF – Stress Factor

Estimation of Energy Requirements Corrected for Hypermetabolism

Disease Accompanying Acute Renal Failure	Stress Factor
Early starvation	0.925
Postoperative (no complications)	1.025
Long bone fracture	1.225
Cancer	1.275
Peritonitis	1.15
Severe infection/multiple trauma	1.425
Burns: 10%–30% body surface area	1.5
Burns: 30%–50% body surface area	1.75
Burns: >50% body surface area	2

Cardiology

Systemic Vascular Resistance = $(MAP - CVP)/CO(L/min)$ (Wood units) $\times 80$ – dynes $\times$ sec $\times$ cm^{-5}

LDL Cholesterol = Total − HDL − Triglycerides/5

Mean BP = $(SBP + 2 \times DBP)/3$

Normal cardiac index = 2.5–3.8 L/min/m^2

EF = Stroke volume/End diastolic volume

Oxygen consumption = Cardiac output $\times$ $(p_aO_2 -$ Mixed venous O$_2)$

CHAD2 evaluates ischemic stroke risk in patients with atrial fibrillation

CHADS2 =

Congestive heart failure (+1)

Hypertension (+1)

Age 75 years or older (+1)

Diabetes mellitus (+1)

Stroke or TIA (+1)

Respiratory

Oxygen consumption: $V_{O2} = CO \times (p_aO_2 - p_vO_2)$ $(p_aO_2 - pv_{O2}$ means arterial minus mixed venous oxygen content difference; CO is cardiac output); $V_{O2} = 130 \div 140 \times$ body surface area

Mixed venous oxygen content: $p_vO_2 = p_aO_2 - (V_{O2}/CO)$

$pCO_2 = CO_2$ production / alveolar ventilation

Alveolar ventilation = minute ventilation − dead space ventilation

Minute ventilation = rate $\times$ TV

A-a gradient = A − a (A is the pO$_2$ of the inhaled air [inside the lungs]; a is arterial pO$_2$ [p_aO_2])

$A = 713 \times FiO_2 - (PaCO_2/0.8)$ or $A = 713 \times FiO_2 - PaO_2 + (pCO_2 \times 1.25)$

On room air: $A = FiO_2 \times 713 = 150$

Hematology

Transferrin saturation (%) = (Iron/TIBC) × 100%

Corrected reticulocytes (what reticulocyte % would be if patient was not anemic): Corrected reticulocytes = (Hct/45) × patient's reticulocytes

Toxicology

Dose of activate charcoal = 1 g/kg of body weight

Distribution volume of toxin = Amount ingested/Plasma concentration

Body Measurements

$BSA = (BW^{0.425}) \times (H^{0.725}) \times 71.84/10{,}000$

BSA – body surface area

BW – body weight (kg)

H – height (m)

$BMI = Weight (kg) \div Height (m^2)$

Abbreviations

A-a gradient – alveolar–arterial oxygen gradient

AAA – abdominal aortic aneurism

AAV – ANCA–associated vasculitides

ABG – arterial blood gas

ABx – antibiotics

AC – assist control

ACE2 –angiotensin-converting enzyme 2

ACEI – angiotensin-converting enzyme inhibitors

ACS – abdominal compartment syndrome

ACS – acute coronary syndrome

ACTH – adrenocorticotropic hormone

ADH – antidiuretic hormone

ADQI – Acute Dialysis Quality Initiative

AFB – acid-fast bacteria

AG – anion gap

AI – adrenal insufficiency

AI – aortic insufficiency

AIHA – autoimmune hemolytic anemia

AIN – acute interstitial nephritis

AKI – acute kidney injury

AKIN – Acute Kidney Injury Network

Akt – serine-threonine protein kinase B

ALI – acute lung injury

ALK – anaplastic lymphoma kinase

ALL – acute lymphocytic leukemia

AMS – altered mental status

ANA – antinuclear autoantibodies

ANCA – antineutrophilic cytoplasmic antibody

ANP – atrial natriuretic peptide

APP – abdominal perfusion pressure

APRV – airway pressure release ventilation

APS – antiphospholipid syndrome

APS1 – autoimmune polyendocrine syndrome type 1

ARB – angiotensin receptor blocker

ARDS – acute respiratory distress syndrome

ARF – acute renal failure

ARF – acute respiratory failure

ARF-D – acute renal failure that required dialysis

AS – aortic stenosis

ASA – aspirin

ASB – asymptomatic bacteriuria

ATN – acute tubular necrosis

AV – arteriovenous

AV – atrioventricular

AVF – arteriovenous fistula

AVG – arteriovenous graft

AVM – arteriovenous malformation

AXR – abdominal X-ray

AZA – azathioprine

BAL – bronchoalveolar lavage

BCR-ABL – breakpoint cluster region–Abelson

BMD – bone mineral density

BRAF – v-Raf murine sarcoma viral oncogene homolog B

BSA – body surface area

BUN – blood urea nitrogen

BW – body weight

CA – catheter-associated

CAA – cerebral amyloid angiopathy

CAD – coronary artery disease

cANCA – cytoplasmic ANCA

CAPD – continuous ambulatory PD

CAPS – catastrophic antiphospholipid syndrome

CaSR – calcium-sensing receptor

CAVH – continuous arteriovenous hemofiltration

CCB – calcium-channel blocker

CCP – anticyclic citrullinated peptide

CCPD – continuous cycling peritoneal dialysis

CDI – *Clostridium difficile* infection

CFA – cyclophosphamide

CFPD – continuous flow peritoneal dialysis

CFU – colony-forming units

CHF – congestive heart failure

CI – cardiac index

CKD – chronic kidney disease

CLL – chronic lymphocytic leukemia

CML – chronic myeloid (myelogenous) leukemia

CMML – chronic myelomonocytic leukemia

CMV – continuous mandatory ventilation

CMV – cytomegalovirus

CNS – central nervous system

CO – carbon monoxide

CO – cardiac output

CoNS – coagulase negative staphylococci

COPD – chronic obstructive pulmonary disease

COVID-19 – coronavirus disease 2019

CoVs – coronaviruses

CPP – cerebral perfusion pressure

CPPD – calcium pyrophosphate dihydrate crystal

CRP – C-reactive protein

CRRT – continuous renal replacement therapy

CRS – cytokine release syndrome

Crs – respiratory system compliance

CSF – cerebrospinal fluid

CT – computer tomography

CTA – CT angiography

CTLA – cytotoxic T lymphocyte antigen

CVC – central venous catheter

CVVH – continuous veno-venous hemofiltration

CVVHD – continuous arteriovenous hemofiltration with concomitant dialysis (continuous veno-venous hemodiafiltration)

CXR – chest X-ray

DBP – diastolic blood pressure

DDAVP – desmopressin (1-deamino-8-D-arginine vasopressin)

DDx – differential diagnosis

DI – diabetes insipidus

DIC – disseminated intravascular coagulation

DKA – diabetic ketoacidosis

DLCO – diffusing capacity of the lungs for carbon monoxide

DNMTi – DNA methyltransferase inhibitors (i.e., azacitidine and decitabine)

DO2 – oxygen delivery

dsDNA – double stranded DNA

DST – dexamethasone suppression test

DWI – diffusion weighted imaging

Dx – diagnosis

EBV – Epstein-Barr virus

ECG – electrocardiogram

ECMO – extracorporeal membrane oxygenation

EEG – electroencephalographic

EGFR – epidermal growth factor receptor

EGPA – eosinophilic granulomatosis with polyangiitis (formerly Churg–Strauss)

ENA-antibodies – extractable nuclear antigen antibodies

EOD – every other day

ESRD – end-stage renal disease

EULAR/PRINTO/PRES – the European League Against Rheumatism, the Pediatric Rheumatology International Trials Organization and the Pediatric Rheumatology European Society

EVD – external ventricular drain

FE – fractional excretion

FEES – fiber-optic endoscopic evaluation of swallowing

FENa – fractional excretion of sodium

FEV1 – forced expiratory volume in one second

FFP – fresh frozen plasma

FGF23 – fibroblast growth factor-23

FiO_2 – fraction of inspired oxygen

FISH – fluorescence in situ hybridization

FSGS – focal segmental glomerulosclerosis

FVC – forced vital capacity

G6PD – glucose-6-phosphate dehydrogenase

GABAA – γ-aminobutyric acid type A

GAVE – gastric antral vascular ectasia

GBM – glioblastoma multiforme

GCS – Glasgow coma scale

GERD – gastroesophageal reflux disease

GFR – glomerular filtration rate

GI – gastrointestinal

GLP-1 – glucagon-like peptide 1

GN – glomerulonephritis

GPA – granulomatosis with polyangiitis (formerly Wegener's)

GST – glutathione S-transferase

GU – genitourinary

HA – headache

HACEK – *Haemophilus* species, *Aggregatibacter* species, *Cardiobacterium hominis*, *Eikenella corrodens*, and *Kingella* species

HAP – hospital acquired pneumonia

Hb – hemoglobin

HCTZ – hydrochlorothiazide

HD – hemodialysis

HDAC – histone deacetylase inhibitors

HELLP – hemolysis, elevated liver enzymes, low platelet count

HFpEF – heart failure with preserved ejection fraction

HFrEF – heart failure with reduced ejection fraction

HHS – hyperosmolar hyperglycemic state

HIF – hypoxia inducible factor

HIT – heparin-induced thrombocytopenia

HIV – human immunodeficiency virus

HLH – hemophagocytic lymphohistiocytosis

HMG-CoA – 3-hydroxy-3-methylglutaryl-coenzyme A (HMG-CoA) reductase (HMG-CoA)

HR – heart rate

HRCT – high resolution CT

HSP – Henoch-Schönlein purpura

HTN – hypertension

HUS – hemolytic uremic syndrome

i:e – inspiratory to expiratory time ratio

IABP – intra-aortic balloon pump

IAH – intraabdominal HTN

IAP – intraabdominal pressure

IBD – inflammatory bowel disease

IBS – irritable bowel syndrome

IBW – ideal body weight

iCa – ionized calcium

ICD – implantable cardioverter defibrillator

ICH – intracerebral hemorrhage

ICP – intracerebral pressure

IDU – injection drug use

IE – infective endocarditis

IFN – interferon

IHSS – idiopathic hypertrophic subaortic stenosis/hypertrophic cardiomyopathy

ILD – interstitial lung disease

IM – intramuscular

IMV – intermittent mandatory ventilation

IP – intraperitoneal

IPPV – invasive positive pressure ventilation

IV – intravenous

IVC – inferior vena cava

IVH – intraventricular hemorrhage

JVD – jugular vein distention

KDIGO – Kidney Disease Improving Global Outcomes

KIM-1 – kidney injury molecule-1

KIR – killer Ig receptor

LAP – leucocyte alkaline phosphatase

LBBB – left bundle branch block

L-FABP – liver fatty-acid binding protein

LMW – low molecular weight

LMWH – low molecular weight heparin

LN – lupus nephritis

LP – lumbar puncture

LQTS – long QT syndrome
LV – left ventricle/left ventricular
LVEDP – left ventricular end-diastolic pressure
MAC – *Mycobacterium avium*-Intracellulare Complex
MAHA – microangiopathic hemolytic anemia
MAP – mean arterial pressure
MAS – macrophage activation syndrome
MCA – middle cerebral artery
MCD – minimal change disease
MDI – metered dose inhaler
MDR – multidrug resistance
MDS – myelodysplastic syndrome
MEK – mitogen-activated protein kinase
MI – myocardial infarction
MIS – minimally invasive surgical techniques
MMF – mycophenolate mofetil
MPA – microscopic polyangiitis
MR – mitral regurgitation
MRA – magnetic resonance angiography
MRSA – methicillin-resistant *Staphylococcus aureus*
MS – multiple sclerosis
MSSA – methicillin-sensitive *Staphylococcus aureus*
mTOR – mammalian target of rapamycin
MTX – methotrexate
N/A – not applicable
NAG – N-acetyl-beta-glucosaminidase
NAVA – neurally adjusted ventilatory assist
NG – nasogastric
NGAL – neutrophil gelatinase-associated lipocalin
NIHSS – NIH Stroke Scale/Score
NIID – non-infectious inflammatory diseases
NIPPV – non-invasive positive pressure ventilation
NMBA – neuromuscular blocking agents
NMES – transcutaneous neuromuscular electrical stimulation
NO – nitric oxide
NOACs – non–vitamin K oral anticoagulants
NPT – sodium-phosphate cotransporter
NS – normal saline
NSAIDs – nonsteroidal antiinflammatory drugs
NSCLC – non–small-cell lung cancer
OGTT – oral glucose tolerance test
OKT3 – murine monoclonal anti-CD3 antibody
P/F – PaO_2 to FiO_2 ratio
PAC – pressure assist-control
PAD – pain, agitation, and delirium
PAH – pulmonary arterial hypertension
PAI-1 – plasminogen activator inhibitor-1
PAN – polyarteritis nodosa
pANCA – perinuclear ANCA
Paw – mean airway pressure
PAWP – pulmonary artery wedge pressure
PC – pressure control
PCC – prothrombin complex concentrates
PCI – percutaneous coronary intervention
PCR – polymerase chain reaction
PCV – polycythemia vera
PCV – pressure-controlled ventilation

PCWP – pulmonary capillary wedge pressure
PD – peritoneal dialysis
PD – programmed cell death
PEEP – positive end-expiratory pressure
PEEPi – intrinsic positive end-expiratory pressure
PET – peritoneal equilibration test
PET – positron emission tomography scan
PID – pelvic inflammatory disease
PKD – polycystic kidney disease
PL – transpulmonary pressure
PML – progressive multifocal leukoencephalopathy
PMN – polymorphonuclear leukocyte
PO – oral
P_{osm} – plasma osmolality
PP – pulse pressure
PPIs – proton pump inhibitors
Ppk – PIP – peak pressure
Pplat – PLP – plateau pressure
PR-3 – protein kinase-3
PRBC – packed red blood cell
PSB – protected specimen brush
PSV – pressure support ventilation
PTH – parathyroid hormone
PTSD – posttraumatic stress disorder
PTU – propylthiouracil
QB – blood flow rate
QD – dialysate flow rate
QID – four times a day
RA – refractory anemia
RA – rheumatoid arthritis
RA – right atrium
RAI – relative adrenal insufficiency
RASS – Richmond agitation–sedation scale
RCC – renal cell carcinoma
RD – rheumatologic diseases
RIFLE – Risk, Injury, Failure, Loss of kidney function, and End-stage kidney disease
RRT – renal replacement therapy
r-RT-PCR – real-time reverse transcription-polymerase chain reaction
RSBI – rapid shallow breathing index (ratio of respiratory rate to tidal volume)
RTA – renal tubular acidosis
RT-iiPCR – reverse transcription insulated isothermal polymerase chain reaction
RT-LAMP – reverse transcription LOOP-mediated isothermal amplification
Rx – treatment
SaO_2 – oxygen saturation
SARS – severe acute respiratory syndrome
SARS-CoV-2 – severe acute respiratory syndrome coronavirus 2
SBP – systolic blood pressure
SCC – squamous cell cancer
SCD – sudden cardiac death
S_{Cr} – serum creatinine
$ScvO_2$ – mixed central venous oxygen saturation (drawn from central line)
SGLT-2 – sodium–glucose cotransporter 2
SIADH – syndrome of inappropriate antidiuretic hormone secretion
SIC – sepsis-induced coagulopathy
SIRS – systemic inflammatory response syndrome
sJIA – systemic juvenile idiopathic arthritis

SLE – systemic lupus erythematosus
S$_{osm}$ – serum osmolality
SRC – scleroderma renal crisis
SSTI – skin and soft tissue infections
STEMI – ST-elevation MI
SV – stroke volume
SvO$_2$ – mixed venous oxygen saturation (drawn from pulmonary artery catheter tip)
TBW – total body water
Te – expiratory time
TEE – transesophageal echocardiography
TEG – thromboelastography
TFT – thyroid function test
TH – therapeutic hypothermia
Ti – inspiratory time
TIA – transient ischemic attack
TIBC – total iron binding capacity
TKI – tyrosine kinase inhibitor
TLC – total lung capacity
TMA – thrombotic microangiopathy
TMP-SMX – trimethoprim-sulfamethoxazole
TNF-α – tumor necrosis factor-α
tPA – tissue plasminogen activator
TPD – tidal peritoneal dialysis
TPE – therapeutic plasma exchange
TSOAC – target-specific oral anticoagulants
TST – tuberculin skin test
TTE – transthoracic echocardiography
TTKG – transtubular potassium gradient
TTP – thrombotic thrombocytopenic purpura
TV – tidal volume
U$_{Ca}$ – urine calcium
U$_{Cl^-}$ – urine chloride
U$_{creatinine}$ – urine creatinine
U$_K$ – urine potassium
ULN – upper limit of normal
U$_{Mg}$ – urine magnesium
U$_{Na}$ – urine natrium
U$_{osm}$ – urine osmolarity
URI – upper respiratory infection
URR – urea reduction ratio
US – ultrasound
UTI – urinary tract infection
U$_{Urea\ nitrogen}$ – urine urea nitrogen
VAC – volume assist-control
VALI – ventilator-associated lung injury
VAP – ventilator associated pneumonia
VC – volume control
VCV – volume-controlled ventilation
VDRL – the Venereal Disease Research Laboratory test
VEGF – vascular endothelial growth factor
V$_{EI}$ – gas exhaled in a ventilated patient during prolonged apnea (lung volume at inspiration V$_{EI}$), includes the tidal volume and the additional volume of gas due to dynamic hyperinflation
VFSS – video fluoroscopic swallow study
VGS – viridans group streptococci
VP – venous pressure
VPC – ventricular premature complex

V-Q mismatch – ventilation-perfusion mismatch
VSD – ventricular septal defect
VSMC – vascular smooth muscle cell
Vt – tidal volume
VT – ventricular tachycardia
VTE – venous thromboembolism

Index

Page numbers followed by *b* indicates boxes, *f* indicates figures and *t* indicates tables.